THE SANITARIANS

THE
SANITARIANS

A History of American Public Health

JOHN DUFFY

UNIVERSITY OF ILLINOIS PRESS
Urbana and Chicago

Illini Books edition, 1992
© 1990 by the Board of Trustees of the University of Illinois
Manufactured in the United States of America
1 2 3 4 5 C P 5 4 3 2 1

This book is printed on acid-free paper.

Library of Congress Cataloging-in-Publication Data

Duffy, John, 1915–
 The sanitarians.

 Bibliography: p.
 Includes index.
 1. Public Health—United States—History. I. Title.
RA445.D84 1990   614.4′4′097309   89–5107
ISBN 0-252-01663-7 (cloth : alk. paper)
ISBN 0-252-06276-0 (paper : alk. paper)

*To my brother, Charles M. Duffy, with
admiration and affection*

Contents

Acknowledgments

I am deeply indebted to many of my former graduate students and research assistants, to my colleagues in the history of medicine and public health, and to a host of librarians in the many institutions I visited throughout the country. My travel and many other expenses were made possible by a grant from the National Library of Medicine. When my project was delayed, Dr. Jeanne L. Brand and her associates at the National Library of Medicine kindly extended the time period allocated for the grant. The University of Maryland, through its History Department, cooperated fully as the sponsoring institution.

Six individuals deserve special mention. Dr. Arthur J. Viseltear of Yale University School of Medicine and Dr. Stuart Galishoff of Georgia State University read the entire manuscript and made many valuable suggestions. My old friend, Dr. Ben Freedman of New Orleans, gave me the benefit of his knowledge and wisdom for the last four chapters. Mrs. Margaret Burkett of the University of Maryland History Department, as she has done for some of my earlier works, carefully scrutinized the manuscript for stylistic errors. My son, James N. Duffy, read sections of the manuscript and made some perceptive comments. As always, my sharpest critic and best editor was my wife Corinne. I should like to take credit for the many confident judgments I have passed, but I suspect the best ones were borrowed from my colleagues.

Introduction

The history of American public health is one that historians have tended to neglect, and since so much research remains to be done, I propose simply to outline its main developments. Essentially I have written a narrative history—a form of history somewhat out of fashion today, but one, I think, that will always be with us.

The major problem in writing a history of public health is to determine precisely what "public health" encompasses. The term is so familiar that we tend to assume its meaning is clearly understood; yet defining it has been a major preoccupation of public health leaders for the past one hundred years or more. Essentially it means—and always has meant—community action to avoid disease and other threats to the health and welfare of individuals and the community at large. To this may be added the current view, which emphasizes a more positive approach—that public health policy should actively promote health rather than simply maintain it.

The changing definition of public health over the years has been accompanied by comparable alterations in the public's perception of what constitutes disease and ill health. Reflecting the nineteenth-century view that the main purpose of public health advocacy was to fight contagious diseases, in 1873 Dr. J. M. Toner wrote that the law of nature gives communities the right to use "an organized medical police" since disease is calamitous to individuals and "a positive loss to the State."[1] Almost fifty years later C.-E. A. Winslow defined the field of public health as "the science and the art of preventing disease, prolonging life, and promoting physical health and efficiency through organized efforts." Recognizing the role of poverty, he added that ensuring public health also required the development of social machinery to guarantee every individual a standard of living "adequate for the maintenance of health."[2] Still later the World Health Organization included the promotion of mental well-being among the objectives of public health advocates.

To complicate the historian's task further, there are few community activities that do not bear, directly or indirectly, upon public health; consequently, the historian must decide whether or not such social factors as tenement conditions, the role of immigration, or even poverty properly belong within his or her purview. Obviously housing and living standards do affect public health, but the question is, How much attention should they receive in a history of public health? While I have sought to show where they impinge directly on public health, as a public health historian I have limited my focus primarily to chronicling organized and in-stitutionalized efforts to improve community health.

Nonetheless, as is evident to anyone working in the fields of public health and social work or to students of the history of these areas, public health is determined to a large extent by the public's standard of living. A well-fed and properly housed population is far more resistant to all of the ailments besetting humanity than one that is impoverished. The reduc-tion in infant mortality and the increase in life expectancy in England during the eighteenth century was helped by the work of reformers, but it rested on the country's increasing general wealth. In the United States today the higher maternal and infant mortality rates and lower life expec-tancy among most minority groups reflect their below-average income levels. And poverty, regardless of race, invariably breeds sickness.

Among the themes that seem to run through American public health history, possibly the most striking one is the constant alternation between apathy and sharp reaction to periodic health crises. Whether or not familiarity breeds contempt, it certainly breeds acceptance. Tuberculosis ranked high among the main killer diseases in the nineteenth century, but it received little attention compared to the more dramatic epidemic disorders. In the American colonial period, smallpox and, to a lesser extent, yellow fever preoccupied public attention; yet the diseases responsible for most sickness and death in this period were malaria, respiratory infections, and enteric diseases. These disorders were accepted as the normal order, one of the more unpleasant aspects of everyday life.

In contrast, yellow fever visited the colonies only rarely; yet, as a strange inexplicable pestilence it invariably aroused the community to take preventive measures. The reverse situation has always seemed to hold true for environmental abuses. Water or air pollution, although common, sel-dom attracts attention until it reaches a crisis stage. Warning voices usually go unheard until enough people are affected directly. A health crisis such as a major epidemic or the "Great Stink" (a time when the stench from the Thames River temporarily forced the British Parliament to adjourn) can arouse the public to demand action. But once the immediate problem is solved or eased, apathy again sets in.

Another theme is the impact of acculturation upon public health. America was built on peoples of diverse cultures, most of whom were integrated into American society within one or two generations. This acculturation process applies equally to native Americans since, over the years, they experienced a population shift from rural areas to urban centers. Since population density creates special sanitary and environmental problems, before the twentieth century public health measures were restricted largely to cities and towns. Throughout American history, whether the newcomers to the cities have been American farmers, black sharecroppers from the South, poverty-stricken Irish, Eastern European peasants, or poor Latinos, they have all had to be taught how to live in an urban environment.

The fight to replace ineffective traditional ways of maintaining health with more effective ones is another constant in public health history. Humans are creatures of habit and tend to shy away from major innovations. Rural immigrants to urban areas, conditioned to accept sickness and death and suspicious of new disease prevention methods, often sought to hide their sick from health officers and on occasion rioted against compulsory vaccination. Even in times of major emergencies, many were reluctant to give up traditional therapeutics or preventive measures. The problem continues today and has been compounded by the insensitivity of many urban health and social workers to language and cultural differences.

Another recurrent theme in American public health is the clash between individual liberty and the public welfare, as government attempts to regulate human conduct in accordance with the prevailing principles of community health. America is a country of vast resources and space, and the discharge of human and industrial wastes into the natural environment was of little consequence for many generations. Over time, industry's befouling of the environment became almost a God-given right, for government interference in business had always been considered on a par with interference in citizens' personal lives. Unfortunately, sanitary and health regulations inevitably infringe on individual rights, a situation compounded by the general American distrust of all laws and regulations. For example, the number of deaths and injuries from drunken driving would be much lower if the average American did not consider driving a right rather than a privilege.

The zealous guarding of individual rights creates major problems for health officials in a democracy. A classic example of this was described to me by Dr. Fred Lowe Soper. (For a more detailed account of Soper's experiences see *Ventures in World Health: The Memoirs of Fred Lowe Soper*.)[3] Soper, with the support of President Getúlio Vargas of Brazil, in the 1930s began a program for eliminating the *Aëdes aegypti* mosquito, the carrier of yellow fever, from Brazil. By presidential edict, Soper's mosquito inspectors were given the right to enter all homes and businesses to inspect and spray for mosquitoes. After achieving success in Brazil, Soper persuaded the other South and Central American countries to join in a mass eradication program. The eradication work moved along smoothly until it reached the southern border of the United States, where the mosquito was endemic. Here it came to an abrupt halt when the federal government was unable to institute an effective eradication program. The result was the gradual reinfiltration of the mosquitoes from the United States into Latin America. In explaining the United States' failure to act, Dr. Soper attributed it to the federal government's lack of jurisdiction and the inability of the American government at any level to enter private premises in search of mosquitoes.

While the foregoing themes run throughout public health history, American public health until the end of the nineteenth century consisted primarily of quarantine and sanitary laws. The organization of the early temporary boards of health and the subsequent emergence of permanent health boards and departments arose from the efforts to strengthen and administer these early laws. Public health today is a firmly structured part of government, but long before health committees, health boards, and other formal community agencies emerged, responsible individuals and leaders recognized that certain conditions were detrimental to the health of the community, and they sought either to eliminate or modify them. Throughout the history of public health, the first and foremost factor in determining what measures to use has been prevailing medical concepts. When sickness was ascribed to the gods or spirits, then prayers, sacrifices, and ceremonies were required for healing, and the proper observance of taboos and rituals was the correct form of preventive medicine. On the other hand, the later assumption that disease arose from miasma, a noxious gas emanating from filth, putrefying vegetation, or the bowels of the earth, necessitated far different therapeutic and preventive measures. In turn, knowledge of the role of microorganisms radically altered the practice of public health.

A second factor determining public health policy has been prevailing social attitudes. If disease is sent by God, then people can do little about it other than resorting to prayer. For example, when a disease is equated with sin, as has been true of venereal disease for the past two hundred years, society will have little inclination to cure it or prevent it. To illustrate this point further, it was not until well into the twentieth century that the subject of venereal disease could be discussed publicly.

A third factor shaping public health has been economics. One of the most telling arguments used by public health reformers was that health and prosperity were closely related. Unfortunately, the public has always had a short memory: once community leaders brought a health problem under control, their constituents saw little need for preventive measures.

Keeping these factors in mind, as well as the general themes raised earlier, it may be well to begin this history by surveying community efforts to preserve health from earliest times to the American colonial period. Primitive peoples, living in a world beset by a host of dangers and subject to many unexplainable forces, attributed them to the world of spirits. To protect themselves they sought to propitiate the spirits by offering food and drink, resorting to rituals, observing taboos, making sacrifices, and wearing amulets and other protective devices—all of which, in their own way, were a form of preventive medicine.

Although the rationale behind these early preventive measures does not agree with modern thinking, many of them were effective. The fear that a medicine man or witch doctor at the behest of an enemy might work contagious magic against them, for example, led many primitives to hide their excreta, saliva, fingernail parings, and so forth. For fear of offending the spirit of the river or lake, many tribes placed a taboo on defecating or urinating in streams and bodies of water. A good many primitive groups isolated the sick or simply fled from an area where sickness was present. The elimination of defective children was quite common, an effective policy from a eugenic standpoint.

The rise of early civilizations brought major changes in terms of public health. The number of medical problems ascribed to rational causes began to increase, although the many inexplicable sicknesses and diseases were still attributed to religious or magical causes. The emergence of villages, towns, and cities, however, created significant environmental problems. As communities became permanent, they had to deal with the problems of garbage and human waste disposal and providing adequate supplies of good drinking water and food. The Egyptians, for example, emphasized personal hygiene, washing and anointing themselves daily. They also protected their food from flies and other insects and washed their clothes. Workmen engaged in the huge Egyptian construction projects were not permitted to relieve themselves near their work, and the straw huts in which they lived were burned down every year.

Sanitary measures and the protection of food and water supplies characterized virtually all of the early civilizations. Wherever cities developed, provisions were made for sanitation and water supplies and for the regulation of food markets. The Minoans, who paved the way for the rise of the Greek culture, developed fairly sophisticated water and sewer systems—systems that included reservoirs, copper pipes, baths, lavatories, and flush toilets.

The main contribution of the Greeks was to lay the basis for Western medicine: for over two thousand years the writings of the Hippocratic physicians literally dominated medical thought and practice. From a public health standpoint, the most significant of these works was one by

Hippocrates, *Airs, Waters, and Places*, which emphasized the role of environment in determining public health. In it, Hippocrates stated that exposure to the sun, the prevailing winds, the water supply, the nature of the soil, and the habits of the people all helped shape their energy and vitality. Ironically, in the eighteenth and nineteenth centuries, precisely at a time when Hippocratic concepts were coming under question, the value of *Airs, Waters, and Places* received a renewed recognition and became the theoretical basis for the sanitary movement—and it is well to bear in mind that public health before the twentieth century consisted largely of sanitation and quarantine. The irony of the revived appeal of *Airs, Waters, and Places* is that in the nineteenth century it provided strong support for the miasmic explanation of disease and thereby delayed acceptance of the germ theory.

The Romans were a pragmatic people who borrowed many of their philosophic concepts from the Greeks. Their chief contribution to public health was made by their architects and engineers, who greatly improved on the water and sewer systems of their predecessors. In the sixth century B.C. they built their first sewer, and around 300 B.C. they began constructing a great system of aqueducts. The water from these aqueducts was separated on the basis of quality, with only the best water used for drinking. The homes of wealthy Romans had excellent sanitary facilities, and public latrines were provided for the populace. In addition, a wide variety of regulations governed the markets and streets. Nonetheless, the living conditions for the great majority of Romans, crowded in dirty tenements, scarcely reflect a bright picture—nor do the many descriptions of open sewers in poorer districts and the accounts of the main sewers frequently being blocked with garbage and refuse.

The decline and eventual downfall of the Western Roman Empire affected medicine and public health in two significant ways. In the first place the movement toward a rational approach to medical problems initiated by the Greeks was halted and replaced in the medieval period by a return to religious, or priestly, medicine. Disease, and epidemic disease in particular, was considered to be either a sign of God's wrath or a form of testing the faithful. Life on earth was considered but a fleeting moment in the eternity of time, and hence there was little incentive to improve it. Second, Western Europe's political and economic problems combined with the impact of the barbarian invasions virtually destroyed the Roman urban centers, and their downfall meant the disintegration of water and sewer systems and the elimination of food and sanitary regulations. Since concern for public health is essentially an urban phenomenon, only the great Arab civilization centered in the Mediterranean continued to make progress in this area, although the Byzantine Empire in the East managed to hold on to some of the gains made by the Romans until it, too, collapsed in the fifteenth century.

The rise of towns and cities in the later medieval period once again forced communities to deal with sanitary problems and water and food supplies. Unfortunately, the history of public health shows that cities tend to grow faster than the ability of municipal officials to cope with health and sanitary matters. In the feudal era the difficulties of maintaining public health were compounded by the necessity for hemming cities in by defensive walls that compressed the growing population and accentuated sanitary problems. Nonetheless, efforts were made to handle garbage and human wastes and to regulate food markets.

A second significant development in the medieval era was the emergence of isolation and quarantine as a defense against contagious disease. The first of the two disorders responsible for this development was leprosy, which spread widely throughout Europe from the twelfth to the fourteenth centuries, probably as a result of the Crusades. This horrible disorder created so much fear that its victims were literally read out of society. In many areas individuals diagnosed as lepers had their burial services read, were forbidden entrance to towns and cities, and were required to wear distinctive clothing. In all probability, the isolation of leprosy patients was a major factor in the sharp reduction in their number by the fifteenth century, although other factors, including the ravages of the Black Death, also contributed to their decline.

The disease that gave rise to the word "quarantine" was bubonic plague, the dreaded Black Death of 1348. Convinced that the infection, as with leprosy, was spread by direct contact, Europeans applied the principle of isolation to it. Venice was the first city to isolate plague victims and to attempt to prevent the introduction of the disease through imported goods, travelers, or vessels. Other cities and states quickly adopted similar measures. In 1377 Ragusa on the Dalmatian coast ordered a 30-day period of isolation for anyone arriving from a plague-infested area. Subsequently this period was lengthened to 40 days—the *quarantenaria*. J. G. C. Hecker, in his classic history of epidemics in the Middle Ages, suggests that the 40-day detention period was based on the doctrine of critical days, which maintained that the fortieth day marked the division between acute and chronic disorders.[4] Whatever the case, quarantine measures of one type or another became basic to public health in the Western world.

The Renaissance, which witnessed a revival of interest in the classical civilizations, helped to advance medical knowledge but did little for medical practice or public health. The same holds true for the seventeenth century, the Century of Genius. The work of Harvey, van Leeuwenhoek,

Santorio, van Helmont, and others in medicine significantly added to our basic knowledge but had no immediate practical application. The most important development during these years from the standpoint of public health was the emergence of what was first described as political arithmetic. Around 1600 the city of London began publishing regular weekly mortality reports. The theory of mercantilism had already postulated that population constituted a form of wealth, and two Englishmen were among the first to see the significance of vital statistics. William Petty (1623–87) recognized that information could be gleaned by analyzing statistics, and he coined the term "political arithmetic." His friend, John Graunt (1620–74), laid the basis for statistical analysis in his work *Natural and Political Observations . . . upon the Bills of Mortality*, published in 1662. Once it became evident that statistics could reveal a great deal about the economic condition of a nation and the health of its people, the basis was laid for developing a national health policy. The application of such a policy, however, required a strong and effective government structure, and this did not come until the twentieth century.

Thus in the years when the American colonies were being established, public health consisted of limited quarantine and isolation measures, sanitary regulations, which were established as much for aesthetic purposes as for public health, and ordinances intended to control markets and the sale of food.[5]

NOTES

1. John M. Toner, "Boards of Health . . . ," in *Selections from Public Health Reports and Papers Presented at the Meetings of the American Public Health Association (1873–1883)* (New York, 1977), 499.

2. C.-E. Winslow, *Man and Epidemics* (Princeton, N.J., 1952), 30.

3. Fred Lowe Soper, *Ventures in World Health: The Memoirs of Fred Lowe Soper,* John Duffy, ed. (Washington, D.C., 1977), 112, 347–57.

4. J. F. C. Hecker, *The Epidemics of the Middle Ages* (London, 1844), 65.

5. Many of the food regulations, however, were motivated by economic concerns dating back to medieval times. Merchant guilds sought to regulate competition within cities and to maintain markets for food shipped out of town by guaranteeing its quality.

1

The Early Years

In the history of American colonial health a startling contrast exists between the descriptions of the early colonial environment and the stark picture, once the colonies were established, of recurrent pestilential epidemics and omnipresent endemic diseases. The early explorers and settlers were unanimous in their praise of the New World. They wrote of the fresh bracing air, the vast acres of fertile land, forests full of game, and streams and lakes of pure water. In particular they mentioned the lack of diseases. The native inhabitants were described as strong and healthy and apparently having none of the common disorders of Europe.

Essentially this view of the Indians was correct, for all evidence indicates that native Americans had no experience with, nor any immunity to, smallpox and the other contagious disorders plaguing Europeans. As the Europeans pushed into the interior, their diseases proved the most potent factor in reducing the Indian resistance. On occasion smallpox—the most deadly of infections for the Indians in the colonial period—virtually wiped out entire tribes. The impact of disease on the Indians without doubt represents one of the most tragic aspects of the white settlement of America.

Even in 1624, when starvation and malnutrition were besetting the population of Plymouth, Thomas Prince, in his *Chronological History of New-England*, wrote that the place was healthful, "for in the 3 last Years, notwithstanding their great want of most Necessaries, there hath not one died of the first Planters."[1] In 1630 John Winthrop reported to his son: "Here is sweet aire faire rivers and plenty of springes and the water better than in Eng[land] here can be noe want of any thinge to those who bring meane[s] to raise out of the earth and sea."[2] Three years later Master Wells described New England as very agreeable to "English bodies." Those who could never "be rid of their head ach, tooth ach, Cough and the like" were much healthier in the colony, and "those that were weake are now well long since."[3]

The settlement of New York evoked the same praises of the land and climate. In 1649 a Dutch writer wrote of the pleasant climate and bracing air, and shortly thereafter another settler reported that the country was "good and healthful" and the inhabitants seldom sick. A visitor in 1670 described the climate as ideal, with seasonable showers, "a sweet and pleasant air, and . . . such Influences as tend to the Health both of Man and Beast."[4] Virginia, the first British colony to be settled, did not produce such paeans of praise from its early colonists, for there death and sickness, due largely to mismanagement, beset the colony for many years. Starvation, which had temporarily troubled the New England colonies, was the basic problem in Virginia. Here starvation and malnutrition continued for almost twenty years and was aggravated by the so-called burning fevers, probably typhoid brought in by the settlers themselves.

As the colonies increased in population, the common infectious disorders of Western Europeans—smallpox, malaria, diarrheas and dysenteries, respiratory complaints, measles, mumps, scarlet fever, diphtheria, and so forth—quickly established themselves. Malaria, which was endemic in sections of England and the Continent, by the end of the seventeenth century was firmly entrenched in the colonies, from New England to the Carolinas. In addition, the sanitary problems engendered by community living and the lack of refrigeration in summer guaranteed the presence of the intestinal complaints that proved so disastrous to infants and so debilitating to adults. In the colonial period people of all countries were well conditioned to sickness and death, and they accepted the chronic diseases such as malaria and the various forms of dysentery with resignation. The malignant disorders that appeared sporadically and swept through the colonies with devastating force were another matter.

Geographic factors determined that the colonies would be isolated both from each other and from Europe. This had the fortunate effect of minimizing the number of major epidemics, particularly in the seventeenth and early eighteenth centuries. When epidemic diseases did strike, however, they proved devastating. The two most feared were smallpox and yellow fever. These highly fatal pestilences appeared mysteriously, killed young and old indiscriminately, and disrupted community activities for months at a time. At this date neither their causes nor their methods of spreading were understood, nor was it possible to effect a cure. Hence the appearance of smallpox, a deadly and painful disorder that often left its victims scarred for life, or yellow fever, with its jaundice, high fever, generalized internal hemorrhages, and vomiting of partially digested blood, caused justifiable panic.

The ravages of these diseases have been well recorded; it is enough to say that on occasion single epidemics in Boston, Charleston, and other towns killed as much as 10 percent or more of the inhabitants. During these outbreaks often entire families were swept away, and few families escaped completely. John Saffin sadly noted in 1678 the deaths from smallpox of two of his sons and his "thrice Dearly Beloved Consort." "And now alas," he added, "there Lyes Interred in one Tombe . . . in Boston my Dear Wife Martha Saffin & five of the Eight Sons She bore unto me." One had died shortly after birth, another at the age of two, and the third one had died of "fflux" (some form of dysentery or enteric disease) at the age of seven.[5]

Yellow fever, which did not arrive until the end of the seventeenth century, and diphtheria, which first struck with devastating force in the 1730s, were as deadly as smallpox, but, fortunately, they made fewer appearances. Although diphtheria had been present early in colonial days, it was not until 1735 that a particularly virulent outbreak began sweeping through the colonies. Known by such names as the throat distemper or the children's disease, it wrought havoc in New England. For example, the town of Hampton Falls, New Hampshire, suffered 210 deaths out of a population of about 1,200. About 95 percent of the victims were children, and in twenty families everyone below the age of twenty-one died. Even infections such as measles—generally considered in the twentieth century to be a mild children's disease—could prove highly fatal to children and adults alike in the colonial period. An outbreak in the winter of 1713–14 cost the Reverend Cotton Mather the loss of his wife, three children, and a maid within the space of two weeks.[6]

By the seventeenth century aesthetics and a vague sense of a connection between sickness and putrefying matter had led all European communities to enact sanitary laws of some form. The early Virginia colonists—who, in addition to their other difficulties, had antagonized the Indians—were compelled to live in a fort. In this crowded condition some sanitary regulations were essential. The governor in 1611 decreed that no one was to wash clothes or create any nuisances within twenty feet of the well, nor was anyone "to doe the necessities of nature" closer than "a quarter of mile from the palisade lest the fort be choaked, and poisoned with ill aires." Citizens were also ordered to keep their houses "sweete and cleane" under threat of court-martial.[7]

The other colonies faced neither the sickness nor the crowding that characterized the Jamestown settlement, and only limited attention was paid to sanitation in the first few years. The earliest health measures sought to place some restriction on medical practice, but most of these had minimal effect. One of the first public health laws enacted in Massachusetts concerned shipboard conditions. This colony was far ahead of its time in recognizing that crowding passengers onto ships added to the dangers of the long ocean voyages. In 1629 the General Court of Massachusetts limited the number of passengers according to the size of the vessel.[8] It should be pointed out that a major factor in the high death rate of newly arrived immigrants was their poor physical condition. Most had endured long voyages in overcrowded ships in which sickness had been rampant and food both scarce and inadequate.

The large-scale emigration to Massachusetts beginning in 1630 probably led to the colony's first sanitary law. In 1634 the rapidly growing town of Boston prohibited residents from depositing fish or garbage near the common landing. According to historian John B. Blake, this was the only sanitary ordinance passed before 1652. The authorities did act against specific nuisances on occasion, but in general sanitary matters were left up to the citizens, who were free to dig wells, construct privies, and make drains where feasible.[9]

The Puritan migrants to New England were highly motivated, relatively well educated, and came from fairly well-to-do backgrounds. The high caliber of the settlers and their sense of community responsibility may account for the lack of sanitary legislation before the 1650s. In any event, by this decade the cleanliness of Boston could no longer be left to individual citizens, and beginning in 1652 a series of ordinances were passed. The first dealt with the construction of privies—a subject that was to be the source of literally thousands of sanitary laws involving every community in America for the next three hundred years. The Boston law prohibited placing privies within twenty feet of a highway or neighborhood house unless its construction included a privy vault six feet deep. Privies, however, remained a perpetual source of complaint in urban areas, and it was not until the introduction of large-scale sewer systems in the late nineteenth century that a start was made toward solving the problem.

Other sanitary regulations soon followed. The inevitable tendency of some individuals to toss garbage and rubbish onto public thoroughfares and vacant lots or into drains, streams, and other bodies of water forced the Boston selectmen to prohibit all such actions. Private industry was (and continues to be) one of the worst offenders in befouling the environment. In colonial days, and continuing to the end of the nineteenth century, the so-called nuisance trades or industries were the special object of a good many sanitary laws. At this early date the butchers and blubber-boilers were the chief culprits; later, slaughterers, tanners, and others would join their ranks. One solution, which Boston and other towns tried, was to designate specific areas in which these trades could operate. The key to any regulation, though, is its enforcement, and Boston soon found it necessary to appoint special officers for this purpose. Regulating businesses is a difficult task for any government, and the city was forced to ask the colonial government for help. In 1684 the Massachusetts General Court ordered butchers and slaughterers to keep their premises clean under a threat of a twenty-shilling fine.[10] The constant succession of decrees, ordinances, and laws on this subject in every town and colony demonstrates that the colonists' solutions to their sanitary problems were, at best, temporary.

In a day when horses were the chief form of transportation and cattle, hogs, chickens, dogs, and cats roamed the streets, dead animals on vacant lots and public thoroughfares were a constant source of irritation, offensive to both sight and smell. In March 1666–67 Boston appointed a scavenger to impound stray cows and horses and remove dead animals and other carrion from the streets.[11] The office of scavenger soon became a standard feature of every good-sized town and city in America. In small towns the usual practice was to require the owners of dead animals to be responsible for them. For example, the selectmen in Marblehead in 1673 ordered that any dead animals within "thirtie pole of any dwellinge house in Towne" be buried within twenty-four hours. Owners failing to do so would be fined ten shillings.[12] This system worked reasonably well in places where the owners were known, but as communities grew larger, it became necessary to appoint a scavenger. The title and duties of the office have varied since then, but the need to have someone responsible for removing dead animals has lasted into the twentieth century.

In the seventeenth century groups of citizens occasionally banded together to dig a well or construct a sewer or drain, but no municipal action was involved. The word "sewer" should not be misconstrued, for at this time sewers were simply intended to carry off surface water or to drain stagnant pools. Whatever the intent, these drains usually became sewers in fact since they were soon carrying off the overflow from privies—in addition to what other wastes and debris were simply dumped into them.

New Amsterdam, or New York City, was founded as a military post in 1625, shortly before the founding of Boston, and it grew slowly. Its first sanitary regulation, issued in 1644, was similar to the one promulgated much earlier in Jamestown. It prohibited anyone from depositing filth and ashes within the fort and provided "that no one shall make water" within it. Four years later an order prohibited New Amsterdam's residents from letting their hogs and goats run loose in the streets.[13] As had been the case with privies and nuisance trades, civic authorities were to pass ordinance after ordinance in an effort to solve the stray animal problem, but keeping animals off the streets was no easy task. The tradition of humans living with domestic animals is such a strong one that milk cows and horses were kept within city limits until well into the twentieth century. Hogs were always accepted, both as scavengers and as a source of food for the poor, and it was the end of the nineteenth century before most major American cities eliminated them. A vestigial remnant of our reliance on domestic animals is the widespread assumption, even in this age of sanitation, that dogs and cats should be free to urinate and defecate on sidewalks and streets.

American settlers, like their descendants in the twentieth century, were exceedingly reluctant to let the government place restrictions on the use of their property. Governor Peter Stuyvesant of New Amsterdam fought for years to force the city's inhabitants to pen their animals. On one occasion he ordered his soldiers to shoot all hogs found within the fort. The only concession he gained before he gave up the fight in 1658 came when city officials ordered residents to put rings on the noses of their hogs—an order that still gave tacit permission to the owners to let their hogs roam at large.[14] Interestingly, none of the objections to hogs, at this time or later, was based on health concerns; the major complaint against them was that they damaged property. In the eighteenth and nineteenth centuries the presence of hogs was criticized on aesthetic grounds, but it took the sanitary revolution of the late nineteenth century to drive them out of the cities for good.

In this day of a widely varied diet, it is difficult to appreciate the significance of the statement that bread is the staff of life. Yet throughout recorded history humans have lived largely on grains, and the earliest food laws were those concerned with the price and quality of bread. The settlers in the New World came from countries where bread regulations were still strictly enforced, and comparable laws were soon enacted in the colonies. Food shortages always presented a temptation to bakers to adulterate their bread, and a series of crop failures in 1649 led to complaints against the bakers of New York City. In response, the governor and the Common Council decreed that bread had to be made from pure wheat or pure rye flour and that loaves must be made in three standard sizes, their price varying according to the cost of flour.

In succeeding years a series of more specific regulations sought to guarantee the quality of bread. A 1656 ordinance required bakers to be licensed. When complaints continued, in 1661 two inspectors were appointed and given the authority to seize any bread not meeting certain specifications. When this still did not end the complaints, the powers of the inspectors were increased, and offending bakers were subjected to fines in addition to the confiscation of substandard bread. By the time the British assumed control of New Netherlands in 1664, the quality and price of bread were effectively guaranteed by the government.[15] The regulations established by the Dutch in New York for the control of bread making were typical of the ordinances and laws enacted in all the colonies. The quality of bread remained quite good until the advent of mass baking and the spirit of free enterprise in the Jacksonian Era. The natural food movement that began in this period arose partly in reaction to the adulteration of bread and its declining quality.

The Netherlands, as the premier trading nation of the seventeenth century, was acutely aware of the need to maintain high-quality merchandise, and since food was a basic item of export, New Amsterdam was the first colonial town to regulate food staples. As early as 1653 it established a public weighhouse and storehouse, and three years later a public slaughterer and three official butchers were appointed. These officials were given a monopoly within the city, but their fees were determined by the authorities.[16] Subsequently two inspectors of beef and pork were appointed, thus assuring a measure of government control over all basic food supplies.

As the export of food increased, inspectors were appointed to oversee the packing of barrels of flour and meat. The meat inspector in 1668 was instructed to see that the meat was of good quality and well seasoned, and that "the beste be not left out." He was also to ensure that the barrels were sound and fully packed. A few years later two deputies were assigned the task of inspecting all flour for export. In the 1680s the city marketing code imposed a fine of forty shillings on anyone selling "unwholesome or Stale Victuall," "Blowne meat," or "Leprous Swine" in the city market.[17] New York City was ahead of the other colonial towns in regulating its food supply, but the basic pattern it set was emulated by every other colonial port of any consequence. Motivated both by paternalism and the economic theory of mercantilism, provincial and town officials throughout the colonial period made conscientious efforts to maintain reasonably priced and good-quality food staples.

The earliest colonial quarantine regulations were enacted almost simultaneously with the first sanitary measures. Epidemic disease, however, was assumed by most colonists to have been sent by God, and days of prayer and fasting usually accompanied—and sometimes preceded—the initiation of quarantine laws. Upon receiving news of a major epidemic in the West Indies during the winter of 1647–48, the General Court of Massachusetts proclaimed a day of fasting, "having cause to feare least our sinnes may provoke the Lord to lay more heavy corrections upon us." At the same time the court ordered all vessels from the West Indies to anchor in the harbor until they were given clearance. These same actions were taken in 1665 when the colony was threatened by the Great Plague of London.[18]

New York City, possibly because it grew more slowly in its first few years, lagged behind Boston in instituting quarantines. A variety of problems in 1649, including sickness, led Governor Stuyvesant of New Amsterdam to proclaim a day of fasting and prayer, but nothing was said about quarantine. In 1668 British Governor Francis Lovelace also announced "a General Day of Humiliation" because of "unusual sicknesse," but he, too, did not order a quarantine. It was not long, however, before the rising threat of smallpox, a disorder often brought in from England or the West Indies, forced New York to begin inspecting vessels for what were known as "pestilential diseases."[19]

One of the major roles of public health authorities is simply to initiate community action on matters pertaining to health. Once the means for controlling a specific problem have become institutionalized, community authorities may then assign responsibility for it to a separate government agency. Street cleaning and garbage removal, initially a health problem associated with the danger from miasma, remained the responsibility of private citizens until the latter part of the seventeenth century. One of the first steps toward community action was taken in 1670 by New York City when cartmen asked for a monopoly on transporting goods within the city. The governor granted their request, agreeing to limit the number of licenses on the condition that the cartmen assume responsibility for filling up "breaches" in the roads and for removing the piles of dirt, rubbish, and garbage from the streets every Saturday. The cartmen's sole obligation was hauling away the dirt and filth; residents were required to sweep it up in front of their houses and load it onto the carts. Complaints of citizens throwing garbage and debris into the streets continued, and a few years later the city constables were made responsible for enforcing the street-cleaning laws. In 1695 the city appointed a scavenger at thirty pounds a year to supervise street cleaning.[20] Although cities such as Boston and New York began moving in the direction of civic responsibility for street cleaning, throughout the colonial period it rested largely in the hands of individual citizens.

Charleston, South Carolina, was the third substantial colonial town to emerge in the seventeenth century. Dating to the founding of the Carolinas in 1670, it grew fairly rapidly, reaching about three thousand inhabitants by 1700. By this date, following the pattern of other colonial towns, it had passed ordinances for cleaning lots and streets and preventing hogs from running loose, and it had set standards for constructing privies. A 1698 statute ordered the removal of all slaughterhouses and cattle, hog, and sheep pens from the town. The preface to a 1704 law dealing with garbage removal and slaughterhouses that began, "The air is greatly infected and many maladies and other intolerable diseases daily happen," clearly shows how these subjects were associated with health.[21]

Whether medical care should be considered within the purview of public health has been hotly debated during the twentieth century, but care of the sick poor has traditionally been a community responsibility. In Virginia the London Company erected a hospital in 1612, but it did not last for long. In 1620, while the colony was still struggling to survive, the Privy Council ordered that "Guest houses" be built for the sick. There is no evidence to show that the order was carried out, and henceforth the sick were cared for in private homes. [22] Physicians often took severely ill patients into their homes, and parish and town records all show local officials paying physicians for treating the sick poor.

In New York the care of the sick poor in the city's early years was left to churches and private charity. In 1685 the Common Council ruled that the alderman in each ward should certify the names of deserving poor. Two years later the city appointed a physician of the poor at a salary of five pounds per year.[23] Eventually, comparable positions were created in all colonial towns, but care of the sick poor generally remained a mixture of private and community concern.

Fire fighting, although it scarcely seems within the province of public health, does have health implications since fires are a major cause of death and injury. For the same reasons that health officials in the late nineteenth century sought to regulate the sale of kerosene and expressed interest in occupational injuries, authorities in colonial times sought to prevent or limit fires. It is true, however, that in colonial days their major concern was danger to property. Wooden frame houses with thatched or shingled roofs, as well as open fires and candles, presented a constant threat of fire, particularly in view of the lack of water systems. As early as 1648 New York enacted the first of a long series of fire regulations. These included prohibitions against thatched roofs and wooden fireplaces and a requirement that residents provide fire buckets, ladders, and hooks at street corners.[24] It should also be pointed out that the danger from fires was a major factor in the development of city water systems in the late eighteenth and early nineteenth centuries.

Another area of importance to public health is statistics. The English had long maintained parish registers of births, marriages, and deaths, and the practice was quickly adopted by the colonies. Moreover, the seventeenth century was one in which an awareness of the value of statistical data emerged, and this awareness gave added impetus to the collection of vital statistics. In 1611, at a time when the Virginia colony was still struggling to survive, the London Company required each minister to keep a record of "Christenings, Marriages, and Deaths," and the first colonial legislative assembly in 1619 enacted a similar registration law, with the added proviso that annual reports be made. Some eighteen years later a specific office of register of the colony was established.[25]

The New England Puritans, too, following the English pattern, began keeping parish registers, but, as Calvinists, they believed that recording marriages and burials was a civil, rather than an ecclesiastical, concern; consequently, the Massachusetts General Court in 1639 ordered the town recorders to keep what essentially were vital statistics. The Massachusetts system was adopted by all the New England colonies and ultimately spread throughout the United States. Thus Massachusetts deserves credit for changing the collection of vital statistics from an ecclesiastical responsibility to a civic one. In addition, the Massachusetts system held individual citizens, rather than clerks or ministers, responsible for reporting vital events occurring within their families.[26] By the time the Carolinas were founded in 1670, the concept of political arithmetic was familiar in intellectual circles, and the elaborate plan for government attributed largely to John Locke, the *Fundamental Constitutions,* specified that a registrar be appointed to record all deaths, burials, and marriages.[27]

By the end of the seventeenth century all the colonies required clerks or ministers to record vital statistics, but, as is always the case, laws without public support or effective enforcement are meaningless. As the colonists pushed out from their original settlements to establish farms and plantations often far removed from ministers, churches, or government officials, few records were maintained. Moreover, the growing disagreement between the colonies and the British government, which began in New England in the seventeenth century, made the colonists reluctant to reveal information about themselves, either collectively or individually. Excellent statistics are available for individual parishes and communities, but for the colonies as a whole, the figures are sparse. The gathering of relatively accurate vital statistics had to await the twentieth century.[28]

By the end of the seventeenth century several colonial towns had reached a stage in their development requiring them to pass basic sanitary laws. With the exception of food regulations, most of the measures were rudimentary, and their enforcement was sporadic. On the other hand, towns were small, and offenders were usually well known; hence public pressure could prove an effective deterrent. Quarantine laws, too, had been enacted, but these were purely temporary; once a health crisis had passed, they quickly lapsed. The rapidly growing colonial population, together with expanding trade with Europe and the West Indies, brought the ever-increasing threat of imported disease, and the eighteenth century would see quarantine laws greatly strengthened.

NOTES

1. Thomas Prince, *A chronological history of New-England in the form of annals . . .* (Boston, 1736), 1:151.

2. John Winthrop to John Winthrop, Jr., Charleston, S.C., July 23, 1630, *Winthrop Papers* (Boston, 1943), 2:306.

3. Master Wells to family in Tarlington, Essex, New England, 1633, Sloane MSS, Library of Congress Transcription, Manuscripts Division, Library of Congress, vol. 922, no. 90.

4. John Duffy, *A History of Public Health in New York City, 1625–1866* (New York, 1968), 6.

5. The Notebook of John Saffin, 1665–1708, New York Historical Society MSS, pp. 9–10.

6. *Diary of Cotton Mather, 1709–1724*, American Classics (New York, n.d.), 2:249–61.

7. Wyndham B. Blanton, *Medicine in Virginia in the Seventeenth Century* (Richmond, Va., 1930), 75.

8. John B. Blake, *Public Health in the Town of Boston, 1630–1822* (Cambridge, Mass., 1959), 1.

9. Ibid., 13–14. I have relied on Blake's excellent study for much of the early sanitary history of Boston.

10. Ibid., 15–16.

11. Ibid.

12. "Marblehead Town Records," *Historical Collections* of the Essex Institute (Salem, Mass., 1913), 69:269.

13. Duffy, *Public Health in New York City, 1625–1866*, 10–11.

14. Ibid., 13.

15. Ibid., 13–14.

16. Ibid., 14–15.

17. Bernard Mason, "Aspects of the New York Revolt of 1689," *New York History* 30 (1939):170–71.

18. Blake, *Public Health in Boston*, 18–19.

19. Duffy, *Public Health in New York City, 1625–1866*, 19, 34–35.

20. Ibid., 24–27.

21. Joseph Ioor Waring, *A History of Medicine in South Carolina, 1670–1825* (Columbia, S.C., 1964), 15.

22. Blanton, *Medicine in Virginia*, 149–55.

23. Duffy, *Public Health in New York City, 1625–1866*, 34.

24. Ibid., 12–13.

25. James H. Cassedy, *Demography in Early America: Beginnings of the Statistical Mind, 1600–1800* (Cambridge, Mass., 1969), 15–18.

26. Ibid., 29–31.

27. Waring, *Medicine in South Carolina*, 14.

28. Cassedy, *Demography in Early America*, 36–37.

2

The Years of Growth and Expansion

Because public health in any era is based largely on prevailing medical concepts, it may be well to survey medical thought in the seventeenth and eighteenth centuries. From the time of Hippocrates, most physicians had operated on some variation of the humoral concept. This theory assumed that there were four basic bodily substances, or humors—blood, phlegm, black bile, and yellow bile—and that diseases arose from an imbalance of these humors or from one or more of them having become corrupted, or "vitiated." In the seventeenth and eighteenth centuries several new theories were set forth, but they had little impact upon medical practice, and physicians continued to bleed, purge, vomit, and blister their patients as they had done from time immemorial. Neither the humoral theory nor any of the newer concepts satisfactorily explained the sudden and mystifying appearance of epidemic diseases. To account for them the theory of epidemic constitutions emerged, based upon the Hippocratic thesis that climate and environment played a significant role in determining health or sickness.

The leading exponent of the theory of epidemic constitutions was Thomas Sydenham (1624–89), the most famous English physician of his day. He accepted the Hippocratic view, but since he was unable to correlate epidemics with specific weather conditions, he became convinced that they were caused by inexplicable changes in the atmosphere. These changes, he believed, resulted from miasmas or effluvia arising from what he termed the bowels of the earth. The concept of miasmas did not negate the old assumption that temperature, humidity, prevailing winds, and other factors affected health, since most physicians managed to incorporate both theories into their view of epidemics. It was obvious, however, that bubonic plague and smallpox were spread by direct contact, and observant physicians considered these disorders exceptions.[1]

Assuming that certain atmospheric conditions promoted sickness and fever, it seemed logical that foul odors and gases arising from the earth or from putrefaction must also play some role. Malaria had long been associated with low-lying marshy land, and when yellow fever struck the colonial port cities, it always appeared first in the waterfront areas. These invariably were the older parts of the city where the poorer citizens lived, crowded together in filthy, foul-smelling housing. In ships, hospitals, army camps, jails, and wherever individuals were jammed together in dirty and unsanitary conditions, sickness was always present. The obvious connection between sickness and filth gave credence to the miasmatic theory, which dominated medical thinking about disease well to the end of the nineteenth century. It held that an invisible, noxious substance, emanating from the earth or from putrefying substances or some other source, contaminated the atmosphere and that this contamination led to widespread sickness.

Dr. William Douglass and a number of other American physicians espoused the views of Sydenham, but the one who had the most influence on public health was Cadwallader Colden, a Scotsman originally destined for the ministry who studied medicine in London, migrated to Philadelphia, and then moved permanently to New York. Although he practiced medicine for only eight years, he continued to take a keen interest in the subject. During the summers of 1741 and 1742 New York City was attacked by several fevers, one of which may have been yellow fever since the disorder was appearing widely in the colonies at this time.

As surveyor general of the province and a member of the Governor's Council, Colden decided to publish his thoughts on yellow fever in 1743. In his previous essay, *Account of the Climate and Diseases of New York,* published in 1720, he had postulated that the various hot-weather fevers in New York were occasioned by the city's poor water supply. He had now come to the conclusion that they arose from the effects of "noxious vapors from stagnating filthy water" on the "animal oeconomy." The various miasmas produced by fermentation in these waters resulted in "different fermentations in the animal fluids"; hence the type of fever was dependent upon the kind of miasma produced by filthy water or putrefying substances.

The nature of fevers had long been a troublesome question to thoughtful physicians. It was recognized that various fevers tended to strike during the summer months and that infants and children were peculiarly liable to them. Arguing against the common belief that most of these deaths were due to eating fresh fruit, Colden pointed out that country children, who had greater access to fresh fruit than city children, did not die in nearly such great numbers. The real cause, he declared, was the deleterious atmosphere and the unsanitary condition of the city.[2]

On this assumption Colden reviewed the history of yellow fever and then turned to the areas in New York City that he considered to be the true breeding grounds of the disease. He pointed out that yellow fever invariably appeared in the vicinity of docks built upon low-lying land, where dirt and filth tended to accumulate. As in the case of other summer fevers, he felt that yellow fever was of local origin and that the way to prevent it was to cleanse the city and remove the foul miasmas. Colden's views were put to practical use in New York City, where a large-scale sanitary program was undertaken, but, more important, they helped establish the miasmatic thesis as a basis for the subsequent public health movement.

A variation of this theory was expounded by Dr. John Jones, a founder of King's College (Columbia University) Medical School and author of the first American work on surgery. In a publication intended as a practical guide for military surgeons during the Revolutionary War, he spoke of the "morbid effluviae" exhaled from the body and lungs of sick and wounded men. These effluvia, he wrote, vitiated the air and, where sick and wounded men were crowded together, could "generate a jail or hospital fever" and carry off patients and attendants alike. He warned that soldiers should not be allowed to relieve themselves in the vicinity of their camps except in privies placed on the lee side so that the prevailing winds would carry the odors away. He also recommended changing campsites frequently.[3]

The miasmatic theory was best expressed by Noah Webster at the end of the eighteenth century. In the preface to his 1796 work, *A Collection of Papers on the Subject of Bilious Fevers . . . ,* he wrote that he was "persuaded that the American may be convinced by *facts* that even in our climate Epidemic and Pestilential maladies may be generated by local causes." Until his fellow citizens learned this lesson, he was afraid, they would continue to bring on sickness and pestilence by wallowing in filth, crowding their cities with dirty houses, neglecting bathing and washing, and "devouring in hot seasons undue quantities of animal food."[4] By this date the miasmatic thesis was firmly established, and its application on a broad scale led to the full blossoming of the sanitary movement in the nineteenth century.

The most significant development affecting public health in eighteenth-century America was the tremendous increase in the colonial population and, as a corollary, the creation of a much more complex society. As communities grew into towns and towns into small cities, intimate relationships between neighbors gave way to the more impersonal contacts characteristic of urban society. As of 1700 New York City had a population of about 4,500, Philadelphia around 4,400, Charleston less than 3,000, and Boston, the largest of all, about 6,700. By 1770 Philadelphia had grown to 28,000, New York to 21,000, Boston to 15,520, and Charleston to almost 11,000. In this same period the total number of inhabitants in the colonies had increased from around 300,000 to almost 2,500,000.

With this growth the health and welfare of citizens could no longer be left solely to individuals or to private charity. Necessity in some cases, and the spirit of paternalism or social consciousness in others, led to an increasing measure of government intervention. Private wells began to give way to public wells, and by the end of the century elementary public aqueducts and water systems began to appear. Ordinances and regulations governing sanitation, food, and water supplies became both more specific and more comprehensive, and the need to provide for the poor and sick led to the appointment of town physicians and the appearance of almshouses and pesthouses.

Since the majority of epidemic disorders are essentially crowd diseases, the expanding colonial population provided an ideal environment for their spread, and the growing trade with Europe, Africa, and the West Indies guaranteed their importation. One geographic advantage the colonies possessed was their relative isolation from each other. The lack of roads in the colonies and the distances between them necessitated traveling largely by sea; therefore, as Boston's example demonstrated, an effective quarantine at the port cities could keep certain diseases at bay or at least limit their spread. On the other hand, the absence of a disorder such as smallpox for a fifteen- or twenty-year period ensured the appearance of a generation of nonimmune individuals, so that once the disease later gained a foothold, it could prove devastating. Moreover, relatively mild childhood disorders such as measles and mumps were anything but mild when they struck a virgin population of young adults and children.

Understandably, the epidemics that aroused the most attention in the colonial period were the two highly fatal pestilences, smallpox and yellow fever. They appeared mysteriously, swept through the community with deadly force, struck down old and young alike, and brought a ghastly death to many of their victims. Diphtheria was a terrible scourge, too, but it reached major epidemic proportions only once in the colonial period. Although local outbreaks occasionally proved deadly to children in a particular family or community, the disorder did not become a serious problem until the latter part of the nineteenth century.

The constant references in colonial letters, diaries, journals, newspapers, and official records to the two great killer diseases, smallpox and yellow fever, speak more for their dramatic nature than for their actual impact upon colonial health. People have always feared strange and unknown dangers far more than familiar ones, and this holds true for diseases. The appearance of a few cases of Legionnaires' disease or bubonic plague in the twentieth century has been enough to cause newspaper headlines and bring demands for action by the federal government. The outcry today about AIDS does not reflect its true impact on morbidity and mortality but rather anxiety due to the fact that we know so little about it. By contrast, the thousands of deaths caused by smoking or drunken driving are familiar and hence acceptable. We may deplore them, but they arouse no fear or consternation among us.

The real threat to health and life in the colonial era came from malaria, generally known as "fever and ague"; various enteric disorders, usually lumped under the terms "flux" or "bloody flux"; and the omnipresent respiratory diseases. These disorders winnowed the infant population, accounted for a major share of the deaths among young people and adults, and, particularly in the case of malaria, debilitated a large proportion of the entire population. Sickness and death, largely associated with these endemic ailments, were recurrent themes in the correspondence and diaries of American colonials.[5] Yet it is well to bear in mind that by the eighteenth century, when the colonies had established sound economies, life expectancy in North America was higher than in Great Britain and Europe, and general health conditions were better.

While physicians and lay intellectuals debated the origin and nature of disease (with the majority convinced that all diseases arose from some one fundamental cause), the public never doubted the contagiousness of the great pestilences. The Black Death in the medieval period had taught people to shun plague victims and to use quarantines to keep the plague at bay. In the colonies Massachusetts led the way in instituting relatively effective methods for preventing the introduction of diseases. As early as 1647–48 the General Court proclaimed a day of fasting and ordered ships coming from the West Indies, the scene of a reported epidemic, to remain anchored in Boston Harbor until inspected. Similar measures were taken in 1665 when bubonic plague was ravaging London.

In 1699 the General Court passed a comprehensive law to prevent "the Spreading of Infectious Sicknesses." Ships arriving from an infected port or with sickness aboard were prohibited from landing passengers or goods without permission from the local authorities. The British government disallowed the measure on grounds that its one-hundred-pound fine and other penalties were too high, but a modified law enacted in 1701 was accepted. This law contained additional provisions that made it possible to isolate individuals with a contagious disorder. If necessary, town authorities could preempt a house and transfer the sick to it. In succeeding years the quarantine and isolation laws were gradually strengthened, and in 1717 a permanent pesthouse was built on Spectacle Island in Boston Harbor. Twenty years later, in 1737, it was replaced by a better one on Rainsford Island. By this date Massachusetts had the most effective quarantine system of any of the colonies.[6]

Charleston was another leader in the quarantine movement, possibly as a result of its warmer climate and closer proximity to the West Indies, the source of yellow fever and other disorders. As early as 1698 ship captains were ordered to report any contagious sicknesses aboard their vessels and were required to make provision for any sick sailors who landed in Charleston. A series of yellow fever attacks that began in 1699 led to the appointment in 1712 of Gilbert Guttery as port quarantine commissioner and to the establishment of a temporary pesthouse on Sullivan's Island in Charleston Harbor. In 1721 another quarantine measure required ship pilots to inquire about the health of the crew and passengers on all incoming vessels.

These quarantine laws—as would remain true of most public health measures until well into the nineteenth century—were either temporary or else tended to fall into abeyance once a crisis was over. In response to several successive outbreaks of yellow fever, the Carolina General Assembly in 1747 passed a quarantine law that revived provisions of the previous law and named six physicians to inspect all ships entering Charleston Harbor. Five years later the quarantine restrictions were applied to Georgetown and Beaufort (Port Royal). Aware that smallpox, yellow fever, and other infections were endemic in Africa, South Carolina required all slaves imported from Africa to serve a ten-day quarantine in the pesthouse on Sullivan's Island.[7]

As early as 1700 Pennsylvania had a quarantine law, but it was relatively ineffective. In the late 1730s and 1740s the arrival of shiploads of Irish and German settlers, many of whom were beset by contagious illnesses, forced the colonial government into taking stronger action. A "malignant distemper," probably smallpox, which spread through Philadelphia in 1738, was attributed to the German and Irish immigrants, and it led to a quarrel between Governor George Thomas, appointed by the colony's proprietors, and the General Assembly. In January 1739 the governor reported to the assembly that he had taken strict measures to enforce the quarantine laws, including appointing a physician to inspect incoming vessels and requiring ship captains to care for the sick outside the city. He then appealed to the assembly to vote funds for a pesthouse, asserting that had one been available the epidemic might have been averted. The assembly was unconvinced and no action was taken.[8]

Two years later the governor again appealed for a pesthouse, noting that German petitioners had protested the loss of lives caused by confining sick passengers on board their ships for lack of a hospital or pesthouse. In his address he acknowledged that many citizens resented the influx of Germans, but he argued that the immigrants represented potential wealth to the community. He denied that the assembly could not afford to build a pesthouse and urged that one be built on the grounds of humanity and "the Health of this City."[9] It is difficult to say how much the opposition represented antipathy to the immigrants and how much it reflected the recurrent clashes between the governor and the colonial legislature. In any event, the legislators, belatedly recognizing that sickness among immigrants represented a threat to themselves and their constituents, established a pesthouse shortly thereafter. Once the immediate crisis was over, though, little attention was given to maintaining it, and, when two shiploads of Palatinates arrived in a sickly condition in 1749, the pesthouse was found in a deplorable condition. The trustees of the pesthouse promised to put it in good order and to build additional temporary quarters. In consequence of this affair the provincial council introduced a bill to prohibit the "Importation of Germans and other passengers in too great Numbers on any one Vessel," but nothing seems to have come of it.[10]

New York followed a pattern similar to that of the other colonies with large ports. Quarantine laws had been enacted as early as the seventeenth century, but it was not until a series of major smallpox and yellow fever outbreaks in the 1730s that more specific quarantine regulations were established. Upon hearing reports of smallpox and yellow fever in the West Indies and Charleston in 1738, the New York City Council established a quarantine anchorage for all vessels coming from infected ports. More significant, Dr. Roeliff Kiersted was made official port physician, the first health officer appointed by the city. Subsequently the Provincial Council of New York entered the picture, and a series of quarantine regulations culminated in 1755 in one that empowered the governor to appoint a health officer and authorized the city to construct a pesthouse. After investigating various sites, the city council selected Bedlow's Island, and in 1760 the city's first pesthouse was opened.[11]

The growth of trade and commerce and the increasing threat from contagious diseases led all of the colonies to enact various quarantine regulations, but they differed widely in effectiveness. As indicated earlier, the colonies with the largest ports faced the greatest danger, and consequently they developed the most elaborate quarantine systems. Even so, in general the absence of disease for several years invariably led to neglect of quarantine procedures, and each new outbreak always resulted in denunciations of officials and the reenactment or strengthening of the previous laws.

Smallpox became an increasing problem as the colonial period advanced. It gave a major impetus to the passage of quarantine measures in colonial ports, and it also led to a series of ordinances and regulations with respect to its spread by land. Fortunately, it was also the first disease for which a relatively effective form of prevention was discovered. A series of letters in the *Transactions* of the Royal Philosophical Society in 1714 and 1716 described in detail a procedure used in Greece and Turkey for preventing smallpox. It consisted of taking pus from the pustules of an active smallpox case and inserting it in an incision made in the arm of a healthy individual. The procedure, known as inoculation, usually induced a mild case in those inoculated, thereby giving them immunity to the disease. The practice was common in sections of Africa and the Middle East and apparently was part of the folklore of Great Britain and the Continent.

The *Transactions* articles did not arouse too much attention until Dr. James Jurin and other physician members of the royal society took an interest in the subject. The inoculation movement received additional help from the wife of the British ambassador to Turkey, Lady Mary Wortley Montagu, who had encountered the practice while in Constantinople. In 1721 she had her three-year-old daughter inoculated, and through her contacts she may have influenced the royal family to experiment with the new technique. Whatever the case, although its use was restricted largely to the upper classes, inoculation became an accepted practice in England.[12]

Meanwhile, in Boston the Reverend Cotton Mather, in the course of querying a newly acquired slave about smallpox, learned about inoculation. Stimulated by the *Transactions* articles, he urged Dr. William Douglass, the only one of the ten physicians in Boston with an M.D. degree, to give the practice a trial. Douglass, a conservative physician, was reluctant to experiment with a deadly disease, particularly one that might kill or scar the subject for life. Fortunately, another Boston physician, Dr. Zabdiel Boyleston, had also heard of inoculation, and when smallpox appeared in Boston in the spring of 1721, he promptly inoculated his and Mather's children. Despite considerable opposition from most of the other physicians, some clergymen, and a good many citizens, Boyleston and two of his colleagues in the Boston neighborhood inoculated almost three hundred persons. Of those undergoing the practice, six died, or approximately 2 percent. Among those who acquired the disease naturally, the death rate ran about 14 percent.[13]

The 1721 epidemic had demonstrated that inoculation could limit the ravages of smallpox, but the procedure remained highly controversial for many years. Unlike the case with vaccinated persons, those inoculated with smallpox were capable of spreading a horrible and fatal pestilence. For the next fifty years the careless use of inoculation was undoubtedly responsible for causing a good many epidemics. Physicians such as Douglass denounced the practice as dangerous and unnecessary; ministers decried it on the grounds that it contravened God's will; and a good many citizens were reluctant to see smallpox introduced into the community under any circumstances. Nonetheless, the practice spread generally throughout the colonies, and by the time of the Revolution it was widely accepted.

At first the tendency was to prohibit inoculation unless the danger from smallpox was imminent. As the technique improved and those undergoing the procedure began to be kept isolated, these laws were gradually relaxed. The complete acceptance of inoculation was demonstrated following the siege of Boston. During the siege, smallpox, both natural and inoculated, had spread throughout the city and the surrounding countryside. Following the British evacuation in March 1776, General Washington ordered that all susceptible troops be inoculated. At the same time, the majority of the town's residents who had not suffered from smallpox resorted to inoculation, too. As a result, only a few individuals died of the disease.[14]

Without doubt, smallpox was the most feared disease in the colonial period, and it is safe to say that the disease inspired the majority of quarantine measures. Aside from the many laws prohibiting inoculation, one can find many similar to a Massachusetts law in 1731 entitled, an act "to prevent persons concealing the smallpox and requiring a red cloth to be hung out in all infected places." Connecticut in 1722 enacted a law "to prevent the small-pox being spread in this colony by pedlers, hawkers, [and] petty chapmen."[15] On one occasion Rhode Island made the penalty for violating the quarantine law death "without benefit of clergy."[16] The colonial records contain literally hundreds of ordinances and regulations prohibiting individuals coming from areas infected with smallpox or other disorders from entering a particular province or town.

Inoculation, in combination with improved quarantine and isolation measures, played a major role in reducing the death rate from smallpox in the eighteenth century. It is ironic that smallpox, one of the viral diseases, the last group to be conquered by the bacteriological revolution, should have been the first disease for which an effective preventive was discovered. More important, smallpox inoculation paved the way for vaccination. In 1798 Edward Jenner's announcement of his discovery that cowpox (vaccinia) was a far safer preventive for smallpox than inoculation was accepted almost immediately. Cotton Mather and Zabdiel Boyleston deserve much credit for introducing smallpox inoculation into Boston, for in addition to saving many lives, the American experience with the practice contributed greatly to its acceptance in the Old World.[17]

For aesthetic, as well as health, reasons, the residents of colonial towns increasingly concerned themselves with sanitary affairs. By the eighteenth century all the major towns had appointed scavengers, who were responsible for the removal of garbage, rubbish, and dead animals from the streets. For example, to ensure that the cartmen and residents complied with the street-cleaning law, New York City in 1695 employed a scavenger at a salary of thirty pounds a year. Citizens were still required to sweep up the dirt and debris in front of their houses and load it onto the carts;

the scavengers were to see that this was done and also were to remove any dirt, rubbish, or dead animals for which the cartmen were not responsible. As the city grew, more scavengers were appointed, but individual citizens continued to be responsible for keeping the streets in front of their homes clean. The only change from the original law of 1670 requiring cartmen to remove the garbage and rubbish every Saturday was a modification permitting the cartmen themselves to load the piles of debris onto their carts for a slight fee. The fee was optional, and citizens who wished to could continue to do the job themselves.[18]

The history of street cleaning in Boston resembles that for New York City. In 1712 scavengers were instructed to hire men with carts to clean the streets, but the city's residents were still required to sweep up the dirt and shovel it onto the carts. In both cities a tradition of civic responsibility made the street-cleaning system work reasonably well. By the second half of the eighteenth century, however, this tradition no longer sufficed, and increasingly complaints were recorded about the condition of the streets. Philadelphia and the other colonial towns lagged somewhat in adopting regulations for street cleaning—Charleston, for example, did not hire scavengers until 1750—but by the Revolution virtually all of them had adopted systems similar to those in New York and Boston.[19]

A major problem in all colonial towns was the lack of adequate drainage. Individual citizens usually took it upon themselves to drain their own property, or groups of them might build a common sewer or drain. In Boston complaints about individuals digging up the streets to make drains led to an ordinance requiring them to get prior permission from the selectmen. New York City had some special problems since its boundaries included a good many low-lying areas, particularly those in the vicinity of docks and slips, and the city reluctantly began constructing drains. The city markets created special sanitary problems, too, and on one occasion the city council, noting that it had gone to great expense to build a drain, or sewer, from one of the markets, forbade all vessels from obstructing the drain outlet by anchoring too close to it. In 1751 the council appointed a committee to investigate the feasibility of constructing an underground sewer in place of the Fly Market drain. The committee, reflecting a view that would prevail until well into the next century, concluded that the project would be far too expensive.[20]

These drains, or open sewers, soon became receptacles for every type of filth, all of which drained into the slips in the harbor. The solid material was deposited on the bottom of the slip; and when the tide was out, the stench, particularly in summer, was almost unbearable. The committee appointed by the New York City Council in 1751 recommended that the slip be dredged so as to leave twelve inches of water at low tide. Although

this recommendation was occasionally followed, the situation steadily worsened with the growth of the city. Not only were the slips the recipients
of the contents of the sewers, but the cartmen and scavengers later employed to empty privies all cheerfully dumped their loads either onto the
docks or into the slips. Conditions were not too bad in colonial days, but
they became acute by the end of the eighteenth century. Other colonial
towns also faced this situation, but, fortunately, to a lesser degree.

The growing urban population in the eighteenth century sharply accentuated the problems caused by nuisance industries such as tanning, bone
boiling, slaughtering, butchering, fishmongering, cloth dying, and starch
making. For example, slaughterers and butchers drained the blood from
slaughtered animals into gutters or drains and piled entrails, refuse, and
hides outside their places of work until the fat-burners, bone-boilers, and
tanners could come to take them away. The hides, complete with bits of
flesh, the entrails, and other refuse were eventually hauled away to the
establishments of the other tradesmen, who then piled them on their own
premises. One can only imagine the odor and flies surrounding these
workplaces. In a process that would repeat itself time after time, as cities
gradually expanded and encircled these industries, local residents demanded action, and the authorities eventually required slaughterers and
others to locate outside of town. The reluctance of town officials to move
against the owners of these businesses arose from the fact that it was
usually the poor who lived in the vicinity of what were termed the "noxious trades"—and the poor rarely have much influence. In consequence,
the situation had to be desperate before city officials would take action.

The eighteenth century also saw civic authorities becoming more concerned about the water supply. The rising population density increased
the demand for water and at the same time threatened its purity. Probably
as a result of the poor quality of its water, New York City was forced into
leadership in this area. As early as 1677 the residents along six streets were
ordered to dig public wells. A few years later the city council ordered the
construction of nine more public wells, with the city paying half the cost
and the adjacent residents paying the rest. The brackish water from New
York's wells was a constant source of complaint from both residents and
visitors. Toward the end of the colonial period a Swedish visitor wrote
that only the "less delicate" drank water from the city wells, and that even
horses were reluctant to drink it. Those who could afford to bought water
from water carriers, who obtained it either from springs outside the city
or from a spring located at Chatham and Pearl streets known as the Tea
Water Pump. By 1761 the city undertook to license these water carriers.[21]

Health was only a minor concern of those who led the fight for an
adequate water supply. The omnipresent danger of fires in an age when

open fires and candles were common provided the real impetus. By 1753 New York City assumed full responsibility for maintaining and repairing all public wells and pumps. In 1774 Christopher Colles, a British engineer who had come to America in 1765, proposed constructing a reservoir and a system to "Convey Water thro' the Several Streets of this City." The city council agreed to purchase land for a reservoir, provided that potable water could be found under it. Colles sank a well, and the well water was pronounced to be of good quality. Work began on the project immediately, and by the spring of 1776 the reservoir was ready for operation. Water was pumped from the reservoir and distributed by means of hollow logs. The water supply proved inadequate, though, and any chance Colles had to rectify the situation was doomed by the start of the Revolutionary War. By this time the project had cost the city some £11,400. Unfortunately, another twenty-five years would elapse before a new water system would be put into operation.[22]

In the majority of colonial towns and villages, the water supply remained the concern of private citizens, who individually or collectively constructed and maintained wells. In the larger cities some regulations were usually enacted with respect to the water supply, and the authorities occasionally assumed responsibility for one or more public wells. The common use of privies and the presence of stables, dairies, and the nuisance industries within towns raise some intriguing questions as to the quality of the water pumped from these shallow wells.

By 1700 most of the larger towns employed a physician of the poor or made provision for individual hardship cases. To care for the homeless poor, almshouses began appearing in the 1730s. Although they essentially provided custodial care for the aged and sick, the almshouses usually had a physician assigned to them. The standard practice was to buy a house to care for the poor, although a building was occasionally erected for this purpose. Since the majority of their residents tended to be sick, the almshouses served as a form of hospital for the poor—a situation that has led to much historical debate over priority in the establishment of hospitals.

Probably the first hospital to be established in the present United States—and certainly the oldest one in existence today—was Charity Hospital in New Orleans, founded in 1736 as "a hospital for the sick." As with many hospitals, Charity tended to fill up with the aged poor, and some historians have argued that it was an almshouse and not strictly a hospital. On the other hand, claims of precedence have been put forth for Blockley in Philadelphia, an almshouse founded at about the same time, which also supplied a measure of medical care. In 1738 Charleston opened a public workhouse and hospital, but it, too, was largely an almshouse.

The best claim to priority in the American colonies is that of Pennsylvania Hospital, established in 1752 under the auspices of Dr. Thomas Bond and Benjamin Franklin. Its function was essentially curative since its first regulation specified that no one considered incurable should be admitted.[23]

Regardless of which hospital in the colonies was founded first, all are evidence that civic leaders were beginning to take some steps toward caring for the sick and poor. Judging from complaints, these measures were far from adequate. Although Charleston had established a place for the sick poor in 1738, a grand jury complained to the legislature in 1765 about the "want of a general hospital or poor-house," explaining that "the place at present assigned for the accommodation [was] insufficient" and "a very improper receptacle for the poor being crowded with criminals, vagrants, sailors, and negroes."[24] The existence of criticisms such as this one at least indicates a growing sense of social responsibility.

This same rising social consciousness can be seen in the establishment of the first institutions to care for the insane. In the seventeenth century most colonies had established regulations providing guardianship or financial support or both for the mentally ill. In the early eighteenth century some mentally ill persons were accommodated in almshouses on a custodial basis. The first institution to offer medical care for the insane was Pennsylvania Hospital, an institution that admitted both charity and private patients. One of the first two patients admitted to the institution in 1752 was a "lunatic," and shortly thereafter another one was admitted as a private patient.[25]

In Boston, Charleston, and other colonial towns appeals were made on behalf of the mentally ill, but nothing came of them. Although hospitals traditionally have been associated with urban areas, the colony of Virginia, which had no major city, was the first one to establish a state institution devoted solely to the care of the mentally ill. Acting upon the request of Governor Francis Fauquier in 1766, the Virginia House of Burgesses began a long process of studying, and finally appropriating funds for, what became the Eastern State Hospital in Williamsburg. It opened in 1773, complete with a keeper, a matron, and an attending physician. According to the law, the institution was open to any "person" in the colony. Although the term excluded slaves, surprisingly the hospital admitted free blacks. Moreover, the directors took it upon themselves to provide needy recovered patients with a small sum of money for travel and clothes. The institution had a difficult time during the Revolutionary War years, but it managed to survive and still serves the state today.[26]

In the eighteenth century lead poisoning, associated with the processing of cider in England and rum in the American colonies, became a fairly serious problem. Physicians discussed and debated the issue, but it was soon recognized that what was known as "the dry belly-ake" arose from the use of lead pipes in the distillation process. Massachusetts in 1723 sought to prevent this practice by passing an act "for Preventing Abuses in Distilling Rum and Other Strong Liquors." As with many of the early laws regulating food, the motive here was probably as much to protect the rum trade as it was to safeguard the public health.[27]

The picture drawn in these past two chapters of colonial life is fairly grim. Epidemic and endemic disorders flourished, infant mortality was high, and death was always close at hand. Compared to modern cities, colonial towns were odorous and lacked effective water, sewer, and street-cleaning systems. Yet if we compare them with similar British and European towns, the picture is much brighter. Nearly all Europeans visiting the colonies in the eighteenth century commented upon the spaciousness, orderliness, and relative cleanliness of American towns. They commended the pure air and noted that many of the main streets were paved and clean. By the time of the Revolution, American towns were beginning to face serious urban problems, but most citizens still had a strong sense of community responsibility. Moreover, land was still relatively cheap, and even the housing of the poor was better than that for those crowded in the ancient fetid slums of Europe. To European visitors, American cities still possessed a measure of charm.

NOTES

1. John Duffy, *The Healers: A History of American Medicine* (Urbana, Ill., 1979), 28.

2. Duffy, *The Healers,* 42–44; Saul Jarcho, "Cadwallader Colden as a Student of Infectious Disease," *Bulletin of the History of Medicine* (hereafter cited as *Bull. Hist. Med.*) 29 (1955):100–103.

3. John Jones, *Plain Concise Practical Remarks on the Treatment of Wounds and Fractures* (New York, 1775), in appendix to James W. Beekman's *Centenary Address Delivered Before the Society of the New York Hospital, Monday, July 24, 1871* (New York, 1871), 12–13.

4. Noah Webster, *A Collection of Papers on the subject of Bilious Fevers prevalent in the United States for a few years past* (New York, 1796), frontispiece entitled "Advertisement."

5. John Duffy, *Epidemics in Colonial America* (Baton Rouge, La., 1953), 237ff.

6. Francis R. Packard, *History of Medicine in the United States* (New York, 1931), 1:166–67; John B. Blake, *Public Health in the Town of Boston* (Cambridge, Mass., 1959), 32–36.

7. Joseph Ioor Waring, *A History of Medicine in South Carolina, 1670–1825* (Columbia, S.C., 1964), 18, 26, 30–31, 60, 63–65.

8. *Pennsylvania Archives,* 4th ser., 1 (Harrisburg, Pa., 1900), 673–75; *Colonial*

Records, Minutes of the Provincial Council of Pennsylvania (Harrisburg, Pa., 1851), 4:507–24.

9. *Pennsylvania Archives,* 4th ser., 1:767–71.

10. *Colonial Records, Minutes of the Provincial Council,* 5:410, 427.

11. Duffy, *A History of Public Health in New York City, 1625–1866* (New York, 1968), 60–62.

12. Genevieve Miller, *The Adoption of Inoculation for Smallpox in England and France* (Philadelphia, 1957), provides the best account of inoculation in England.

13. Duffy, *Epidemics in Colonial America,* 23–42; Blake, *Public Health in Boston,* 52–73.

14. Blake, *Public Health in Boston,* 126–27.

15. Packard, *History of Medicine in the United States,* 1:166–67.

16. Ernest Caulfield, *A True History of the Terrible Epidemic Vulgarly Called the Throat Distemper which Occurred in His Majesty's New England Colonies Between the Years 1775 and 1740* (New Haven, Conn., 1939), 3.

17. Genevieve Miller, "Smallpox Inoculation in England and America," *William and Mary Quarterly: A Magazine of Early American History,* 3d ser., 13 (1956):476–78, argues that the deaths in New England and the prohibition of inoculation there actually delayed the spread of inoculation in England.

18. Duffy, *Public Health in New York City, 1625–1866,* 24–26, 41–42.

19. Waring, *Medicine in South Carolina,* 68.

20. *Minutes of the Common Council of the City of New York, 1675–1776* (New York, 1905), 5:145–46, 343–44, 369.

21. Per Kalm, *Travels into North America,* John R. Forster, trans. (London, 1770–71), 1:249–50.

22. Duffy, *Public Health in New York City, 1625–1866,* 48–50. For a description of the water system see Isaac N. P. Stokes, *The Iconography of Manhattan Island* (New York, 1915–28), 4:926.

23. John Duffy, ed., *The Rudolph Matas History of Medicine in Louisiana* (Baton Rouge, La., 1958–62), 1:103–11; Duffy, *The Healers,* 58–59.

24. *South Carolina Gazette,* June 8, 1765, cited in Newspapers of South Carolina, Toner Collection MSS, Library of Congress.

25. Gerald N. Grob, *Mental Institutions in America: Social Policy to 1875* (New York, 1973), 13–25.

26. Norman Dain, *Disordered Minds: The First Century of Eastern State Hospital in Williamsburg, Virginia, 1766–1866* (Williamsburg, 1971), 5–20.

27. Jacqueline K. Corn, "Historical Perspective to a Current Controversy on the Clinical Spectrum of Plumbism," *Milbank Memorial Foundation Quarterly* (Winter 1975):99.

3

The Appearance of Health Boards

The outbreak of the Revolutionary War disrupted civic life in every major city and led to widespread epidemics of infectious disorders. The mobilization of civilians and the subsequent movement of troops increased both the incidence and spread of enteric and respiratory infections, while smallpox, which had been on a slight decline, flared up in serious proportions. As for malaria, as the eighteenth century had advanced, it had gradually receded from the New England colonies. One result was that, as the fighting moved into the southern colonies, the New England troops suffered heavily from the ravages of malarial fever. The Boston area, scene of the initial fighting, was the first to feel the weight of a major smallpox epidemic. In June 1776 John Adams wrote almost in despair: "The small pox! The small pox! What shall we do with it? I could almost wish that an inoculating hospital was opened in every town in New-England."[1] Fortunately, the general use of inoculation gradually brought smallpox under control, but during the first two or three years of the war it remained a serious problem in all sections of the country.

One reason for the surge in infectious diseases at the onset of the war was that the majority of recruits came from country areas, where isolation provided a measure of safety from epidemic diseases. Once they were brought into crowded army camps, where sanitary precautions were minimal, they fell prey to a host of infections. Accustomed to relieving themselves in any convenient spot, the men proceeded to befoul their camp sites at a rapid pace. Many of the officers were little better than their men in this respect, and the lack of discipline in the early years made it difficult even for conscientious and informed officers to enforce sanitary regulations. The result was that diarrheas, dysenteries, typhoid fever, and other intestinal disorders compounded the medical problems of the Continental armies. As has been true of all wars for the past three centuries, the value of strictly enforced sanitary regulations was eventually recognized, and with better discipline, the condition of the camps gradually improved. Yet sickness and disease, aided and abetted by inadequate and poorly cooked food, killed nine or ten times as many men as did battle injuries.

The Revolution itself, by pitting citizen against citizen, disrupted normal services in the port cities, and this disruption was compounded by successive military occupations. Each of these military operations resulted in mass flights by the civilian population. New York City, which was held by the British from 1776 to the end of the war, probably suffered the worst setback. Earlier clashes between Patriots and Tories that had taken place before the British conquest had already destroyed some property and reduced the level of city services. The capture of the city by the British forced thousands of Patriots to flee, reducing the population by half. In the wake of the occupation forces came an influx of Tories and a consequent looting of Patriot homes. Public buildings and a number of large private ones were commandeered by the army for use as barracks and other purposes. To add to New York City's difficulties, two major fires in 1776 and 1778 devastated large areas. Under normal circumstances the many volunteer fire companies might have been able to minimize the damage, but their ranks had been greatly diminished.

The breakdown of civilian government forced the British army to assume some measure of control, and efforts were made to restore normal city services, but with limited success. As the war dragged on, damage from the fires and the influx of Tories and their sympathizers resulted in a severe housing shortage; huts, shanties, and shoddy buildings erected by unscrupulous contractors gradually filled in many areas destroyed by fire. Little if any maintenance was done on public buildings, and Colles's water system, already in difficulty, was completely abandoned. Out of necessity some street cleaning was performed, the public wells were kept in operation, certain of the bread laws and other food laws were enforced, and a little care was provided for the sick and the poor.[2]

When the British evacuated New York in the spring of 1783, the population was again reduced to about twelve thousand. At this time many areas of the city were still fire-blackened, and the municipal buildings, the medical school, and other structures requisitioned by the British were in poor repair. The revived city government faced an enormous task in restoring municipal services and in repairing civic buildings, docks, slips, and equipment. The job was made no easier by a massive influx of former New Yorkers who had fled the British occupation and of thousands of others seeking economic opportunities.

While New York City, possibly because of the length of its occupation, felt the ravages of war more than most American cities, all of them experienced bitter factionalism, destruction of property, and a general dislocation engendered by wartime conditions. Despite these difficulties, recovery from the British occupation was usually quite rapid. Boston, the first to be occupied, was relieved of the British in March 1776. Although its recovery was hindered by the continuing war, it was functioning reasonably well by 1780. This same situation held true for most other towns and cities. Even during occupation the sanitary situation was never too bad since the work of the celebrated eighteenth-century English army physician, Sir John Pringle, had made British officers conscious of the need to enforce sanitary regulations. If anything, the war may have increased public awareness of the need for personal and community hygiene—but if this was true, the lesson was soon lost.

In the years following the Revolution, American cities witnessed a strong growth in population. The most extreme example was New York City, where the population jumped from about 12,000 following the British evacuation in 1783 to 23,614 by 1786. By 1790 the population was over 33,000. Philadelphia, which had not suffered as severely as New York, also witnessed a rapid increase in the same period, and by 1800, with a population of almost 80,000, it had become the largest city in America. Boston's population increased by about 60 percent between the Revolution and 1800, and other cities showed commensurate growth.

In terms of street cleaning, garbage collection, and water supplies, little change ensued for the first few years following independence. The basic pattern of sanitary regulations established in colonial days was modified only slightly. Individual citizens were still responsible for cleaning their premises and the streets in front of their homes. A number of towns, however, began to employ or contract cartmen to remove street dirt. In addition, more scavengers and other officers were appointed to enforce the regulations regarding street cleaning, the nuisance industries, and the removal of carrion and debris from vacant lots and public places. Despite conscientious efforts by many civic leaders, American cities and towns were outgrowing their governmental structures, and sanitary problems continued to increase well beyond the capacity of city officials to cope with them.

Food regulations, too, remained relatively unchanged, but the growing population brought some fundamental changes in the processing and distribution of food. These years saw the transitional growth of towns into cities, and with this growth came middlemen and food processors. Effective as the introduction of food processing on a larger scale may have been from an economic standpoint, it also opened the way for the increasing adulteration of food. Complaints began to appear in newspapers about "hogslard and tallow" being added to butter, and a New York dairyman's advertisement that he intended "to supply the town with good Milk, unmixed with water" speaks for itself.[3]

As New York City expanded, its municipal abattoir could no longer handle all slaughtered animals, and butchers were once again permitted to slaughter at their places of business. In response to outraged cries about the butchers throwing offal and other offensive substances into the streets, the city council passed an ordinance strictly forbidding the practice. The growing demand for food also created profitable opportunities for sharp businessmen such as John Jacob Astor, who on one occasion sought to corner the beef market by buying all cattle coming into New York. His action reflected this period's rising spirit of free enterprise, which clashed with the traditional regulations designed to protect the consumer.[4] The result was a gradual weakening of the laws designed to control the quality of bread and meat.

Although New York City made some efforts to revive the water system project, its citizens, and those of all other towns and cities, continued to rely on public and private wells. The old regulations for maintaining and protecting the pumps and wells remained in effect, and, although some laws were reworded to strengthen their enforcement, no progress was made until the yellow fever crisis of the 1790s. In the meantime growing population density, combined with the use of privies and the presence of stables and dairies in town, did little to improve the quality of water drawn from shallow wells.

For the first ten years or so after the Revolution Americans were preoccupied with establishing state constitutions and a federal government, and health concerns were given little consideration. This situation changed abruptly in 1793 when the first of a series of devastating yellow fever epidemics hit virtually every port city and town on the East Coast—and ranged as far as New Orleans on the Gulf Coast. Fortunately, up to this date the young nation had escaped a major pestilence; but the negative side of this good fortune was that the quarantine laws had tended to fall into abeyance. Although yellow fever was no stranger to America, its terrible attacks, beginning in the 1690s, had gradually tapered off by the mid-eighteenth century; after one final outbreak in Philadelphia in 1762, it disappeared for over thirty years. In the meantime an entire generation had grown up with no experience of this deadly disease; hence its sudden and mysterious reappearance in 1793 understandably aroused terror and consternation. For over ten years following the Philadelphia yellow fever epidemic, this dreaded pestilence ravaged American coastal cities, giving a major impetus to the early public health movement. From the standpoint of American public health, the period from 1793 to 1806 deserves to be known as the yellow fever era.

Cases of yellow fever first appeared in Philadelphia early in August 1793, but it was not until August 19 that a definite diagnosis was made. By the end of the month the number of deaths was in the hundreds, and the town was in a state of panic. Members of the College of Physicians were unable to agree as to the disease's cause or cure, and the beginning of September witnessed a mass flight of townspeople. Although Philadelphia had a port health officer (who was responsible for enforcing the quarantine regulations and managing the quarantine station) and a port physician to care for sick crewmen and passengers, unfortunately, no funds were available to support them. Consequently, as late as September 5, 1793, ships from the West Indies, where yellow fever was rampant, were still entering the port without being inspected. The Pennsylvania state legislature, urged on by the governor, on this same day granted him emergency powers, revived a former quarantine law, and promptly adjourned so that its members could leave town. On September 10 President Washington left the city, and by the middle of the month most federal, state, and civic officers had fled. Fortunately, Philadelphia had a courageous and conscientious mayor, Matthew Clarkson, who remained on the job throughout the epidemic.

Clarkson faced an enormous task. The governor had allocated some emergency funds to the city, but the official responsible for them had left. The mayor himself had very limited resources and was forced to rely largely on voluntary help. The only agency available to care for the sick was the Guardians of the Poor, a volunteer group. By September 10 the weekly death toll was running into the hundreds; the Guardians of the Poor and the African Society, as well as various church groups and other voluntary organizations that were trying to help the sick, were literally overwhelmed. On this day Mayor Clarkson issued an appeal for volunteers. Four days later a committee of some twenty-six citizens was formed, with Clarkson at the head. It promptly arranged to borrow money and then set to work organizing hospitals, arranging for physicians, providing for the sick, and caring for the poor and orphaned.[5]

Significantly, the committee had no legal status, and in this time of crisis Philadelphia was forced to rely upon the voluntary action of its citizens. With the municipal government in complete disarray, the volunteer committee became in effect an extralegal government. Its appeal for funds, food, and supplies was quickly answered. From neighboring towns came cartloads of food and other contributions. A committee in New York City raised $5,000, and smaller amounts of money came in from other towns and individuals. This epidemic, which virtually paralyzed the city and killed over 5,000 of its residents within less than four months, shocked the entire country and promoted a widespread sense of civic responsibility. Although volunteer effort continued to be the main support during times of epidemic crises, increasingly throughout the United States municipal and state governments began to play a role.

Yellow fever returned to Philadelphia the next year, 1794, and continued its attacks until 1805. In 1794 it appeared in Baltimore and New Haven, and in 1795 New York City felt its full force. For the next ten years it ravaged the entire East and Gulf Coasts, relaxed its grip slightly, and then returned briefly to the Northeast Coast around 1820. Henceforth, except for an occasional outbreak of a few cases, yellow fever concentrated its attack upon America's coastal regions from Norfolk, Virginia, southward.

As news had spread of the first arrival of the pestilence in Philadelphia in 1793, quarantine measures in every town and state were revived and enforced. Baltimore called out the militia to guard the roads against sick refugees from Philadelphia, and local and state officials along the entire East Coast were given extraordinary powers to prevent the entrance of the disease. New York City tightened its quarantine regulations, and its mayor and council voted to appoint as many inhabitants as necessary in each ward to carry "into strict execution the Law for preventing Nuisances in this City." This city's physicians could not agree as to whether the contagion was generated locally or imported, but government officials chose the cautious route of resorting to both quarantine and sanitary measures.

New York City was more fortunate than Philadelphia since it had two years of warning before experiencing its first major epidemic in 1795. Upon receiving the first news of the presence of yellow fever in Philadelphia, the New York City Council discussed the matter but was reluctant to authorize any expenditures to protect the city. Its failure to act led to the formation in 1793 of a voluntary citizens' group similar to Philadelphia's. It promptly took upon itself the responsibility for employing two physicians to assist the city's health officer in inspecting incoming vessels, hired additional inspectors to patrol the wharves and ferries to prevent anyone landing from Philadelphia, and then sent representatives to meet with the mayor and city council. The latter, happy to be relieved of responsibility, established a seven-man committee to work with the citizens' group and invested the joint body with full power "to do everything which may become necessary."[6]

This "Health Committee," as it was called, immediately established a rigid quarantine around the city, hired a boat to help the health officer check on incoming vessels, arranged for a quarantine hospital on Governor's Island, and appealed for volunteers to patrol all entrances to the city. A widespread belief at this time held that disease could be transmitted by fomites, that is, particles of contagious matter attached to clothing or other articles. In accordance with this view the committee published a broadside warning of the danger of infection from imported goods such as wool, silk, and cotton. The broadside also gave instructions that all baggage and cargoes from infected areas were to be unloaded, purified, and ventilated. Clothing was to be "smoked with the fumes of brimstone [sulphur] for one day." The committee also pressured the city council into hiring twenty-four additional watchmen to augment the volunteer patrols. Cold weather finally ended the threat of yellow fever, and in December the committee concluded its work. Its final action was to make a series of recommendations to the state government.[7]

The New York state legislature responded to these recommendations the following spring in 1794 by extending the quarantine law to include all vessels entering New York Harbor, providing a salary of about $5,000 a year for the city's health officer, and making Governor's Island the state quarantine station.[8] When yellow fever threatened again in the summer of 1794, Governor George Clinton proclaimed a quarantine against all vessels from the West Indies and New Orleans and reappointed the fourteen-man Health Committee that had acted so decisively the previous summer. The committee was now an official agency of the state and, as such, was the forerunner of a permanent health office. As a result of the committee's work, or else by sheer luck, New York once again escaped.

In April 1795 the Health Committee reported the presence of a malignant fever in the West Indies and ordered all vessels arriving from there to be kept a quarter mile from shore until inspected by the health officer. Early in August the committee issued a statement conceding the presence of a few cases of yellow fever but assuring the public that these cases had been safely isolated. It cautioned against "the imprudent use of Cold Water," urged moderation and personal hygiene, and declared: "The cleanliness of the Streets, Yards, Cellars, & Markets & the removal of all putrescent matter are objects of very great importance and ought to be particularly attended to—especially in those parts of the City which are contiguous to our Eastern Rivers."[9] This statement is significant, for up to this time the Health Committee had concerned itself primarily with quarantine and isolation.

The committee's concern with sanitation reflected the growing division in medical opinion as to the cause of pestilential fevers. The public never doubted the contagiousness of malignant diseases, but observant physicians saw too many instances in which individuals in close contact with fever victims did not catch the disease. They had noted that this was especially true of patients who were nursed in homes away from infected areas. To the physicians, who lacked any knowledge of pathogenic organisms and insect vectors, the miasmatic theory, which attributed disease to a gaseous substance arising from stagnant water or putrefying matter, seemed a logical explanation. By this date, too, the medical profession was beginning to achieve a measure of recognition. Local physicians had been called upon occasionally in colonial times for advice during epidemics; by the time of the Revolution, however, medical societies began appearing on the scene, giving the profession some cohesion. Although these were local groups and most were short-lived, they encouraged physicians to assert their authority on health affairs.

The physicians' views on disease causation brought them into conflict with the Health Committee. During the epidemic of 1795, when the committee insisted on removing all yellow fever cases to Bellevue Hospital, members of the medical profession opposed it. Dr. Charles Buxton, secretary of the College of Physicians, wrote that isolation was harmful to patients, distressing to their friends, and needlessly alarming to the public. Some doctors refused to report yellow fever cases, providing an early example of a perennial complaint of public health officials—health professionals' refusal to report cases of infectious disease. In view of the danger of transporting seriously ill patients in horses and carts over rough streets to a crowded fever hospital, the defiant New York physicians had a valid complaint. More important, however, few of them believed the disease was contagious. On September 5, 1795, the New York Medical Society passed a specific resolution to this effect and sent it to the Health Committee.[10]

By the time the yellow fever epidemic ended, about 750 New Yorkers, out of a population of 40,000, were dead. The city council, in support of the Health Committee, had spent thousands of dollars and assumed a high degree of responsibility for the health of its constituents. The following spring, in 1796, the New York Medical Society, convinced that local conditions were the main factor in transforming the normal summer fevers into epidemic pestilences, urged the council to clean up the city. Among the dangers cited by the society were the "intolerable stench" around the city's docks and wharves, putrefying carrion and other substances in streets and vacant lots, and the filth around slaughterhouses and other establishments of the "noxious trades." The council ordered the society's report to be published and asked the state legislature for authority to comply with the recommendations.[11] The legislature responded promptly and in April 1796 enacted a comprehensive health law.

The first ten provisions of this health law established a permanent health office to enforce the quarantine system. The New York City Health Office was to consist of several appointed health commissioners, one of whom, a practicing physician, was to serve as health officer. The law also required all vessels coming from infected ports and all those carrying forty or more sick passengers to perform quarantine. Another important provision gave the health officer a permanent source of income—an inspection fee of three pounds from each foreign vessel and thirty-two shillings from each domestic ship. The law also provided for a suitable pesthouse, or quarantine hospital. The last few sections of the law authorized the city to pass sanitary ordinances affecting streets, vacant lots, nuisances, and the obnoxious trades. These ordinances, however, could not remain in effect for more than one year without the specific approval of the governor, and the city could not force owners of nuisance establishments to move without compensating them.[12] The council, even when given authority to make general laws about unsanitary conditions, was hesitant about using this power, preferring to deal with individual abuses.

Yellow fever continued to strike each summer, and the Health Office, aided by appropriations from the city council, conscientiously strove to keep the disease under control or to minimize its effects. In 1798 another major epidemic disrupted economic life and caused thousands of residents to flee the city. The Health Office now assumed the functions of the former Health Committee; but with the sick and destitute running into the thousands, the council appointed a special committee with almost unlimited authority to deal with the crisis. This committee erected two temporary hospitals, hired three full-time physicians, and began the major task of caring for the poor. It established three centers, where up to 2,000 persons were fed on a daily basis and where rations were distributed to 500 families. The committee used the almshouse, which was caring for another 800 persons, as a headquarters; here its members interviewed applicants for help and heard complaints. The city also undertook a large-scale drainage and cleanup campaign. Additional scavengers were hired to remove garbage, cellars were inspected and limed, and lime was spread to remove all offensive odors.[13]

The 1798 outbreak killed between 1,500 and 2,000 residents and caused considerable soul-searching among physicians and responsible citizens. In November, following the epidemic, the city council appointed a special committee to investigate the origins of the fever. The committee conferred with the city's medical society, the Health Office, and the chamber of commerce, and submitted its report in January 1799. The report clearly showed that in the argument between the contagionists and sanitationists, the latter had won the day. The entire focus of the report was on the local causes of disease and the need for a continuous effort to keep the city clean. Every sanitary problem of the day was listed among the contributing causes to disease—damp cellars, undrained lots, foul-smelling slips, and overflowing sinks and privies; the miasmas from pickled and dried fish, salt beef and salt pork, imported hides and skins, and burials within the city during hot months; and, finally, the city's narrow streets, which impeded air circulation. Apropos the miasmas mentioned in the list, the report declared that the exhalations from putrefying food are "not only calculated to spread disease, but from the most unequivocal evidence, did produce it in the course of the last season."[14]

To solve these problems the special committee recommended that the city government be given authority to enter and inspect all buildings and grounds, to regulate the condition of privies and their construction, to require lots to be filled or drained, to prohibit the storage of pickled or salted food in densely settled areas, and to deal with any other sanitary issues. Recognizing that the responsibility for street cleaning could no longer be left to individual citizens, the committee urged the municipality to hire carts and laborers and assume full responsibility for the job. In terms of the prevailing views on municipal responsibility these were radical ideas, but the committee went even further. It recommended that the city build underground sewers and plan for a water system. The latter was needed since "a plentiful supply of fresh water" was "one of the most powerful . . . means of removing the causes of pestilential diseases." In addition to making specific proposals, the members of the committee generalized upon the role of government in public health. They recognized that the proposed measures would cause much inconvenience, but they felt that the public good must come first. Only by investing the municipal authorities with "strong discretionary power" could the city be restored to its former healthy state. This report is significant, for implicit in all its recommendations is the principle that public welfare takes precedence over individual property rights.[15]

Within two weeks of receiving the committee's report, the city council drafted a bill for the legislature, which was then enacted with minimum changes. In consequence, the city appointed two street commissioners to carry out all laws for "the cleansing of the City and promoting the Health thereof." One of the commissioners' first discoveries was that some slum housing had been erected on lots so small that there was no room for privies, compelling the inhabitants to make the cellars "receptacles of filth and dirt." In what may have been the first slum clearance project in the United States, the city asked for, and was given, authority to buy these buildings and destroy them. In the next two or three years the city succeeded in strengthening its authority to regulate streets, slips, wharves, and building construction. The municipal government now proceeded to take full control over sanitary matters and left the health commissioners free to administer the quarantine program.[16]

In surveying developments in New York City from 1794 to 1800, it is clear that health needs literally forced the municipality and the state to assume greater responsibilities. During the yellow fever epidemic of 1798 the city government appropriated $11,600, and the state another $45,000. In 1799 when the disease returned, the city council ordered the evacuation of many blocks in the dock areas and provided tents on high ground for housing the poor. These same procedures were resorted to in 1803 and

1805 when the fever again reached epidemic proportions. At the same time temporary hospitals were established, and visiting physicians were employed to care for the sick in their homes. The threat of fever each summer created an awareness of many sanitary abuses and led to attempts to clean up the city. Unfortunately, these problems were insurmountable, and, despite temporary gains, the sanitary condition of New York, as with other rapidly growing towns and cities, grew steadily worse.

Although yellow fever today is usually associated with warmer climates, the disease struck widely along the New England coast beginning in 1794. Hartford, Providence, New Haven, and Boston all witnessed outbreaks of yellow fever, although their cooler climate kept casualties to a minimum. The news of the havoc caused by the fever in more southerly ports along with the presence of a few local cases was enough to stimulate civic and state authorities into tightening quarantine restrictions covering both land and sea.[17] In 1793 Boston, which already had an effective harbor quarantine, appointed a health officer to guard land entrances to the city and asked the governor to assist in enforcing the land quarantine by providing military forces. At first the authorities placed their main reliance upon quarantine, but as the epidemics continued and medical opinion swung toward domestic causation, an increasing concern with sanitary matters developed.

The continuing threat of yellow fever and a minor outbreak in 1796 strengthened the hand of Boston's public health reformers, and in 1797 the General Court of Massachusetts gave municipalities the power to enact limited sanitary regulations and to appoint health officers. Instead of establishing a separate board of health, the Boston selectmen simply declared themselves a health committee and assumed its powers, a practice that was to be followed by councilmen in most American cities for the next fifty or more years.

In 1799, following a more severe yellow fever epidemic that may have killed as many as three hundred Bostonians, a twelve-man board of health was established. Reflecting a growing suspicion of the medical profession fueled by the disagreement among physicians as to the cause of yellow fever, not a single physician was named to the board. The board members, however, did consult with leading physicians as to what sanitary measures they should take. At first the board was relatively ineffective since its powers over sanitation were restricted, with quarantine matters still in the hands of the selectmen. To remedy this situation the selectmen strengthened the board and gave it authority over both quarantine and sanitary affairs. Significantly, the board was authorized to make whatever rules and regulations on health matters it deemed necessary. Since the board members were primarily concerned with yellow fever, once the crisis passed, the work of the board was sharply reduced. Moreover, because the members were elected, a high degree of political influence affected the board's activities. Nonetheless, as John B. Blake has pointed out, Boston had created a permanent health organization and had firmly established the principle that health was a matter of public concern.[18]

Baltimore, a town of about 15,000 or 16,000 in 1793, had relatively little self-government. To meet the threat of yellow fever the governor of Maryland appointed two quarantine physicians in Baltimore, one to check on communication by sea and the other by land. The following year a seven-man committee on health was appointed, and in 1795 the state provided for the election of a board of health and a port health officer. Two years later, in 1797, Baltimore was given a city charter and authorized to enact sanitary and quarantine ordinances. Under the charter a new board of health was created, but its chief functions were to enforce the quarantine laws and manage the quarantine hospital, or pesthouse. It could draw attention to sanitary abuses but could neither prevent nor correct them since these matters were left in the hands of the city commissioners. As in many other cities, the residents were responsible for cleaning and removing nuisances from their property, although garbage was collected once a week by the city. To ensure that the latter job was performed, in 1798 a superintendent of street cleaning was appointed.[19]

Charleston, the American city closest to the yellow fever centers in the West Indies, had a population of over 16,000 by 1790, approximately half of whom were slaves. Yellow fever, however, was a frequent visitor to Charleston and did not arouse quite the alarm it did in the North. Epidemics occurred in 1790, 1792, 1794, 1797, and 1799, but they brought about no major public health reforms other than to transfer quarantine responsibility for Charleston from the state to the city in 1796. In 1797 the Charleston Medical Society formed a volunteer group of medical inspectors to search out cases of yellow fever, but after the epidemic of 1799 it concluded that paid health inspectors were necessary. Convinced that the disease arose from local conditions, the society this same year also urged a complete sanitary program, but little came of its recommendations.[20]

On the Gulf Coast New Orleans, with a population of about 9,000, suffered its first significant outbreak of yellow fever in 1796. The city already had a reputation for filth and dirt, and the epidemic brought the usual demands for sanitary reform. Neither the public nor the government was unduly concerned, though, and nothing was done until 1799, when a second epidemic brought a temporary cleanup. Faced by a rising threat from yellow fever, in 1802 the Spanish governor appointed a board of health to supervise the establishment of a quarantine system. The board was not particularly effective, and further health measures awaited the incorporation of Louisiana into the United States.[21]

The growth of towns and cities inevitably resulted in the pollution of the shallow wells that supplied so much of the water for drinking and other purposes. The growing awareness of this problem alone, as the case of New York City demonstrated, undoubtedly would have forced municipal authorities to seek outside water sources. The association of yellow fever with dirt and filth, however, forced the issue. When Boston began a sanitation program in 1795, one of the city government's first measures was to charter the Boston Aqueduct Corporation to bring water from Jamaica Pond in Roxbury to Boston. By 1798 the aqueduct was carrying water through wooden pipes to the center of the city. The availability of "pure" water was hailed as a means of promoting health and personal cleanliness and preventing "putrid and pestilential fevers, and other fatal diseases."[22] Baltimore, too, contemplated constructing a water system in 1792, but it was not until 1806 that work began on the project.

Philadelphia went one step further by appointing the celebrated architect and engineer, Benjamin Latrobe, to design its water system. The project involved building an aqueduct and a distribution system of wooden pipes through which water was pumped by a steam engine. The water system, which began operating in January 1801, was the most advanced one in America. The appointment of Frederick Gaff as engineer in 1805 enabled Philadelphia to maintain leadership in supplying its citizens with good water for many years. Gaff, who served for forty-two years, was acknowledged in his day as the leading American expert on water systems.[23]

New York City already had constructed a water system in the 1770s only to see it fall prey to the vicissitudes of the Revolutionary War. The unusually poor quality of the local well water, combined with the reappearance of yellow fever in the 1790s, stimulated the city council to investigate anew the possibilities for bringing water into the city. At this time the local well water was so bad that most citizens bought drinking water from the Tea Water Pump, a source of water associated with the Collect, a small lake that had formerly been outside the city limits. By the 1790s the city was already encroaching on its borders, and the Collect was becoming fouled with the garbage, carrion, and refuse dumped into its waters. An outraged citizen in 1798 spoke of "the *nasty wash and slops* carted about from the Collect," which, he asserted, contained "all the leakings, scrapings, scourings, p—s—gs, & ——gs, for a great distance around." A physician about the same time appealed for a good water system on the grounds that pure water would wash away pestilence.[24]

In 1798 the city council, after approving a report suggesting that water be brought into the city from the Bronx River, recommended building a municipal water system. Unfortunately, Aaron Burr, whose reputation for chicanery is well deserved, was chairman of the legislative committee to which the city's petition was sent. Burr and his Republican associates wanted a bank charter, which the Federalist-dominated legislature was not willing to grant. The story is somewhat involved, but basically Burr persuaded the legislature to charter a private water company, and he managed to insert a clause in the charter that permitted the Manhattan Company to invest its surplus capital in "moneyed transactions or operations." Thus he was able to use the water company's charter to establish his bank. To their sorrow, the civic authorities discovered that the charter said nothing about supplying the city with water for municipal purposes, nor did it even contain a provision requiring the company to repair and repave the streets dug up to lay pipe. For the next forty years the water company concentrated on banking and supplied only enough poor water to maintain its charter.[25]

What is clear from examining the reaction of American cities to the yellow fever onslaughts of the 1790s is that fear of the disease provided a major impetus to the movement for sanitary reform. Since the fever usually arrived in midsummer, when long hot days and nights intensified the foul odors from rotting garbage, carrion, overflowing privies, and the wastes from the nuisance industries, its timing seemed to justify the miasmic theory on epidemics. Cleanliness now was no longer purely a matter of aesthetics but essential to the preservation of life and health. The need for pure air, pure water, and pure food was repeatedly stressed in pamphlets and other publications. Spurred on by the threat or presence of yellow fever, town after town began major efforts to drain foul-smelling pools, clear gutters or drains of carrion and refuse, require citizens to empty their overflowing privies, and clean the streets and public and private lands. To prevent miasma lime was used extensively in streets and gutters, and residents were forbidden to disturb the land during hot months. Since miasma was suspected of arising from the bowels of the earth, excavation in summertime was considered dangerous.

Regardless of medical theories, the connection between bad drinking water and gastrointestinal disorders was obvious, and it was equally clear that the quality of the water from local wells and streams was steadily worsening. A good water supply was not only needed for drinking purposes but also for fire fighting, for flushing the gutters and streets, and for personal hygiene. Hence the epidemics, directly and indirectly, contributed to the emergence of city water systems.

Although the foregoing discussion is essentially correct, it should not leave the impression that a major sanitary revolution had occurred. First, disregarding the prevailing medical opinion that pestilential fevers were of local origin, most laypersons were convinced that diseases could be, and often were, imported. The major emphasis behind preventing epidemic pestilences was always on quarantine measures and on isolating disease victims in pesthouses. Quarantine had an additional advantage in that its costs could be placed upon the owners of, and passengers aboard, incoming vessels. Second, financial support for health officers or port physicians often came from their inspection fees. In most cities these positions became sinecures, and quarantine inspections were purely nominal. Once an epidemic started—and when it was too late—the inspection system would be tightened and demands would be made for the head of the local health officer. Fortunately for these officials, the public's memory was short, and most managed to survive.

The major objection to quarantine laws came from businessmen, particularly those dependent upon trade and commerce. A rigid inspection system delayed entrance of their goods into cities, and a firm quarantine proclaimed against any particular port or country severely interrupted their activities. The power to hold a ship in quarantine for thirty or sixty days could prove exceedingly costly to shipowners and importers and provided a temptation to unscrupulous officeholders. John Jones, the health officer for Philadelphia, was accused of illegally collecting fees in 1789. A subsequent inquiry dismissed the charge, placing the blame on his deputy or clerk.[26] Regardless of the reason for quarantine restrictions, businessmen understandably resented them. The city's commercial leaders constituted a powerful vested interest, and health boards and health officers were always reluctant to clash with them. As a result, quarantines were usually not proclaimed until they were too late to be effective.

In retrospect, the two difficulties with sanitary programs have always been their cost and the fact that they go against human nature. One has only to view the refuse and debris cast upon the streets, alleys, and public and private lands of American cities today, on our highways, and in the countryside to realize that neatness and cleanliness are scarcely normal human attributes. Urban America can condition individuals to accept community hygiene, but it takes considerable time. Cities such as New York and Chicago that have had to absorb generation after generation of rural immigrants from overseas or from the United States itself have battled valiantly but unsuccessfully in their attempts to maintain civic cleanliness. The American free enterprise system itself scarcely encourages a clean environment. It is obviously far more profitable to pour industrial wastes into local rivers, streams, and ponds than to provide for their proper disposal—and for every conscientious entrepreneur there is at least one who is not so conscientious. Under the immediate threat of a terrible pestilence, civic leaders and the public are easily persuaded to make unusual efforts toward both civic and personal hygiene. Once that threat is removed, however, enthusiasm for this sort of activity quickly wanes. Not surprisingly, as the danger from yellow fever receded from northern cities in the years after 1800, the appeals of the sanitary reformers went largely unheard.

Another factor that worked against sanitary reform was its relatively large cost. Paving streets; constructing drains, sewers, and water systems; replacing inadequate privies and cesspools; and providing manpower to remove garbage, carrion, and rubbish from the streets required both large amounts of capital and higher taxes. Higher taxes, as the American Revolution and the Reagan revolution demonstrate, have always been anathema to the American public, and leading citizens have always been happy to espouse the ideas of sanitationists and environmentalists while dismissing them as impractical.

What is impressive about the reaction of American cities to the yellow fever epidemics is the way in which residents joined together to meet the crisis. Once the initial panic was over, volunteer groups and municipal leaders collaborated to minimize the damage. Sanitary campaigns and belated quarantine measures may have been of limited use against yellow fever, but at least citizens were applying the prevailing medical concepts. Physicians and nurses were hired to care for the sick, temporary hospitals were opened, and major welfare programs were established to care for the families of the sick and for the surviving dependents of the dead. The mass removal of residents from affected areas, as was carried out in New York City, and the provisions made for the housing and feeding of those who needed it were unprecedented in American history. So, too, were the unlimited powers given to health boards and committees at this time. Much of what was done probably reflects the paternalism of the eighteenth century, but it also shows the beginnings of social consciousness among the middle and upper classes. Volunteerism was to remain basic to American efforts on behalf of the poor, but pestilence, a community health problem, helped to restructure American municipal government. Neither quarantine nor sanitation could be safely left to individual initiative, and as the public health movement evolved, moving toward institutionalization through the first temporary boards of health, it helped to strengthen the role of government in providing for the public welfare.

NOTES

1. *American Archives*, ser. 4, 6 (Washington, D.C., 1846), 1083.
2. Duffy, *A History of Public Health in New York City, 1625–1866* (New York, 1968), chapter 4.

3. New York *Daily Advertiser,* January 16, 30, 1786, November 20, 1788.

4. Sidney Pomerantz, *New York: An American City, 1783–1803* (New York, 1938), 173–74.

5. For the best account of the yellow fever in Philadelphia see J. H. Powell, *Bring Out Your Dead: The Great Plague of Yellow Fever in Philadelphia in 1793* (Philadelphia, 1949).

6. New York City Health Committee, Minutes, 1793–1796, New York Historical Society MS, pp. 1–6.

7. Ibid., 7–23, 41–42, 53–54, 74, 94–98, 112, 114–21.

8. *New York State Laws,* 17th sess., chap. 53, March 27, 1794, 3:525–26.

9. New York City Health Committee, Minutes, 190–92.

10. M. L. Davis, *A Brief Account of the Epidemical Fever which lately prevailed in the City of New York* . . . (New York, 1795), 27–31, 35–37.

11. *Minutes of the Common Council of the City of New York, 1784–1831* (New York, 1917–30), 2:212–13, 217; James J. Walsh, *A History of Medicine in New York: Three Centuries of Medical Progress* (New York, 1919), 1:60–62.

12. *New York State Laws,* 19th sess., chap. 38, April 1, 1796, 3:682–86; Susan W. Peabody, "Historical Study of Legislation Regarding Public Health in the States of New York and Massachusetts," *Journal of Infectious Diseases,* supp. 4 (February 1909):6–7.

13. Duffy, *Public Health in New York City, 1625–1866,* 107–9, 134–35.

14. *Minutes of the Common Council,* 2:481, 494–97, 501.

15. Ibid., 498–99.

16. Duffy, *Public Health in New York City, 1625–1866,* 137–39.

17. For an account of yellow fever in Connecticut in these years see Linda Ann McKee, "Health and Medicine in Connecticut, 1785–1810" (Ph.D. diss., University of New Mexico, 1970).

18. John B. Blake, *Public Health in the Town of Boston, 1630–1822* (Cambridge, Mass., 1959), chapter 8.

19. William T. Howard, *Public Health Administration and the Natural History of Disease in Baltimore, Maryland, 1797–1920* (Washington, D.C., 1924), 47–49, 63.

20. Joseph Ioor Waring, *A History of Medicine in South Carolina, 1670–1825* (Columbia, S.C., 1964), 113–15.

21. Duffy, *The Rudolph Matas History of Medicine in Louisiana* (Baton Rouge, La., 1958–62), 1:207–12.

22. Blake, *Public Health in Boston,* 156–57.

23. Russell Wigley, ed., *Philadelphia: A 300-Year History* (New York and London, 1982), 226–28.

24. New York *Commercial Advertiser,* August 28, 1798; *Commercial Advocate,* September 5, 1798.

25. For an account of Burr's role in the Manhattan Company see Beatrice G. Reubens, "Burr, Hamilton and the Manhattan Company," *Political Science Quarterly* 72 (1957):578–607, and 73 (1958):100–125.

26. *Colonial Records of Pennsylvania, Minutes of the Supreme Executive Council of Pennsylvania* (Harrisburg, Pa., 1853), 16:133–34, 171–72.

4

From Paternalism to Rugged Individualism

From the standpoint of the role of the American government and the development of public health, the period from 1800 to 1830 is an interesting one. The Renaissance and the Protestant Reformation had ended the association of sanctity with poverty; and by the eighteenth century acquiring wealth, presumably to use it wisely, had become a Christian virtue. Accumulated wealth was taken to be a sign of thrift, hard work, and noble character. In 1776 Adam Smith spoke for his age when he wrote that the possession and accumulation of property was a natural right. By the early nineteenth century this view of property led logically to the assumption that poverty, rather than being a sign of holiness and of Christian virtues, represented the opposite, or, at best, was a sign of a weak moral character. Societal changes occur slowly, and the harshness of the Protestant ethic was mitigated by the traditional concepts of Christian charity and noblesse oblige. So long as communities were relatively small and their members were tied together by personal relationships, there was a general recognition that poverty often arose through circumstances beyond individual control. The rise of almshouses in American colonial towns, the employment of physicians to care for the sick poor, and the development of various outdoor or home relief programs attest to a sense of community responsibility.

The remarkable way in which citizens in every American town and city aided the victims of the yellow fever epidemics from 1793 to 1806 clearly illustrates this point. Workers deprived of their jobs by the ravages of the epidemics, poor families forced to evacuate their homes, and widows and orphaned children could scarcely be held accountable for their benighted condition. Consequently, the community rallied to their support. By providing this support, the community strengthened local governmental structures—a process that was further stimulated by efforts to prevent or mitigate the epidemics. Whether a disease was imported, necessitating quarantine laws, or of local origin, requiring major sanitary programs, municipal and state governments had to create new agencies and offices. The health boards and other offices that came into existence at the turn of the century were nearly all temporary, and most were ineffective, but they laid the basis for better state and local government later in the century.

Even as the yellow fever epidemics were bringing forth a high degree of individual philanthropy and communal responsibility, the early stages of the industrial revolution and the beginnings of what later became known as the philosophy of rugged individualism were tending to undermine them. The growth of cities brought with it a loss of personal relationships between community members and merged the poor into a faceless mass. The widening income gap between economic classes also led to a corresponding separation in terms of their residential areas. At the same time, the economic dislocations engendered by the industrial revolution concentrated the impoverished class in city slums. In the early years of the nineteenth century all these factors gradually changed the attitude of the middle and upper classes toward the impoverished. In the first place, the loss of personal contact meant that the poor became an abstraction, and as such they could easily be stereotyped. In the second place, their support required increasing taxes—an abhorrent thought to the vast majority of Americans. Under these circumstances, the concept of the deserving poor was gradually replaced by that of the lazy, idle, and immoral poor. Despite all studies for the past three hundred years demonstrating that the majority of those requiring public assistance have always been—and still are—the aged, the infirm, and women and children, the taxpaying public still tends to assume that most of them are healthy individuals who refuse to work.

This is not to say that in these years philanthropy disappeared or that no government action was taken to help those in need. Assistance, however, was kept to a minimum. Yellow fever receded from the North after about 1805, and no great pestilences threatened America again for over twenty-five years. As a result, government efforts to promote public health and social welfare were sharply reduced. With only a few exceptions, the temporary health boards disappeared, and the quarantine and sanitary laws enacted in the late 1790s fell into abeyance. These developments demonstrate how governments, and democratic ones in particular, respond largely to crises, and this fact is especially true when it comes to public health measures. The enormous mortality among infants and the omnipresence of malaria, typhoid, tuberculosis, and a host of other infectious disorders at this time were accepted as the normal tribulations of life; hence they aroused no general consternation. The public was further reassured by the confident way in which physicians immediately recognized these disorders and proceeded to treat them with the traditional methods of bleeding, purging, vomiting, blistering, and sweating.

The one disease that did stimulate governmental action in this period was smallpox. This most feared disease had been brought under some measure of control in colonial days through the use of inoculation, and in 1798 Jenner's introduction of vaccinia opened the way to its prevention. Within a few years, as we have seen, the use of vaccine matter became widespread throughout the United States and sharply reduced the incidence of smallpox. The medical profession, however, by virtue of the nature of its work, tended to be conservative, and a good many practitioners—and many laypersons, too—clung to inoculation until it was prohibited by law. Dr. Thomas Cook, who had studied under Valentine Seaman, claimed that Seaman's introduction of vaccination into New York City "was not accomplished without great opposition, both from the profession and the community."[1] This support for inoculation was strong enough to require New York State to enact a law on February 16, 1816, stating that "no physician, surgeon, or other person shall communicate the small pox by inoculation to any person or persons." While vaccination generally won quick acceptance, many individuals remained reluctant to accept the new smallpox preventive, and some never accepted it. The state of Maryland had to prohibit inoculation as late as 1850.[2]

The first state in which positive governmental action was taken to promote smallpox vaccination was Massachusetts. Of the several Boston physicians who sought to obtain vaccine material, the first to succeed was Dr. Benjamin Waterhouse. Waterhouse, who actually tried to monopolize vaccine matter, persuaded the Boston Board of Health in 1802 to sponsor a public test of vaccination. Despite the test's successful results with nineteen volunteers, the public remained hesitant about switching from inoculation. Gradually the medical profession and intelligent laypersons became convinced of the efficacy of vaccine, and the movement for its use received a major impetus when the town of Milton in 1809 embarked on a program to vaccinate all its residents. The program's success led the town's officials to introduce a bill into the Massachusetts legislature to promote the statewide use of vaccination. The legislators responded with a law requiring each town without a board of health to appoint a vaccination committee. Either these committees or the local health boards were to supervise the vaccination of all residents, with the town paying all or part of the cost. Since the law carried no penalties, it had only a limited impact. Even the Boston Board of Health, probably the best city health agency in the United States at that time, was content to give moral support to vaccination.[3]

Fortunately, in Boston and elsewhere medical societies took the initiative in promoting vaccination. Members of the Boston Medical Association in 1811 agreed to administer vaccinations at a reduced fee and to vaccinate the poor free of charge. In the absence of the immediate threat of an epidemic, however, the public showed little interest. It took a major smallpox epidemic, which swept through the United States from 1815 to 1817, to arouse Boston's citizens and their board of health to take advantage of vaccination.

New York City's experience with vaccination closely resembled Boston's. The New York City Board of Health was primarily concerned with yellow fever and paid no attention to smallpox. Responding to this lack of concern, a group of physicians, led by Dr. Valentine Seaman, organized the New York Institution for the Inoculation of the Kine-Pock in 1802. Its purpose was to provide free vaccination for the poor, to maintain a supply of fresh cowpox vaccine, and to educate physicians in the vaccine's use. Shortly after its founding, the officers of the institute asked the city council for an appropriation of $200 for the vaccination of the inmates of the city almshouse. The councilmen were agreeable to the proposal but were not willing to fund it. After the Kine-Pock Institute had gone ahead on its own and vaccinated about five hundred children, the council reconsidered and voted to appropriate a sum of $200 per year to the institute.[4]

With the blessings of the city council, the institute was absorbed into the New York Dispensary, a private agency that received both state and city funds. The vaccination program, however, languished until a mild outbreak of smallpox, which also affected Boston, occurred in 1809. The dispensary appealed for a general vaccination, but, as had been true in Boston, the public was largely apathetic. Public apathy continued until the major smallpox outbreak of 1815–17 struck. On this occasion the city council voted to appropriate an additional $1,000 to cover the cost of vaccinating the poor, and, in collaboration with the New York City Board of Health, it began an educational campaign to encourage the use of vaccination. The occurrence of a good many smallpox cases and deaths in these years provided the incentive for municipal authorities in Boston, Charleston, and other cities to begin similar educational campaigns.

Smallpox was never a major threat in the United States in the nineteenth century, but because it was such a deadly and disfiguring disease and a preventive was at hand, it received far more attention than did the more disabling and fatal disorders. The Spanish government in 1802 sent vaccine matter to its provinces in New Spain, and the governors of the territories now comprising Texas and New Mexico made repeated requests for vaccine matter in the early nineteenth century.[5] In St. Louis an advertisement in the *Missouri Gazette* in 1809 announced that a local physician had vaccine matter and would vaccinate paupers and Indians free of charge.[6] An outbreak of smallpox in New Orleans in 1804 led the city council to rebuke some of the city's doctors for inoculating several children without first notifying the city health officer. A few days later the council urged citizens to delay inoculation until the results of vaccination, "which had just been tried on a great number of subjects," could be determined. In 1808 the city requested that the territorial legislature create a bureau of vaccination to provide free vaccination for all who wanted it. When the legislature failed to act, a local physician offered his services free of charge. The reappearance of smallpox in 1817 induced the city council first to provide free vaccination for the poor, and then to employ a physician to vaccinate any person applying for it.[7]

One of the earliest national public health laws resulted from the smallpox vaccination movement. Thomas Jefferson, after learning about vaccination from Dr. Waterhouse, actively promoted its use in Virginia, and his influence undoubtedly contributed to the passage of a federal law to encourage vaccination, which was approved on February 27, 1813. The measure authorized the president of the United States to appoint an official vaccine "agent to preserve the genuine vaccine matter" and send it through the post office to anyone who applied for it. Dr. James Smith, the state vaccine agent for Maryland, was appointed to the position. In 1822, however, reflecting the accepted view that government should only intervene in health concerns in times of emergency, the law was repealed.[8]

By 1830, although the use of smallpox inoculation had not disappeared, vaccination was generally accepted. Whenever cases of smallpox occurred, state and local authorities took measures to make vaccination available to all who wanted it. By this date most states had appointed vaccine agents. Unfortunately, the success of vaccination in drastically reducing the incidence of smallpox during the first thirty or forty years of the nineteenth century proved almost self-defeating. With the rise of a generation of Americans who had never experienced this horrible disease and thus were less resistant to it, vaccination was neglected; consequently, beginning in the 1840s the incidence of smallpox began rising in the United States.

The story of smallpox vaccination illustrates the growing involvement of local government in public health. This involvement in the years from the yellow fever epidemics in the 1790s to the first great Asiatic cholera epidemic of 1832 is best typified by the development of public health in New York City. The institutionalization of public health in New York began with the voluntary health committee organized to meet the threat of yellow fever in 1793. This committee became an official agency of the municipal government the following year. In 1796 the state created a permanent health office in New York City to deal with quarantine matters. In addition, the state legislature authorized the New York City Council to enact sanitary ordinances, with the proviso that these measures were valid for only one year unless specifically approved by the governor. Meanwhile, the city council had appointed a committee of its own members to deal with health matters. During emergencies these agencies worked quite well, but, when the city council lacked a sense of immediate danger, it was reluctant to use even the limited powers granted to it. It seldom passed general sanitary ordinances, for example, preferring to deal individually with specific cases. Under normal circumstances strong vested interests and personal relationships inhibited council action, and it usually took a major crisis to build enough political pressure to force it into action.

In 1798, following a series of yellow fever outbreaks, the existing New York health laws were repealed and a new health office, consisting of three commissioners, was created. In addition to enforcing a much-strengthened quarantine code, the Health Office was authorized to make sanitary regulations, but these regulations required the concurrence of the mayor and council. As long as yellow fever threatened or was present each summer, the city council collaborated quite effectively with the Health Office. In addition to this new health agency, the city was given broader powers over sanitary conditions.[9]

With the exception of the Health Office, which had jurisdiction primarily over quarantine affairs, the health committees were all temporary agencies. The first permanent office concerned with general sanitary matters was that of city inpector, established in 1804. The city inspector was required to see that all city ordinances were enforced, to gather information about public nuisances, and to report any abuses to the city council. John Pintard, an outstanding citizen, was appointed to the position. Pintard was interested in statistics, and he was probably responsible for an ordinance, passed shortly after he assumed office, requiring sextons to send weekly returns of all burials to the City Inspector's Office. The chief weakness of the office was that the inspector could report abuses but had no authority to correct them. In ensuing years, when enthusiasm for public health measures waned, a succession of able city inspectors served as the community's conscience, constantly reminding the authorities of the city's worsening sanitary condition.

Beginning in the early 1790s, New York City had been assuming more control over its internal affairs. Since the Health Office was a state agency, the city council decided to establish a municipal board of health. A temporary board was established first, which then drafted a proposed state law to create a new board with broad powers. The council passed this on to the state legislature, which in turn authorized the city to appoint a board and invest it with all powers pertaining to public health. The first New York City Board of Health, appointed in March 1805, consisted of the mayor, the recorder, five aldermen (one from each of the five wards), and, as ex officio members, the commissioners of health (the three officials from the Health Office). The last of the series of yellow fever epidemics struck in the summer of 1805 and fully tested the new board. By this date the city had experienced ten years of the pestilence and was fully prepared; hence the ravages of the disease were minimized. Infected districts were evacuated, medical care was provided, temporary hospitals were erected, and rigid quarantine and sanitary measures were enforced.

While the actions of the board in 1805 gained it strong public support, it was designed to function primarily during emergency situations. With the disappearance of yellow fever in ensuing years, the board's duties gradually became purely nominal; the quarantine system was in the hands of the Health Office, and sanitary matters were usually handled by the city inspector, the street commissioners, or directly by the council. Each year the mayor appointed a board, but since its chief purpose was to prevent or minimize pestilential diseases (and yellow fever was the only one of major concern at this time), the appointments were usually made shortly before the onset of warm weather. Since no serious health crises occurred for a number of years, the board members contented themselves with occasionally reminding the public of the sanitary regulations or, even more rarely, suggesting a new one. The board's declining role in municipal affairs is shown by the steady reduction in the funds allocated to its budget. In 1805 the city appropriated $8,500; by 1809 the amount was down to $1,000; and in 1819 the board received only $900.[10] These figures are even more significant in light of the city's rapidly increasing population.

As with every major port city, New York maintained a reasonably strict quarantine during the yellow fever era. With the medical profession divided over the issue of causation, however, the opponents of quarantine became more vocal each year that passed without the appearance of the disease. Shipping and commercial interests consistently opposed interference with their livelihood, and they could always find support from some of the physicians who argued against quarantine laws on medical grounds. President Jefferson's attempt to maintain American neutrality during the Napoleonic Wars by means of an embargo seriously damaged maritime commerce and strengthened demands for easing quarantine regulations. In New York the state legislature responded to this pressure by giving the state health officer more discretionary power. This rising opposition to quarantine was felt in other port cities, with the result that, with one or two exceptions, the quarantine laws in America became far less effective. In addition to this general relaxation of the regulations, in many cities the position of health officer of the port often became a sinecure, with the officeholder far more interested in collecting fees than in inspecting vessels.

By 1830 three administrative agencies in New York City dealt with health affairs: the state-appointed Health Office, with jurisdiction over quarantine, consisting of a health officer, resident physician, and a health commissioner; the City Inspector's Office, which was concerned with the sanitary condition of the city; and the Board of Health. This last body ordinarily consisted of the mayor and aldermen acting in a health capacity during a health crisis. The City Inspector's Office was unique to New York, but virtually every port city had a health officer of the port (the title varies) to enforce quarantine regulations and some type of local health board. In a few cities the board was appointed every summer, but in most cases it came into existence only when a major pestilence threatened. In some instances the health board consisted of a group of physicians acting in an advisory capacity and had no authority.

New York City followed the usual pattern of appointing only laymen to its health board. Oddly enough, in 1811 three physicians were placed on the board, but this was an exception to the general rule. The first half of the nineteenth century was characterized by widespread distrust of the medical profession, and throughout the United States nearly all the early boards were controlled by laymen. The bitter arguments over disease causation within the medical fraternity convinced most of the lay public that a health board consisting of physicians would be too divided to take action. On the other hand, health boards often called on the local medical society or leading physicians for advice.

Without doubt, the most effective health board in these years was the one in Boston. When the first board was authorized by Massachusetts in 1797, the Boston selectmen simply assumed this function themselves. A yellow fever epidemic in 1798, however, convinced the town's citizens that they needed a formal board of health, and the following spring the General Court passed the necessary legislation. The new Boston Board of Health, which consisted of one man elected annually from each of the city's twelve wards, was given fairly broad authority, including the power to order nuisances removed from a business or property at the expense of the owner. As might be expected, the threat of yellow fever for a few years guaranteed the board strong support from city officials, and it took an active role in both quarantine and sanitary affairs.[11]

The end of the yellow fever outbreaks inevitably weakened support for public health measures, but the Boston board members, who represented individual wards, were more responsive to public opinion than were their counterparts in cities that relied upon appointed boards. No matter what physicians thought, the lay public always supported quarantine regulations; this fact may help explain why the democratically elected Boston Board of Health was far more successful in resisting pressure from commercial interests to relax the town's quarantine regulations. On the other hand, the better-educated Boston upper classes, including its businessmen, appear to have had a greater awareness of the need for sanitary and public health measures than the board members responsive to the lower socioeconomic classes. Whatever the case, although the regulations were eased slightly, on the whole, Boston maintained an effective quarantine system.

In terms of quarantine regulations, the experience of New Orleans was far more typical than that of Boston. Although occasional quarantines had been declared under the Spanish regime, a formal quarantine system had never been established. In 1804 the first city council organized under the American regime, urged on by Territorial Governor William C. C. Claiborne, established a health board consisting of two physicians and three laymen. It was given wide authority over quarantine and sanitation, but its actions were subject to the approval of the city council. Outbreaks of yellow fever and smallpox that year led to considerable activity on the part of the board, but by the following year it apparently died a natural death.

Despite complaints of worsening sanitary conditions and a mild yellow fever epidemic in 1809, no efforts were made to revive the New Orleans Board of Health. The crisis that provided the impetus for action was a major flood in 1816. It was assumed that once the water receded and the sun's rays struck the wet ground, the resulting miasma was certain to precipitate a pestilential fever. After consulting the local medical society, and after much soul-searching, in March 1818 the city authorities and the state legislature established a five-man health board consisting of three physicians and two laymen. Its primary function was to act as a quarantine agency, but it was also given a measure of authority over sanitary matters. In attempting to enforce quarantine regulations, the board immediately clashed with powerful business interests. To make matters worse, when it sought to remedy unsanitary conditions, it also clashed with the city council. The net result was that one year later, in 1819, the act creating the board was repealed, and the governor of Louisiana was ordered to sell the quarantine station.

Two successive yellow fever attacks in 1819 and 1820 and the steadily deteriorating sanitary condition of the city led to the establishment of a third board of health in 1821. This one consisted of five aldermen and seven citizens appointed by the governor. It was given wider powers than its predecessor, but its chief responsibility was to establish and maintain a quarantine. This board seems to have been more effective than the earlier ones, but it survived only four years before foundering on the issue of quarantine. New Orleans was the entrepôt for the entire Mississippi Valley, and trade was the lifeblood of the city. With strong support from the anticontagionists in the medical profession, in 1825 the city's business interests were able once again to abolish the board and order the governor to dispose of the quarantine station. So strong was the opposition to quarantine that another sixteen years elapsed before the health board was revived.[12]

To New Orleans' credit, the city at least tried to establish quarantine regulations. Most American ports made little effort in these years to enforce the quarantine laws, using the prevailing anticontagionist views of the medical profession as justification. Baltimore established a nine-man board of health in 1797, which functioned largely as a quarantine agency. Legally it had authority over sanitary matters, but in practice these were left to the city council. Within a few years after the last yellow fever epidemic the quarantine system virtually collapsed. The Baltimore Board of Health, too, fell on hard times, but it managed to survive, although its membership on one occasion was reduced to two. Coincident with the brief reappearance of yellow fever in northern ports beginning in 1820, the board was briefly revived and strengthened, although it concentrated upon relieving the domestic causes of yellow fever, that is, eliminating the foul miasmas.[13]

Philadelphians, too, rapidly lost their zeal for quarantine after 1805, but the governor and state legislature applied constant pressure upon the city to maintain its quarantine. The chief work of the Philadelphia City Board of Health, created in the 1790s, was to enforce the quarantine. Following a mild yellow fever outbreak in 1803, Governor Thomas McKean credited the rigid enforcement of the quarantine regulations with minimizing the epidemic and urged that the laws be strengthened. Since imported contagions such as yellow fever usually entered the state through its major port, Pennsylvanians, like citizens in other states, suspected that the authorities in their major port city were not overly zealous in enforcing the quarantine laws, and the outspoken opposition of businessmen to quarantine restrictions did little to allay public apprehension. In addition, Pennsylvania's health acts were usually valid only for a limited time, and the health board had to be reappointed annually. In succeeding years, although governor after governor stressed the need for a health board and urged that its quarantine authority be strengthened, on two occasions governors vetoed supplementary health acts. These vetoes were made on the grounds that these measures would have taken the power to appoint subordinate officials away from the governor and given it to the Board of Health.[14] Whether this reflected the governor's suspicion of local board members or a reluctance on their part to give up some patronage is difficult to say.

It is well to bear in mind that state executives and legislatures kept a great deal of control over cities and towns. Rural-dominated legislatures have traditionally distrusted urban centers, and this was particularly true of early state legislatures. In nearly every case the health officer, the head of the health office, was a state appointee, as were his associates or subordinates. Moreover, his authority over quarantine matters was never statewide, extending instead over a particular port. The health boards, too, had jurisdiction only within their own cities. The one major difference between the health office and the board of health was that, while the state usually controlled health office appointments, cities were often given the right to select health board members. But here, too, state officials frequently were unwilling to surrender opportunities for patronage. One other point worth noting is that before the Civil War no board of health had statewide authority; the first state board, established in Louisiana in 1855, was essentially a board of health for the city of New Orleans.

With the exception of the Boston Board of Health, the health boards appointed from the 1790s to 1830 were all temporary. They varied widely in terms of membership, ranging from city councilmen acting in a public health capacity to physicians. Most of the boards in times of crises requested help from the local medical profession, and many included the port health officers as ex-officio members. In almost every instance the boards were dominated by laymen. Dr. Peter S. Townsend of New York wrote in 1823 that he was firmly convinced that health boards should be in the hands of a few distinguished citizens. Were a health board "exclusively made up of medical gentlemen, there is too much reason to fear that their different opinions might lead, as too often happens, to interminable disputes, and to most disastrous consequences."[15] The main purpose of these health boards was to enforce quarantine laws, but, in accordance with prevailing medical thought, they all advocated sanitary measures. Rarely did these boards have any real authority, and they could usually count upon support from their respective city councils only in emergencies. In the period from 1800 to 1805 yellow fever was still a serious threat, and this period marks the high point for the early boards; shortly thereafter most of them disappeared. A few were revived briefly, but they played no significant role in public health.

Ironically, at the time when governmental concern with public health was diminishing, health conditions in America were beginning to deteriorate. American cities were mushrooming at a rate that exceeded the capacity of municipal officials to govern them. The crude methods for removing garbage and debris and for emptying privies could not keep pace with the accumulation of waste matter, and neither the technology nor the engineering skills to provide adequate water supplies and sewer systems was available.

As the well-to-do gradually built their homes on higher ground, the older areas they left behind quickly filled with newcomers, often with entire families jammed into one or two rooms. The rising demand for homes induced jerry-builders to step in and cram poorly constructed housing on every inch of available space. The only water supply for most slum housing was a corner well or a standpipe (if the city had a water system) one or two blocks away. To compound the problem, often one or two privies served a half-dozen or more families. Under these conditions cleanliness was impossible, and diseases of all sorts flourished. The upper classes, who had distanced themselves from these conditions, salved their consciences by blaming the poor for having to live in filth and in degraded circumstances. Before the major cities could adjust to these changing conditions, the massive influx of Irish and other immigrants in the 1840s and 1850s made the situation far worse.

Sanitation in small towns and in the countryside was only slightly better than that in the metropolitan areas. While yellow fever was restricted largely to major ports, smallpox, diphtheria, measles, scarlet fever, and a host of other infections steadily worked their way through America. The westward movement carried all the diseases of the East into the Transappalachian area, and newly arrived settlers in the West quickly encountered new strains of enteric and respiratory complaints and struggled with the perennial malarias.

No single disease aroused so much complaint throughout America as malaria. It had largely disappeared from much of New England, but it was endemic everywhere else, and it followed the advance of the western frontier all the way to California. No part of the Mississippi Valley escaped its ravages; the first settlers were enthusiastic about health conditions, but it did not take long for malaria to become endemic. Governor John Reynolds wrote in his memoirs that during the first years of the nineteenth century Illinois was thought to be a "graveyard." In the 1820s "miasmatic" fevers wiped out 80 percent of the residents in one county.[16] Erwin Ackerknecht, in his study of malaria in the Upper Mississippi Valley, asserts that malaria was nearly epidemic in southern Illinois from 1770 to the 1840s.[17]

The southern states, where the anopheles mosquito could survive year-round, suffered even more from malaria. South Carolina was notorious for its malarial fevers, and, while New Orleans' reputation as a pesthole was based largely on yellow fever, endemic malaria was a far greater threat to the health of Louisianians. In his medical history of Alabama, Howard L. Holley states that around 1820, as the land was cleared and settled, the severity and incidence of malaria greatly increased. The disease became so bad in certain areas that it forced the abandonment of two of the state's early capitols.[18] In discussing the disorders of the Mississippi Valley, Timothy Flint stated that the fevers and agues, "when often repeated and long continued, gradually sap the constitution, and break down the powers of life."[19]

Without adequate statistical information for the 1800–1830 period, one cannot say whether urban conditions were more unhealthy than those of towns and rural areas, although this was true later in the nineteenth century. Dysentery, typhoid, and other enteric disorders were widely prevalent in all areas of the United States, particularly in summer, but the crowded and filthy conditions of urban life undoubtedly provided them with an ideal environment. Whatever the case, the rapidly increasing American population and the explosion of urban areas created major sanitary problems. At the same time urban living tended to sharpen class lines and bring about a decline in the traditional paternalism and sense of personal concern for the welfare of the poor.

NOTES

1. Thomas Cook, inaugural address to the New York Academy of Medicine, April 7, 1852, New York Academy of Medicine MS, p. 4.

2. *An Act, To prevent the destructive ravages of the Small Pox, February 26, 1816* (n.d., n.p.), broadside, Americana, New York Academy of Medicine; Eugene F. Cordell, *The Medical Annals of Maryland, 1799–1899* (Baltimore, 1903), 46–47.

3. John B. Blake, *Public Health in the Town of Boston, 1630–1822* (Cambridge, Mass., 1959), chapter 9.

4. John Duffy, *A History of Public Health in New York City, 1625–1866* (New York, 1968), 245–46.

5. Myrtle Greenfield, *A History of Public Health in New Mexico* (Albuquerque, 1962), 9–11; Texas State Department of Health, *A History of Public Health in Texas* (Austin, 1950), 3–4.

6. Robert L. Kirkpatrick, "History of St. Louis, 1804–1816" (M.A. thesis, Washington University, 1947), 141.

7. Duffy, *The Rudolph Matas History of Medicine in Louisiana* (Baton Rouge, La., 1958–62), 1:372–75.

8. Ralph Chester Williams, *The United States Public Health Service, 1798–1950* (Washington, D.C., 1951), 69–70.

9. For this material, see Duffy, *Public Health in New York City, 1625–1866,* chapters 6 and 7.

10. Ibid., 162.

11. Blake, *Public Health in Boston,* 161, 167.

12. Duffy, *Matas History of Medicine in Louisiana,* vol. 1, chapter 7.

13. William T. Howard, *Public Health Administration and the Natural History of Diseases in Baltimore, Maryland, 1797–1920* (Washington, D.C., 1924), 48–53.

14. *Pennsylvania Archives,* 9th ser., 6 (Harrisburg, Pa., 1931), 4656–59.

15. Peter S. Townsend, M.D., *An Account of the Yellow Fever, as it prevailed in the City of New York, in the summer and autumn of 1822* (New York, 1823), 235.

16. Thomas N. Bonner, *Medicine in Chicago, 1850–1950* (Madison, Wis., 1957), 7.

17. Erwin H. Ackerknecht, *Malaria in the Upper Mississippi Valley, 1760–1900* (Baltimore, 1945), 30.

18. Howard L. Holley, *The History of Medicine in Alabama* (Birmingham, Ala., 1982), 6.

19. Timothy Flint, *The History and Geography of the Mississippi Valley* . . . (Cincinnati, 1832), 1:38–39.

5

The Early Sanitary Movement

The initiative for the sanitary movement in the United States came largely from Europe. The transformation of society by the industrial revolution compounded virtually every urban social problem, and, as living conditions steadily worsened, a humanitarian movement emerged. In Great Britain the movement began in the eighteenth century under the leadership of men such as Thomas Coram, John Howard, and William Wilberforce. In the nineteenth century it was continued by Michael Sadler, Lord Ashbury, Edwin Chadwick, and a host of others. Edwin Chadwick's report in 1842 on the atrocious living conditions of British workers gave a major impetus to the British sanitary movement and was largely responsible for the creation of England's national board of health a few years later.

While the sanitary movement was sweeping through Western Europe, it made surprisingly little progress in the United States. Obviously, the relatively late rise of American cities helps to account for this lag. Yet by the 1830s other American reform movements were in full swing; temperance, the abolition of slavery, women's rights, and other reform issues were gaining strong support. Health and diet reforms, too, were among those championed, but their emphasis was upon individual health rather than community health. Although most of the social evils that horrified British reformers were present in major American cities in these years, the sanitary movement made little headway.

One explanation for this situation lies in the ineffectiveness of church leaders. The American religious revival movement in the early nineteenth century concentrated on individual salvation, unlike the evangelical movement in Britain with its emphasis upon social concerns. Moreover, the insistence on personal salvation and on the Bible as the sole religious authority led to a decline in the general educational level and social authority of the clergy. The one group of professionals who came in direct contact with poverty and misery were the physicians working in city hospitals and dispensaries. Hence it is not surprising that the medical profession supplied a large proportion of the early public health reformers. Unfortunately, the first half of the nineteenth century was a period marking the nadir of the profession. It had neither public support nor an effective organization and was thus unable to supply the necessary leadership to make community health a public concern.

Possibly the deciding factor in America was the abolition movement, which gradually absorbed the energies of most leading reformers. Between 1830 and 1860 it became an all-consuming issue in American public life, relegating other reform movements to insignificance. Whatever the reasons, only limited progress was made in public health. Virtually nothing was done at the national level, and not much more at the state level. Only the major cities moved tentatively to provide for the health of their citizens, and even these cities, as the mortality statistics show, were losing ground in the battle for health.

The American sanitary movement arose, at least in part, from efforts to account for the omnipresent epidemics that periodically scourged the population. While the humoral concept, or variations of it, and the newer medical theories of the seventeenth and eighteenth centuries offered fairly reasonable explanations for individual sicknesses, they could not account for the mysterious appearance and rapid spread of the major pestilential disorders. The association of warm weather with the "summer" fevers and intestinal complaints, and of cold weather with respiratory infections, clearly implicated weather as a causal factor in epidemics. The assumption of a correlation between the two is evident in a number of books dealing with weather and diseases that emerged as early as the 1700s. Typical of these works are Lionel Chalmers, *An Account of the Weather and Diseases of South Carolina* (1776), and William Currie, *An Historical Account of the Climates and Diseases of the United States of America . . .* (1792).

The connection seemed so obvious that almost every early medical society of any consequence appointed a series of committees to study the role of weather. For example, the Medical Society of New Jersey appointed a standing committee for this purpose in 1810 and ten years later asked it to include birth and death records in its studies.[1] Individual physicians, too, frequently kept daily meteorological records during epidemics. At the beginning of outbreaks health boards often appointed a physician to correlate daily temperatures with morbidity and mortality rates or else requested the local medical society to do the job. As the nineteenth century advanced and the search for disease causation grew even more desperate, the number of studies attempting to correlate epidemics and weather vastly increased.

Another common factor that seemed to correlate with the rise and fall of disease was the impact of sunshine on damp or swampy ground. From earliest times to the closing of the western frontier in the 1890s, the first settlers had invariably commented upon the healthfulness of newly settled regions. Within a generation, though, malaria and other endemic disorders became firmly entrenched; with the exception of those living in well-drained areas, settlers constantly complained in their diaries and letters of the perennial fevers. The widely accepted explanation for this phenomenon was that clearing the land exposed damp ground to the sun's rays, thereby releasing miasma. Supporting this belief was the fact that once the land was cultivated and drained, the incidence of malaria tended to decline. A leading Creole physician in New Orleans wrote in 1820 that the "number of Europeans who became victims of the emanations from newly cleared land, and heated for the first time by the rays of the sun, is incalculable." Cutting down forests, he explained, destroyed the protective shade which nature used "to prevent the miasmas from rising and poisoning the atmosphere."[2]

City dwellers, too, firmly adhered to this theory. Throughout the entire nineteenth century, newspaper editors and physicians complained about the danger of city workers and private contractors disturbing the soil during the summer months. In urban areas where garbage, human wastes, and other substances were simply dumped on undrained vacant lots, river banks, slips, and shorelines, the appearance of summer fevers was invariably attributed to the effect of the sun's rays on this matter. The tendency of epidemics to concentrate in low-lying, poorly drained areas occupied by the poor gave further credence to the association of sunshine, dampness, and disease.

While the medical profession in general did not accept the specificity of disease, being convinced that diseases were merely symptomatic of some constitutional imbalance, a good many physicians paradoxically believed, along with the public, that certain diseases could be kept out of the community by quarantine. To observant physicians, regardless of their views on quarantine, it was clear that diseases were not all directly transmissible from one person to another, and the miasmatic thesis provided a logical explanation for the apparent spontaneous appearance of epidemic disorders. The two great pestilences of the nineteenth century, yellow fever and Asiatic cholera, lent proof to the belief that diseases were locally generated, since the evidence clearly showed that some factor other than direct contact with disease victims was necessary for their dissemination. This same theory helped to explain why on some occasions the normal summer fevers led to a major epidemic. Convinced that miasma from putrefying organic matter played a major role in causing disease, a number of prominent physicians in America took leadership in urging sanitary measures.

As Americans pushed westward across the Appalachians, the towns and cities of the Mississippi Valley developed much as their counterparts had in the East. Pittsburgh, one of the first industrial cities to emerge, was more fortunate than most cities in the Mississippi Valley since its terrain was not suitable for the anopheles mosquito. Visitors and residents alike all agreed that the place was singularly free from the intermittent and remittent fevers that plagued the rest of the country. The ready availability of coal for industrial and household use early led to its name as the Smoky City. In 1800 a traveler approaching the town wrote, "we were struck with a peculiarity nowhere else to be observed in the States: a cloud of smoke hung over it in an exceedingly clear sky."[3] The population at this date was about 2,500, and already the town was experiencing sanitary problems. Hogs, dogs, cows, and other animals roamed the streets, no garbage collection system existed, and the townspeople relied on the river for drinking water.

The evolution of public health measures and policies in Pittsburgh and other cities in Transappalachian America during the nineteenth century closely followed the pattern set by eastern cities during the colonial period. Pittsburgh's first regulations, when it became a borough in 1794, dealt with hogs and other animals running at large and with the food supply and public market. In 1800 an ordinance decreed that no one was to slaughter any animals within the public market "or lay any garbage, dung or offal therein."[4] Three years later another regulation provided a twenty-cent penalty for permitting one's horse to roam at large, although nothing was said about hogs or other animals.[5] A few years later another ordinance proposed to pave the public square and the surrounding streets, but for some years after only one street was paved.[6]

City newspaper editors were always in the difficult position of having to praise the healthfulness of their city in order to promote economic growth while at the same time trying to reflect citizen complaints about unsanitary conditions. Pittsburgh's 1800 sanitary ordinance regulating the public market was followed by another one that forbade citizens to toss garbage and other noxious substances into the streets and public places. In response to outcries against this law from freedom-loving citizens, the Pittsburgh *Gazette* observed sarcastically that "some folks have no objection to the smell of warm tripe and garbage, to wading through puddles of green stagnant water, or to skating over dabs of ordure. What if a few citizens should be carried off by fluxes and fevers? It would be of no consequence, as our population is rapidly increasing."[7] Flagrant violations of the first sanitary ordinances led to the enactment of a more stringent one in 1807 threatening offenders with a fine of from ten to twenty dollars.[8] This one, too, seems to have been cheerfully disregarded.

Street cleaning and garbage removal at this date was still left in the hands of the residents, which in practice meant that the dirt remained in the streets. According to Leland D. Baldwin, historian of Pittsburgh, the streets became so bad that finally "the custom arose of having the aged or otherwise superannuated men of the town hitch themselves to scrapers and clear the streets. From the fact that they usually worked eight or a dozen abreast they were commonly known as the 'Twelve Apostles.'"[9] By the late 1820s American newspapers were closely following the advance of Asiatic cholera through Asia and into Eastern Europe. More than likely, the threat of this disease stimulated the city government to appoint a street commissioner in 1830 to supervise street cleaning. As the cholera approached closer to the United States, Pittsburgh organized its first health agency.

Despite conceding that smoke and grime characterized the city, and that its streets, vacant lots, and public lands were filthy, Pittsburgh's residents stoutly maintained that their city was unusually healthy. A survey and directory of the city in 1826, however, admitted that the "atmosphere is darkened with a 'sulphurous canopy' which nearly conceals the place from view" and gives the traveler a "dark and melancholy aspect of men and things." In this same work the city's leading physician, Dr. William H. Denny, extolled the healthiness of its residents. There was scarcely any fever and ague, no yellow fever, and less bilious fever and cholera infantum than in other western cities. He attributed this good record to the fact that "no local sources of disease" existed and to the supposed antimiasmatic effect of the omnipresent smoke. "It is sulphurous and antiseptic," he wrote, "and hence it is, perhaps, that no putrid disease has ever been known to spread in the place." Although strangers with weak lungs found their coughs aggravated, he reported that "asthmatic patients have found relief in breathing it."[10] This last comment of Denny's contrasts sharply with an article in 1828 on the diseases of western Pennsylvania, which stated that disorders of the chest and lungs were "increasing among the sedentery population of our towns with fearful strides."[11]

The story of the nation's new capital of Washington, D.C., also illustrates how the public conceived of health in the early nineteenth century. Ten years elapsed from the time the decision was made to locate the capital on the Potomac River until the federal government officially moved there in 1800. Washington grew rapidly, and in 1802 its first public health ordinance was enacted, which established a public market and forbade the sale of "unsound, blown or unwholesome meat." That same year a law providing for an overseer of the poor was passed that required the mayor to contract a physician to care for the poor. In 1803 the presence of yellow fever in neighboring Alexandria on the Virginia side of the Potomac led to the creation of a superintendent of police for Washington, whose chief duty was to see to the removal of nuisances and stagnant pools.[12] President Thomas Jefferson was a firm exponent of the miasmatic theory, and his influence undoubtedly helps to explain the Washington City Council's willingness to vote money in these years to eliminate stagnant pools and swampy areas.

Two ordinances in 1809 speak for the sanitary condition of the town: one forbade citizens from cleaning fish in the streets; the second ordered owners to remove the dead carcasses of their animals from the streets and public places within twenty-four hours. In this same year residents living south of Massachusetts Avenue were ordered to keep their hogs in enclosures, and six years later the same rule was applied to geese. While nothing seems to have been done about horses and cattle, a measure in 1819 authorized the police and other residents to kill "any animal of goat kind" found loose in the streets.[13] Along with hogs, packs of dogs also roamed the city's streets, as they did in all major towns and cities. Periodically cases of rabies would be discovered among them, and the civic officials would order that all dogs be confined. Later in the century municipalities would take much stronger action against dogs.

As was true in a good many other cities, the local medical society in Washington took the lead in urging the establishment of a board of health. The society's members were assisted in this by Mayor James Blake, a medical graduate of the University of Maryland, who appealed to the city council to appoint a health officer in 1814. It was not until 1819, after steady pressure from the Medical Society of the District of Columbia, that the council finally acted. The duty of the health officer was to inform the mayor of any serious nuisances, the presence of any contagious disease, and the sources of that disease. The officer was to receive a maximum of fifteen dollars for expenses in the performance of his duties.

In 1822 a formal board of health was established consisting of one physician-resident and one layman from each ward. In fact, the board members were usually all physicians, a rather unusual arrangement for that time. The board was primarily an advisory body and was given virtually no budget. It was reappointed annually in the late spring, when the threat from "summer" fevers usually approached. Unless smallpox or some other disease broke out, the board remained inactive for most of the year.[14] Since no formal program existed for cleaning the streets, the board of health occasionally reminded citizens to clean up their yards and places of business and the streets in front of them.

Washington, D.C., and Pittsburgh were still relatively small, and although their sanitary problems were growing rapidly, they paled into insignificance beside those of New York City. New York first established a municipal street-cleaning system in 1798 with the appointment of two street commissioners. City residents were still responsible for sweeping the streets in front of their homes, but city employees were to remove garbage, manure, and rubbish from the streets. The process was assumed to be self-supporting since the sale of manure was expected to pay all collection costs. Shortly thereafter conflict between the two commissioners led to their dividing the work. Street cleaning was placed in the hands of a single "Commissioner of Streets," and a "Superintendent of Scavengers" was appointed to supervise the emptying of privies and the removal of nuisances. The system worked reasonably well until 1807, when the city council decided to turn the collection of street dirt over to a private contractor.[15]

Since the profit arose from the sale of manure rather than rubbish, private contractors invariably neglected to pick up the latter. Moreover, the contracts were political plums, which meant that the qualifications of the bidders had little to do with who received the contract. When the dirt and filth in the streets reached a crisis level, temporarily the city would take over the job of street cleaning. To add to these problems, in New York, as in all other cities, street sweeping was only done during the summer months, on the assumption that there was no danger from miasma during cool weather. Another important factor behind the increasingly unsanitary condition of the city was the change in the city's population and its governmental structure. The rising egalitarian spirit of the time meant that the traditional governing elite began to be replaced by nouveau riche businessmen and industrialists and by politicians who were far more responsive to the public—and the public, unless immediately threatened by an epidemic, had little interest in sanitation.

By 1830 nearly all major American cities had taken some responsibility for cleaning the streets. If a city had no street commissioner, then its board of health assumed responsibility. In all cases individual residents were still expected to sweep the dirt in front of their homes or business establishments. Scavengers or cartmen employed by the city, private contractors, or even local farmers (since manure constituted much of the street sweepings) then collected this material. Boston and New York City probably had the most effective method for removing street dirt, but their systems operated primarily during warm months. In addition to the garbage, rubbish, and manure, the streets were also the recipients of dead animals and the refuse from a wide variety of nuisance industries. For example, the blood from slaughterhouses was often drained into the gutters. Periodically efforts were made to eliminate these offenses to the nostrils and eyes—and health—but any successes were fleeting.

The basic problem was that few citizens had any sense of communal responsibility. Sanitary standards are gauged by the lowest common denominator, and a refusal to accept sanitary regulations by even a relatively small percentage of the population can negate an entire sanitary code. In addition, New York and other cities were expanding through an influx of rural immigrants accustomed to leaving the disposal of their wastes and garbage to nature. Sanitary practices that created only minor problems in rural areas proved almost disastrous in densely crowded cities. In consequence, sanitary conditions in American cities in these early years steadily worsened.

A major sanitary problem in urban areas was the disposal of human wastes. Overflowing cesspools and privies were a constant aesthetic outrage and menace to health. In many slum areas one privy often sufficed for twenty or more families. As a result, slum residents resorted to using tubs and bowls, which were simply emptied into the gutters. Since the majority of residents in most cities relied upon shallow wells for their water supply (and this was true even in those cities with a water system at this date), the overflowing privies and drains guaranteed that the wells seldom ran dry. New York required privies to be at least five feet deep and built of stone or brick, and a regulation published in 1829 prohibited building a privy within thirty feet of a public well—a rule that may help to explain the poor reputation of New York's water supply.[16] Yet the city's sanitary regulations were among the best in the country.

Both Boston and New York licensed scavengers or cartmen to empty privies and required the use of special carts, but citizens constantly complained about the contents of these carts slopping onto the streets and docks and of cartmen unloading their malodorous cargoes onto the nearest vacant lot. A good many towns made no provision respecting the emptying of privies, simply leaving it up to private enterprise. By 1830 most of the larger towns regulated the construction and location of privies. For example, Baltimore in 1817 prohibited the building of new privies in the main part of town, and three years later specified that all new ones have brick vaults.[17] Since the existing ones continued to be used for many years, one can only wonder what effect they had upon the city's well water. New Orleans was almost in a class by itself with respect to sanitary problems. The city's high water table prevented the widespread use of privies, and human wastes were either dumped into the streets and canals or else carried to the docks or unloaded on the batture, the section of the river bank between the high and low water marks. As might be expected, New Orleans, along with Charleston, had no system for collecting garbage. Not surprisingly, the general filth in and about the city was a standard complaint of local citizens and visitors alike.[18]

Another sanitation problem involved burials in church graveyards. With cities' increasing population, graveyards tended to fill, creating space problems. Until well into the nineteenth century in many cities bodies were still being interred in church and family crypts; when these became crowded, the churches often petitioned for the right to extend their crypts under adjacent streets and public property. By the late eighteenth century repeated complaints about the nauseating odors emanating from burial grounds and church crypts were appearing in the newspapers of major cities. The yellow fever epidemics of these years, as might be expected, intensified public outcries and led local medical societies to take up the issue.

The thirty-year struggle by New York City authorities to regulate burials that started in 1798 was repeated in one form or another in every major city. That year the New York Medical Society recommended eliminating burials in populated areas, and its proposal soon won support from the chamber of commerce and the city council. No action was taken at that time, but in 1807, when one of the city health commissioners reported an offensive smell arising from the vault of a black church, the city council promptly prohibited any further interments there. Two years later, however, when two white Presbyterian churches requested permission to extend their crypts, they were allowed to do so. In the meantime residents living near church crypts continued to complain about the foul smells that arose whenever the vaults were opened. In their fight to prohibit these interments, the residents found strong allies among physicians and early sanitary reformers. On the other hand, burials were an important source of income for churches and sextons—one they were reluctant to surrender. The New York City Council generally favored restricting burials but was understandably reluctant to clash with the churches.

For the next few years the issue was widely debated, with the council hesitantly moving toward limiting interments within the city. The last yellow fever epidemic of 1822 brought matters to a head, and the city council, after establishing yet another committee to study the matter, proposed to prohibit all burials south of Canal Street. News of this proposal united virtually every church in the city in opposition. When the council remained firm in its decision and enacted an ordinance to this effect in 1823, the churches turned to the courts, claiming the ordinance abrogated the original grants given to them by the city and deprived them of private property. A series of moves and countermoves ensued, but suffice it to say that in the fall of 1827 the New York State Supreme Court upheld the legality of the 1823 ordinance.[19]

The two worst abuses taking place in city graveyards in general were the failure to bury bodies deeply enough and the disinterment of remains in order to make room for new burials. Potter's fields were a focal point of complaint in nearly every city. Too often grave diggers would make a grave large enough for ten or twelve coffins and then leave it open until it was filled. In winter this practice created minor problems, but in warm weather it filled nearby neighborhoods with pungent odors. In several cities complaints were made that bodies were barely covered with dirt and that dogs and hogs often rooted them out. One of the worst offenders in this respect was New Orleans, whose high water table limited the depth of graves. Considering the Christian attitude toward burial, it is surprising to find so many complaints about the neglect of graveyards—and not only potter's fields—during these years. Ironically, it was public health leaders and not church leaders who fought to correct this situation.

As the accumulating dirt and filth in cities increasingly polluted local wells and adjacent streams and rivers, the need for adequate city water supplies became more evident. An ample supply of water was essential for fighting fires and cleaning the streets, and good water was necessary for personal hygiene and human consumption. Those major cities that had already established water systems by 1800 gradually expanded them in the early nineteenth century. Philadelphia, which led the way in providing good water, first used spruce logs reinforced at the ends with wrought-iron bands for its water mains. Aside from not being durable, these wooden mains tended to leak at the joints, causing a loss of water when pressure was high and threatening to cause pollution when it was low. In 1818 Philadelphia took the radical step of installing cast-iron pipe, the first city to do so. Baltimore also turned to cast-iron mains and lead service pipes beginning in 1820, and, as iron pipe became cheaper and more available, other cities gradually followed suit.[20]

Not all cities were successful in establishing a water system. In 1816 the town of Madison constructed the first water system in the state of Indiana. It consisted of a series of wooden pipes with plugs installed at street intersections. Residents wanting water were to pull out a plug and fill their buckets or other vessels. Unfortunately, the men who had previously carted water around town for sale destroyed sections of the logs, thus putting an end to the system, and the town had to wait over thirty years before another system was built.[21]

The city of New Orleans was almost as unfortunate. Its location on the natural levee along the Mississippi River, with low-lying land in the rear, meant that once a pumping station was erected, it would be possible to flush the city's streets and gutters by gravity flow and at the same time supply water for household purposes. A private company under the direction of the noted architect Benjamin Latrobe undertook the project, and in 1813 construction began on a steam-powered waterworks. The remoteness of New Orleans from manufacturing centers made it difficult to obtain equipment, unfortunately, and the project's skilled workmen imported from the North soon fell prey to fevers and dysentery. In 1817 Latrobe's son, who had been directing the project, died of yellow fever.

Latrobe reorganized the company and came to New Orleans to take charge. Beset by problems, the project dragged on until 1820, when Latrobe himself was felled by yellow fever. Two years later the city council assumed control of the unfinished water system, promising to complete it within a year. Its success can be judged from the recommendation of a new board of health in 1846 that the city provide pumps to supply good drinking water and flush out the streets.[22]

Pittsburgh first authorized the digging of public wells in 1802, at that time also agreeing to contribute to the cost of private wells if the owners made them available to the public. By 1820 the city's water problem was becoming acute, with individuals queuing up at the available wells or else buying river water from water carriers. As the situation worsened, in 1824 the city council proposed to build a water system and appointed a committee of five prominent citizens to raise the necessary funds. The work progressed slowly, and it was 1828 before the system was reported ready for operation. An 84-horsepower steam engine raised water from the Allegheny to a reservoir 116 feet above the river. The system worked poorly at first, but by 1832 Pittsburgh was well supplied with good water, the same year that a water system began operating in St. Louis.[23]

While the city reservoirs acted as settling basins, none of the early water systems provided filtered water. The quality of the water depended upon its source, and, as city boundaries enlarged and new communities developed in neighboring areas, water purity steadily deteriorated. It is well to keep in mind, too, that in these years, and for many to come, only the well-to-do could afford to have water piped into their homes; the majority of citizens relied upon standpipes or hydrants located at intervals on street corners. Along the Gulf Coast, where the average rainfall was around sixty inches, many families relied upon cisterns. Although the cisterns provided a breeding ground for mosquitoes, the water from them was safe for human consumption. It was the common use of cisterns combined with access to river water that enabled New Orleans to get along without a water system for so many years.

The development of water systems intensified another perennial problem, that of drainage. Cities and towns grew haphazardly, with no provision made for draining rain water, springs, and household wastes. Drainage was left largely to individual householders, who usually poured their wastes into the nearest street or stream. Boston, by the early nineteenth century, required householders to convey water by underground drains to the nearest sewer. The word "sewer" was often used interchangeably with "drain" and referred to both covered and uncovered drains. In most cases these drains were simply open ditches. The Boston Board of Health kept a fairly close watch over drainage problems, and on occasion ordered the construction of a common sewer. In the older cities, drains or sewers, which ran through the main part of town, were occasionally enclosed as a matter of aesthetics. One other point is worth noting: virtually every city had ordinances forbidding the discharging of human wastes into the sewers. Sewer systems, as we know them today, came into existence in the latter part of the nineteenth century.

The growth of cities inevitably led to the filling in of low-lying land, which in turn created new drainage problems. In 1826, for example, the New York City Council agreed to fill in Stuyvesant's Meadow, a low-lying stretch of land along the East River. As the cost of the project rose, the city considered simply draining the land by means of a canal or underground drains. A public outcry arose on the grounds that an open canal would become the repository of all sorts of offensive materials and that underground drains would be even worse. The objection to underground drains was well founded; the few existing ones were usually poorly planned and rarely had enough gravity fall to drain their contents. Also, the public tendency to toss everything into the streets, including dead animals, led to the frequent clogging of these sewers. Trapping devices were not common at this time, with the result, particularly in summer, that the odors from sewer openings made life unbearable for people living near them. In the case of Stuyvesant's Meadow, the New York City Council backed down and agreed to continue filling in the land.[24]

The first third of the nineteenth century saw limited advances in municipal government—the emergence of garbage collection and street cleaning, temporary health boards, quarantine systems, city or private water systems, nuisance inspectors, regulations controlling the construction and emptying of privies, and restrictions on intracity burials. Countering these advances was the rapid expansion of city populations. As the well-to-do moved away from the low-lying riverbank and dock areas to higher ground, their former homes became jammed with newcomers, who often came from rural areas. Homes designed for single families now were occupied by several families, compounding the problem of human waste disposal. Tenements were built on occasion with no provision for privies, and shoddy housing was erected on every available inch of land. By 1830 the urban slum was firmly established.

Logically, sewer systems should have preceded water systems, but such was not the case. Vast quantities of water were conveyed into cities with little provision made for their drainage. The introduction of piped water into larger homes made possible the increasing use of water closets at a time when no true sewer system existed. Although in the larger cities it was illegal to pour human wastes into sewers or drains, it was almost impossible to prevent this practice. As of 1830 little thought had been given to the problem of disposing waste water. With slum dwellers crowded together in damp, filthy housing, in some cases lacking even elementary sanitary facilities, and in all cases drinking highly polluted water, the stage was set for the first of the great Asiatic cholera epidemics.

NOTES

1. Morris Saffron, "A Sketch of Medicine in New Jersey to 1825," *Journal of the Medical Society of New Jersey* 81 (1984):714.

2. N. V. A. Gerardin, *Mémoires sur la Fièvre Jaune* . . . (Paris, 1820), 84–85.

3. John Bernard, *Retrospections of America, 1797–1811* (New York, 1887), 182.

4. *Pittsburgh Gazette,* April 5, 1800.

5. Ibid., May 20, 1803.

6. Ibid., June 16, 1807.

7. Leland D. Baldwin, *Pittsburgh: The Story of a City* (Pittsburgh, 1937), 155.

8. *Pittsburgh Gazette,* June 2, 1807.

9. Baldwin, *Pittsburgh: The Story of a City,* 239.

10. S. Jones, *Pittsburgh in the Year Eighteen Hundred and Twenty-six, Containing Sketches . . . Together with a Directory of the City* . . . (Pittsburgh, 1826), 31–32, 39.

11. L. Callaghan, "Topography and Diseases of Western Pennsylvania," extract from the *American Medical Journal,* in *The Register of Pennsylvania* 2 (1828):265–67.

12. Betty L. Plummer, "A History of Public Health in Washington, D.C., 1800–1890" (Ph.D. diss., University of Maryland, 1984), 21–22.

13. Ibid., 24–27.

14. Ibid., 27–32.

15. John Duffy, *A History of Public Health in New York City, 1625–1866* (New York, 1968), 181–93.

16. *Address of the Board of Health, of the City of New-York, to their Fellow Citizens, 1829* (New York, 1829), 19–22.

17. William T. Howard, *Public Health Administration and the Natural History of Diseases in Baltimore, Maryland, 1797–1920* (Washington, D.C., 1924), 66–67.

18. John Duffy, *The Rudolf Matas History of Medicine in Louisiana* (Baton Rouge, La., 1958–62), 1:393ff.

19. Duffy, *Public Health in New York City, 1625–1866,* 218–22.

20. J. J. Cosgrave, *History of Sanitation* (Pittsburgh, 1909), 81; Russell Wigley, ed., *Philadelphia: A Three-Hundred-Year History* (New York, 1982), 228–29; Howard, *Public Health Administration in Baltimore,* 125–26.

21. Indiana State Board of Health, *Monthly Bulletin* 26 (1923):114.

22. Duffy, *Matas History of Medicine in Louisiana,* 1:406–8, 2:170–71.

23. *Pittsburgh Gazette,* August 13, December 17, 1802; *Pittsburgh Gazette, And Manufacturing & Mercantile Advertiser,* February 20, 1824; *The Register of Pennsylvania* 3 (1829), 64; and 7 (1831), 281; *Pittsburgh, Commemorating the Fiftieth Anniversary of the Engineers' Society of Western Pennsylvania* (Pittsburgh, 1930), 39; Thomas E. Parks, "The History of St. Louis, 1827–1836" (M.A. thesis, Washington University, 1948), 30.

24. Duffy, *Public Health in New York City, 1625–1866,* 405–8.

6

The Impact of Asiatic Cholera

Following the shock waves induced by the series of yellow fever epidemics at the turn of the eighteenth century, limited sanitary measures were taken, a number of temporary health boards came into existence, quarantine laws were strengthened, and a few individuals became aware of the need for governmental action to avoid epidemic diseases. Medical societies, representing at that time the elite of the profession, began expressing their concern with the growing filth that characterized towns and cities alike, but the medical profession carried little weight. The inability of physicians to cure or prevent the great epidemic infections of the day frustrated them and contributed to the public quarrels that literally tore their profession apart. The endemic disorders responsible for the high morbidity and mortality rates were all too familiar, and without the stimulus provided by a strange and highly fatal pestilence, the average citizen had little interest in—and even less inclination to spend money for—public health. Out of sheer necessity slow progress was made in developing water supplies, garbage and waste disposal systems, drainage systems, and other essentials, but the problems created by the rapidly expanding urban population were outgrowing these hesitant steps in the direction of sanitation and hygiene.

By the 1820s civic officials and the public itself were largely apathetic with respect to community health. This apathy was shaken later in the decade, when news came that Asiatic cholera was spreading westward from the Far East. By 1830 the epidemic wave reached western Russia and threatened Europe. Despite the deployment of military forces in an attempt to create a *cordon sanitaire,* cholera quickly spread from country to country. It appeared in Great Britain in 1831, and in the early summer of 1832 it crossed the Atlantic and was diagnosed in Quebec, Montreal, and New York City.

Asiatic cholera, a highly fatal disease when untreated, was (and is) an acute disorder of the intestinal tract caused by a comma-shaped bacillus. It was a filth disease, spread by contact with the intestinal discharges from its victims. Thus contaminated water and food and a lack of personal hygiene were the principal means by which cholera spread. Its vomiting, agonizing intestinal cramps, and violent diarrhea could bring death to its victims in a matter of hours by dehydrating them and disrupting their electrolytic balance. The pinched blue faces and dark drawn skin of those affected added to the horror and apprehension with which cholera was viewed.

Ironically, the same industrial and transportation revolutions that transformed the Western world in the nineteenth century set the stage for the brief career of Asiatic cholera in Europe and North America. This disease, which struck in three successive waves during the nineteenth century, found a favorable milieu in the crowded, dirty cities created by industrialism. Limited water supplies made personal hygiene virtually impossible for the lower economic classes, and contaminated water affected all segments of society. Under these circumstances, once cholera was introduced, it spread like wildfire. And in the prebacterial era, cholera was one more strange and deadly pestilence for which there seemed no cause nor cure.

To add to the dread aroused by cholera, no disease in history had been so widely heralded. European and American newspapers began reporting its advance from the East in the late 1820s, and by 1831, as it pushed into Western Europe, Asiatic cholera was a major item of interest. American newspapers carried detailed accounts of its ravages in Russia and Europe, and editorials and medical articles advised readers how to avoid the disease or minimize its hazards. The association of sickness with dirt and filth led popular magazines and medical journals to join with newspapers in urging local authorities to embark on large-scale sanitary programs. By the time the pandemic wave reached Great Britain in 1831, a rising air of tension and alarm was widespread, reflected in the news items and features on cholera that preoccupied American newspapers.[1]

In the fall of 1831 all major Canadian and American ports instituted quarantine measures against ships and goods from infected ports, but they proved of little avail. News of cholera in Quebec and Montreal in June of 1832 confirmed the public's worst apprehensions. Although many religious and political leaders affirmed that the superior health of Americans and their Christian way of life would preserve them from the diseases affecting the decadent Europeans, a lurking fear underlay many of these pronouncements. Moreover, when they looked at their cities—where hogs, dogs, and goats roamed at will; where manure piles, garbage, dead animals, and refuse from the nuisance industries festered in the streets and on vacant lots; where the contents of privies often flowed directly into gutters; and where the inadequate funds provided for sanitation were reduced by corruption and inefficiency—even the most loyal Americans must have had some qualms.

By the time New Yorkers heard on June 15 that cholera was present in Canada, it had already spread into Upstate New York. The governor promptly called a special session of the state legislature, which immediately empowered him to quarantine the Canadian border, and he required all towns and villages bordering lakes, rivers, and canals to appoint health boards. Vermont and other states, too, took similar action. Following a pattern set in early colonial cities, well-to-do citizens began a mass exodus from towns and cities, literally jamming the roads with carriages and wagons.

The New York City Board of Health, composed of city officials acting in a public health capacity, remained unmoved by the growing threat. When late in June 1832 the first few cases of cholera were diagnosed, the mayor and the health board refused to admit that the disease had entered the city. The New York Medical Society, recognizing the need for immediate action, on July 2 publicly announced the presence of Asiatic cholera and consequently brought a torrent of abuse upon itself. Many businessmen promptly denounced the society for needlessly disrupting the economic life of the city. One of them complained that the public would scarcely have noticed the disease had it not been forewarned, and John Pintard, a prominent merchant and banker, called the announcement "an impertinent interference" with the board of health.[2]

In defense of New York's municipal officials, it should be pointed out that admitting to the presence of a pestilential disease was certain to cause panic and invariably resulted in many residents fleeing, in neighboring communities raising quarantine barriers, and in a breakdown of economic activity. Moreover, in the days before bacteriological laboratories it was only rarely that a city's physicians could agree on the diagnosis of the first few cases of an epidemic disease. Under these circumstances, health boards and other city officials never admitted to the presence of an epidemic disease until it was obvious.

The action of the New York Medical Society forced the city's board of health to face up to the crisis. It agreed to meet daily, appointed a seven-man "Special Medical Council" to serve in an advisory capacity, opened several temporary cholera hospitals, began removing nuisances and filling in stagnant pools, and instituted a general cleanup of the city. Expressing the accepted belief that poverty and disease arose from vice, intemperance, and laziness, the Special Medical Council proclaimed that "the disease in the city is confined to the imprudent, the intemperate, and to those who injure themseves by taking improper medicines." Acting on this assumption, the board of health promptly began a campaign to raise the moral standards and personal hygiene of the poorer classes. Public notices warned them against intemperate eating and drinking, advised personal cleanliness, and urged them to avoid laboring in the heat of the day. Precisely how fifteen to twenty families sharing one hydrant and two or three overflowing privies could be expected to practice personal hygiene, or how poorly paid laborers could avoid working in the heat of the day, was never made explicit.[3]

The cholera epidemic in New York City lasted about six weeks, peaking in July. In this time the board of health spent about $118,000 on sanitation, hospitals, medical care, and public education. The death toll from the epidemic amounted to about 3,000, falling largely on poorer citizens.

One of the tragedies of public health is that the poorer citizens who stand to benefit most from public health measures are often anything but cooperative. In New York City the poor, who shared the general public's suspicion of hospitals, objected to temporary cholera hospitals in their neighborhoods and fought to keep their sick at home. Having little understanding of the need for public or personal hygiene, they strenuously opposed health regulations such as those calling for the immediate burial of cholera victims and frequently attacked the health board's physicians and health workers.

From New York State, cholera spread through the entire eastern part of the United States. It followed water and stage coach routes, striking here and there in an aimless fashion, often reaching the remotest communities. It skipped lightly over some towns, missed many completely, and devastated still others. On the Atlantic coast only Boston and Charleston escaped. It did not reach New Orleans until late October. By this time the city's newspapers had been filled with stories on cholera, and its appearance caused thousands to flee. The epidemic lasted less than a month, but within this period between 4,500 and 5,000 people died. Approximately 15,000 of New Orleans' 50,000 inhabitants fled the city at the beginning of the outbreak. Of those who remained, almost 15 percent perished within a month.

The refugees took so many vehicles with them that the city was forced to requisition every remaining available carriage and cart to help take the dead to the graveyards. A shortage of grave diggers caused bodies to pile up in the cemeteries, forcing mass burials. All economic life was disrupted as those who remained concentrated on caring for the sick and burying the dead.[4] It is possible that New Orleanians were too accustomed to repeated yellow fever epidemics and the omnipresent dirt to feel any necessity for a sanitary program or for strengthening its board of health. Whatever the case, the first cholera epidemic had no residual impact upon New Orleans' public health.

Wherever the disease struck in the United States, in city or town, the pattern remained the same. A good share of the population fled, and, of those remaining, a high percentage of those infected died. Philadelphia suffered only lightly, but some of the towns in the interior of Pennsylvania took heavy losses. The governor, George Wolf, proclaimed a day of fasting and prayer that God "might mitigate the afflictions of the epidemic."[5] In Cincinnati the first cholera cases were diagnosed on September 24, and by November 20 the death toll amounted to 571. An estimated 5,000 of the town's 30,000 residents left, and approximately 20 percent of those remaining fell victim to the disease.[6] From Locust Grove, Kentucky, George Hancock wrote: "The cholera has made dreadful havoc in the country around us, on Mr. Brown's farm 12 men died in 36 hours." Four days later he wrote: "You can conceive nothing to equal the gloom spread over the country here. No one leaves home. Crops of wheat standing uncut, corn fields abandoned to winds. . . ."[7] As the disease coursed along the rivers and bayous of the South, it proved devastating to the slave population. One plantation in Louisiana lost 83 of its 104 slaves.[8]

St. Louis took heavy losses in relation to its population, and Wheeling, Virginia (West Virginia), suffered explosive epidemics in 1832 and 1833.[9] Pittsburgh was fortunate enough to escape with only a few deaths both years. The mildness of the Pittsburgh outbreaks probably can be attributed to the city's supply of good water and to energetic action on the part of the mayor and city council. Shortly after hearing of the arrival of cholera in New York, Pittsburgh's city officials transformed themselves into a "Sanitary Board," with authority "to adopt and direct all such measures as [the members] think necessary for averting the introduction of the frightful epidemic disease, which has approached the borders of our country." These measures included a complete sanitary program, temporary hospitals, and other provisions for the care of patients. The city was divided into districts, with an inspector in each one to check for all "offensive, foul, or mouldy vaults, cellars, privies, or other nusances [*sic*] of any Kind." All city employees and private citizens were instructed to obey the written orders of the Sanitary Board, and, more important, the board was given a special fund of $10,000 for sanitary purposes.[10]

With the advice of leading Pittsburgh physicians, a board of medical consultants was also appointed. As too frequently occurred, the two boards clashed, with the physicians claiming that the Sanitary Board had disregarded some of their advice. The exact issue is not clear, but it may have had to do with the Sanitary Board's practice of inspecting river vessels to prevent the landing of sick passengers or crewmen. Whatever the problem, the civic authorities in Pittsburgh deserve credit for taking every action possible to avert the spread of cholera or at least to minimize its effects. The disease did enter the city in the fall of 1832, but it resulted in only a few scattered cases and about thirty deaths.[11] Cholera continued to strike sporadically throughout the United States during 1833 and 1834 and then disappeared for about fifteen years.

Although the cholera epidemic of 1832 shocked the country and literally panicked many citizens, insofar as public health was concerned, its impact was fleeting. The prevailing American spirit in the era of Jacksonian democracy was antigovernment, antimonopoly, and anti-intellectual. All professions, and medicine in particular, were held in suspicion. President Jackson (1828–36) epitomized the American faith in free enterprise and the belief that the least government was the best government. His veto of the Maysville Bill, which proposed a federal road subsidy, and his destruction of the first national bank of the United States were welcomed by most Americans. The role of the government was to provide minimal services and leave economic matters to individual citizens. Regulating nuisance industries, requiring private citizens to clean their premises, or ordering them to remove their hogs from the streets were considered infringements upon individual liberty and private property rights. Although an increasing number of health reformers, most of whom were physicians, pleaded for sanitary reform, as of the 1830s they were voices crying in the wilderness.

The boards of health that had been created thus far in America were essentially emergency bodies designed to restore cities and towns to normalcy. The few that met annually functioned only in summertime, the season of fevers. Those established during the cholera years quickly disappeared or lapsed into inactivity. In New Orleans, where civic leaders insisted that only strangers and the intemperate poor fell prey to pestilential disorders, the city's experience with cholera merely reinforced their belief. In the nation's capital, the board of health functioned quite effectively during the first cholera outbreak, aided by a substantial grant from Congress, but once the crisis had passed, it virtually ceased to function. As of 1848 the Washington Health Board's annual budget was only $15.[12] Pittsburgh, which had spent $10,000 for sanitary purposes during the 1832 epidemic, authorized its mayor to borrow $6,000 when cholera returned in 1833. The city's budget for 1835, however, listed only $144 for removing garbage, $261 for cleaning the markets, and $9.75 for "taking hogs." Another $450 was allocated for the "Hospital and Sanitary Fund."[13] In September 1841, the editor of the Pittsburgh *Morning Chronicle* complained that people were throwing their garbage and dirty water into the streets, where it combined with the dead bodies of cats, dogs, and pigs to make the atmosphere unbearable.[14]

The New York City Board of Health, although it acted somewhat belatedly, performed reasonably well during the cholera epidemic, but for the next few years it was content to simply report breaches of the health code. As the city's population soared, the board's annual budget reached a peak of $14,000 in 1837, most of which went to pay the salaries of sixteen district health wardens. In ensuing years the budget steadily declined, until by 1847 it was only $2,000. In a commentary upon the state of municipal affairs, in 1839, when only $12,000 was allocated to the board, city officers spent $3,200 on champagne, other wines and liquors, and "segars"—a slush fund amounting to one-fourth of the board's total budget.[15] In Chicago the first board of health was appointed in 1834 in response to the threat of cholera. A more permanent board was appointed in 1835, but there is no record to show that it accomplished anything.[16] Although physicians occasionally served on American health boards during this period, most board members were city councilmen. With the public apathetic, health appropriations were generally negligible, and even these small appropriations were usually considered a source of political patronage.

While city residents at best were only vaguely aware of the need for governmental action with respect to health, they could not avoid the nauseous odors arising from festering garbage, carrion, and other substances, which literally surrounded them and made the streets at times almost impassable. New York's problems with garbage were on a larger scale than those of other American cities, but its efforts to deal with them were little different from those made by other cities. Early in the nineteenth century New York had tried hiring one contractor to collect the entire city's garbage. When this arrangement proved unsatisfactory, the council had divided the city into ten districts, on the assumption that a number of small contractors would be more efficient. This method of organization achieved even worse results, and in 1826 the city appointed a force of its own to remove garbage and debris from the streets, but by 1829 the old complaints reappeared. Under the threat of Asiatic cholera, in 1831–32 the city council enacted an ordinance providing that the city both sweep and remove dirt and other matter from the streets. Within a few more years the perennial complaints about filth in the streets were sounded, leading to a review of the situation. The street-cleaning superintendent blamed much of the problem on the city's failure to enforce the laws against throwing offal, garbage, and debris into the streets, but it is clear that his department had become involved in politics. In 1842 street cleaning was once again turned over to private contractors. In succeeding years the city alternated between private contractors and a municipal system, neither of which seemed to work.

In 1855 New York's street commissioner contracted a private company to sweep the streets with machines. Later this same year a grand jury indicted some of the city contractors and officials. In August 1856, the street commissioner requested an additional $100,000 for his department, although, according to the *Daily Times*, some $280,000 had already been spent. Despite this huge expenditure, the newspaper stated, "the streets have been and still are scandalously and dangerously filthy." The basic problem lay in the city's too-rapid expansion and in its lack of an effective governmental structure. Added to this was the tendency of most newcomers to the city to practice outmoded rural sanitary practices ill suited to urban living conditions. The newcomers were not only victims of the slums but were also responsible in part for the city's political problems.[17]

New Orleans in the pre–Civil War period relied upon a street commissioner and private contractors to remove dirt and filth from the streets, but this system was no more effective than New York's, and possibly less effective. Periodically a severe yellow fever or cholera epidemic would result in the establishment of a board of health and a drive to remove the worst nuisances; but, once the outbreak was over, the emergency measures would lapse, and the recommendations of the board of health would be disregarded. Similarly, Washington, D.C., gave its health board responsibility for street cleaning but unfortunately appropriated little money for this purpose. Whenever the situation became too bad, a special appropriation was made. For example, in the summer of 1837 the city council appropriated $1,500 for "purging the streets and alleys of the accumulated filth and garbage" and for the removal of nuisances. Most of the time, the filth and garbage simply accumulated.[18]

Garbage and slops were only part of the offenses to the sight and smell of city inhabitants all over America. Street contractors usually piled manure and garbage on docks or other transfer points; dairies and stables had their own manure piles; and horses, hogs, and other animals roaming the streets contributed an added share to the omnipresent manure. Theoretically scavengers or other city officers were responsible for removing dead animals from the streets, but this responsibility was taken lightly. City planning simply did not exist, and drainage was largely in the hands of property owners. Complaints about stagnant water and undrained filthy pools were a constant in the newspapers. Streams, rivers, canals, and harbors were the respository of everything from human wastes to debris. Most cities had ordinances prohibiting dumping, but they were almost impossible to enforce. A humorous report in a Pittsburgh newspaper in 1848 could have been written about any city in the United States at the time: A young woman attempted suicide by jumping into a local canal, but the water was so bad that she quickly climbed out. She then contemplated jumping in again, but, after "beholding its filthy condition, and inhaling its foetid odor, she concluded to postpone drowning until she could meet with cleaner water."[19]

By the 1830s ordinances existed that prohibited large animals in general from running loose, but their enforcement was at best sporadic. In 1831 a motion to prohibit cows from the streets of New York City was defeated when an alderman explained that the cows were "the entire support of some of the poorer classes in the upper wards." The motion passed the following year, no doubt because the councilmen were confident it would not be enforced. An ordinance in 1839 specified that no swine or cattle could go abroad in the area south of Fourteenth Street. The law did not apply above Fourteenth, and in any event it does not appear to have been enforced. Cows were eventually required to be penned, but frequent complaints were made of injuries resulting from slaughterers driving their cattle through the streets.

Hogs presented an even more difficult problem for civic authorities. In 1842 the New York *Daily Tribune* blamed the filthy condition of the streets upon the presence of about ten thousand hogs.[20] The cholera epidemic of 1849 led to a crackdown on hog owners aimed at requiring them to keep their pigs in sties. Several years later a drive began against the piggeries, resulting in an 1855 measure to force the larger ones out of the main part of town. Small pigsties with not more than three pigs, however, were still allowed in the city, and tenement dwellers continued to keep pigs in their basements, and occasionally in their rooms, until well after the Civil War. In the large eastern cities hogs consumed much of the cities' garbage and were a source of meat for the poorer classes, a fact that made councilmen reluctant to ban them. New York was not alone with its hog problems; the newspapers of every city and town in these years were replete with news items and editorials denouncing the failure of authorities to keep hogs off the streets. Stories of hogs knocking people over or entering homes can be found in newspapers throughout the United States.

Packs of stray dogs occasionally attacked humans and domestic animals and periodically aroused fears of rabies. License and muzzle laws for dogs were enacted early in the colonial period, but, as with other ordinances affecting domestic animals, they were rarely enforced. In the nineteenth century rumors or reports of rabies frequently led to drives to kill all stray dogs. In New Orleans the usual method was to distribute poisoned sausages in the streets. It was quite effective, but since no one took responsibility for removing the dead animals, they soon became an outrage to city residents' olfactory organs. An 1831 ordinance enacted by the town of Allegheny, Pennsylvania, typifies the laws relating to rabid dogs. It provided that whenever a mad dog was reported, the authorities were to notify the public to confine their animals and to employ one or more persons to kill and remove all strays at a rate of fifty cents per dog.[21] It was not uncommon for a city or town to pay a fifty-cent bounty for the killing of stray dogs. New York City tried it on one occasion, with the result that gangs of children went around clubbing to death any dogs they could find. The councilmen quickly repealed the ordinance and employed official dog killers.

Probably no single subject so occupied the attention of public officials, newspapers, and citizens as that of general nuisances. Included in this category were the enormous manure piles, slaughterhouses, dairies, stables, obnoxious trades, overflowing privies and cesspools, and filthy gutters common for that time and a wide range of other annoyances. To visualize nineteenth-century cities, one must bear in mind that horses were omnipresent in the streets and that stables, dairies, and piggeries were scattered throughout business and residential areas. With hogs roaming loose, butchers, fishmongers, and other tradesmen were encouraged to throw their refuse into the streets. In the summertime the manure piles, carrion, and offal bred clouds of flies and must have created an unbearable stench. The New York city inspector reported that during the month of May 1853 some 439 large dead animals had been removed from the streets, along with the bodies of 71 dogs, 93 cats, 17 sheep, 4 goats, and 19 hogs.[22] When, as too frequently happened, the contractors or officials responsible for carrion removal were negligent, the situation must have been grim indeed.

Privies presented one of the most difficult of all sanitary problems. In the poorer districts landlords were reluctant to spend money to have them emptied, with the result that they frequently overflowed. And even when this was not the case, the very emptying of privies created nuisances. Scavengers responsible for this task frequently overloaded their carts and bumped through the rough city streets, scattering their nauseous loads, or else left a trail of the carts' liquid contents as they passed. Large hospitals and hotels frequently poured the contents of their privies into the street gutters or open drains. Scavengers usually unloaded their cargoes of human wastes into the nearest water body or onto the most accessible piece of empty land. In larger cities, a series of ordinances regulated the work of the scavengers, including one requiring them to have covered, watertight carts, but, since the men worked at night, the regulations were difficult to enforce. In New York and the eastern ports, the scavengers were accused of fouling the slips and docks; in New Orleans and other river ports they were charged with defiling the waterfront and river banks. Although several mechanical methods for cleaning privies were introduced and stricter regulations were enacted, privies remained a major health hazard and aesthetic offense until the advent of effective sewer systems during the late nineteenth century (which in turn created massive problems of waste disposal).

Although private citizens were responsible for constructing drains or sewers on their property, towns and cities soon found it necessary to use public funds for this purpose. They did so reluctantly and only to solve particular problems. For example, a city market might start to strain the limited drainage provided by nearby gutters or an adjacent small stream, and the authorities, usually under pressure from neighboring residents, would then authorize the digging of a drain. Or a stream running through the center of town would become so fetid as to force the municipal officials to turn it into a covered sewer. Over the years the drains in the main business sections were gradually enclosed, and feeder drains or sewers were added. The process was piecemeal and sporadic, without any central planning. Sanitary engineering was in its infancy, and only limited attention was paid to gradation. Where main sewers were constructed of brick, their floors were usually flat, and unless an unusually heavy rain flushed them out, they tended to fill with solid matter. Since these sewers were not properly graded, water also tended to stand in them. Few if any of them in the first half of the nineteenth century had traps, and repeated complaints can be found in the newspapers and municipal records of this period about the foul odors emanating from the drains and sewers.

Theoretically the drains and sewers were designed to carry off surface water and not the contents of privies and cesspools. In practice, a good part of this waste material did find its way into the sewers. The problem was aggravated by the introduction, first, of water systems, which added to the strains on the inadequate drainage systems, and, second, of water closets or flush toilets. Ideally, the engineering skills related to water and sewer systems should have developed simultaneously, but unfortunately the technology and design of sewer systems lagged at least fifty years behind those of water systems.

The development of relatively good water supplies was one area of sanitation where significant progress was made in the first half of the nineteenth century. Improvements in steam power and the introduction of cast-iron pipes made it possible to increase water pressure and thus supply far more homes and large buildings. Cast-iron pipes were less likely to leak, a feature that was particularly important since contamination occurred when ground water leaked into pipes during times of low water pressure. Better engineering, too, made it possible to tap more distant and better water sources. Boston, for example, which had originally transported water 4½ miles through wooden logs from Jamaica Pond, was able to tap a much larger and better supply of water from Lake Cochituate in 1848.[23]

The expansion of water systems in these years is demonstrated by the case of Philadelphia. In 1803 the private water company serving the city had a total of 77 customers; by 1835 the number had risen to 14,395, with 2,500 families using public hydrants. At this date the system was supplying the city with 3,400,000 gallons of water a day and distributing it through more than eighty-two miles of cast-iron pipe.[24] Pittsburgh, which spent relatively large amounts of its tax revenues on its water supply, boasted in 1857 that its waterworks distributed "the pure sweet water of the Allegheny" throughout the city.[25] Due to the machinations of Aaron Burr (discussed earlier in chapter 3), New York, which possibly had the most inadequate, and also the poorest, water supply of any major U.S. city, did not solve its water problem until 1842. In the meantime, its residents relied on well water or on the limited number of hydrants provided by Burr's Manhattan Water Company. A major fire in 1829, made much worse by a shortage of water, led to a series of petitions and resolutions urging the city take over the water company. The 1832 cholera epidemic provided further impetus to the movement, and in 1834 the New York state legislature authorized the city to draw up a plan for an aqueduct and water system. Pushed on by the notoriously poor quality of the city's water—even the brewers complained about it—the project steadily advanced. On October 12, 1842—a day celebrated by parades, fireworks, and the ringing of church bells—the city system bringing water from the Croton River was officially opened.[26]

Aside from bringing the health benefits of improved drinking water to New Yorkers, the new water system vastly increased the amount of water brought into the city. The increase stimulated the installation of water closets, and, as these closets multiplied, it became imperative to make some provision for sewerage also. In 1845 the city council for the first time permitted the owners of privies or water closets to connect them to public sewers. In the meantime, the number of private sewers was rapidly growing. Suffice it to say, after several years of detailed surveys and various committee studies, in 1849 the council assigned responsibility for the construction, repair, and cleaning of all sewers and underground drains to the Croton Aqueduct Department. This department, possibly the most efficient one in the city government, promptly began constructing new sewers, complete with receiving basins and culverts; by 1853 New York City had 105 miles of sewers. Just as the 1832 cholera epidemic had increased public demand for better water, so the epidemic of 1849 provided an impetus to the sewer program that began in that year. It is more than a coincidence that the construction of sewers was sharply reduced after 1854, the end of the second epidemic wave of cholera.[27]

The major deterrent to the construction of sewers was the relatively large expense involved. In St. Louis, at the mayor's suggestion, the city council's Committee on Streets and Alleys considered building a common sewer in 1839, but the council decided it would be too costly. Five years later the subject again came up in the council but, once more, was voted down on the grounds of cost.[28] When a New Orleans sanitary commission (appointed after the great yellow fever epidemic of 1853) recommended a complete sanitary program, including building a sewer system, a prominent local physician argued that yellow fever flared up because of the "inexorable law of accumulative mortality" and denounced the sanitary program as an effort to waste the public's money.[29]

The Asiatic cholera epidemic of 1832 clearly had little permanent impact on American sanitation and public health. Cities and towns, particularly those affected by the outbreak, temporarily remedied the worst sanitary abuses, but within a year or two sanitary conditions were even worse than before. None of the health agencies that came into existence as a result of the epidemic continued to function once the danger was past. Cholera did stimulate a demand for better water supplies, though, and probably contributed to the expansion of municipal water systems. That expansion, in turn, forced authorities to give some attention to the development of sewers. On the other hand, improved technology, a higher standard of living, and the pressures of urbanization itself were bound to bring these changes, epidemic or no epidemic.

NOTES

1. John Duffy, "The History of Asiatic Cholera in the United States," *Bulletin of the New York Academy of Medicine,* 2d ser., 47 (1971):1152–68. For the best study of Asiatic cholera in the United States see Charles E. Rosenberg, *The Cholera Years: The United States in 1832, 1849 and 1866* (Chicago, 1962).

2. *Diary of William Dunlop, 1766–1839,* vol. 3, in *New York Historical Society, Collections* (New York, 1930), 64:602; *Letters from John Pintard to His Daughter,* vol. 4, *Collections* 73 (New York, 1941):66.

3. Duffy, *A History of Public Health in New York City, 1625–1866* (New York, 1968), 283–86.

4. Duffy, *The Rudolph Matas History of Medicine in Louisiana* (Baton Rouge, La., 1958–62), 2:138–42.

5. *Pennsylvania Archives,* 4th ser., 4 (Harrisburg, Pa., 1900), 30–32, 41–42.

6. Daniel Drake, "Epidemic Cholera in Cincinnati," *Western Journal of the Medical and Physical Sciences* 6 (1832–33):338.

7. Eugene H. Connor and Samuel W. Thomas, "John Croghan (1790–1849): An Enterprising Kentucky Physician," *The Filson Club History Quarterly* 40 (1966):215.

8. Duffy, *Matas History of Medicine in Louisiana,* 1:142.

9. Robert Moore, "Notes Upon the History of Cholera in St. Louis," *American Public Health Association Papers and Reports* 10 (1884):337; *Niles Weekly Register* 44 (1833):258, 417.

10. *Pittsburgh Gazette,* June 29, 1832.

11. Communication from Sanitary Board to the Board of Consulting Physicians, July 27, 1832, and Communication from Board of Consulting Physicians to the Sanitary Board, July 28, 1832, Western Pennsylvania Historical Society MSS; John Duffy, "The Impact of Asiatic Cholera on Pittsburgh, Wheeling, and Charleston," *The Western Pennsylvania Historical Magazine* 47 (1964):205.

12. Betty L. Plummer, "A History of Public Health in Washington, D.C., 1800–1890" (Ph.D. diss., University of Maryland, 1984), 62–63.

13. *Daily Pittsburgh Gazette*, August 8, 1833, January 5, 1836.

14. Pittsburgh *Morning Chronicle*, September 21, 1841.

15. Duffy, *Public Health in New York City, 1625–1866*, 288–90.

16. Thomas N. Bonner, *Medicine in Chicago, 1850–1950* (Madison, Wis., 1957), 176.

17. Duffy, *Public Health in New York City, 1625–1866*, chapter 15.

18. Plummer, "Public Health in Washington, D.C.," 67.

19. *Pittsburgh Daily Gazette*, April 28, 1848.

20. Duffy, *Public Health in New York City, 1625–1866*, 385–86.

21. *Pittsburgh Gazette*, August 2, 1831.

22. New York *Daily Times*, June 8, 1853.

23. George C. Whipple, *State Sanitation: A Review of the Work of the Massachusetts State Board of Health* (rpt., New York, 1977), 16–19.

24. *Hazard's Register of Pennsylvania* 15 (1835):176–80.

25. *The Pittsburgh Quarterly Trade Circular* 1 (1857):79.

26. Duffy, *Public Health in New York City, 1625–1866*, chapter 17.

27. Ibid., 409–15.

28. Herbert T. Mayer, "History of St. Louis, 1837–1847" (M.A. thesis, Washington University, 1949), 45.

29. M. Morton Dowler, "On the Reputed Causes of Yellow Fever, and the So-called Sanitary Measures of the Day," *New Orleans Medical and Surgical Journal* 11 (1855):58.

7

The Sanitary Reformers

The years from 1830 to the start of the Civil War are important ones for American public health, not so much for what was accomplished during them, but for the basis they laid for the sanitary movement in the latter part of the nineteenth century. These antebellum years witnessed the emergence of vital statistics as a public health tool, the increasing role of medical societies in promoting community health, the appearance of a number of dedicated and intelligent leaders in the area of health reform, and two major Asiatic cholera epidemics. Interestingly, these two cholera outbreaks, in 1832–33 and 1849–54, although far more severe than the subsequent relatively mild ones, had far less direct impact on the development of public health than the later epidemics. Yet they were one of several factors that helped awaken public consciousness to the need for community medicine. As the last chapter indicated, health conditions in urban areas grew steadily worse as the nineteenth century advanced. Statistics on life expectancy and infant mortality, and all other indices of public health, crude as they were, indicate a steady deterioration in urban health after about 1820. It may be that social problems can be seen only when they become acute, and certainly by the mid-nineteenth century urban health conditions were demanding attention.

Improving public health first requires some understanding of community health problems. This understanding could not be achieved in America until the collection of vital statistics had become a function of government. Some statistics had been gathered on population and trade during the colonial period, but their purpose had been primarily economic. Health reformers, all too aware of the atrocious conditions in city slums, had difficulty refuting the Pollyannaish assertions of businessmen and civic leaders, and they were among the first to advocate state registration laws. Interestingly, among the health reformers were a number of southern physicians who began gathering statistics in order to disprove northern charges that New Orleans, Memphis, and other southern cities were unhealthy, only to discover that the accusations were all too true.[1]

Western Europe, which experienced the industrial revolution ahead of the United States, first began collecting vital statistics. The work of European statisticians soon attracted the attention of a number of Americans. The first indication of this interest was the incorporation in 1836 of the New York Statistical Society. Although this organization quickly foundered for want of members, its work was picked up and given a major impetus by Lemuel Shattuck, Dr. Edward Jarvis, and other prominent figures in Massachussetts. Shattuck, a schoolteacher, bookseller, and publisher, was one of the first to recognize that vital statistics could demonstrate the extent of health problems and at the same time help convince civic leaders that sanitary reform was sound economics. In these years Boston was engaged in a series of major reforms—improving its schools, water system, and hospitals—and Shattuck found a congenial environment for his work. He and Jarvis were two key figures in the organization of the American Statistical Association. Essentially a local society for many years, this organization made a major contribution to the advancement of vital statistics and public health. Jarvis was active in politics, serving as a member of the Boston City Council from 1837 to 1841, and his knowledge of politics enabled him to play a major role in pushing through the Massachusetts Registration Act of 1842. Once the law was enacted, he assisted the secretary of state in devising a method for collecting vital statistics, and in succeeding years he helped to improve it. The Massachusetts system, for which Shattuck was largely responsible, became a standard for registration systems in other states.[2]

Physicians, traditionally leaders in the natural sciences, had been collecting statistical information on weather and diseases for many years, and they were among the first to recognize the importance of vital statistics to public health. The medical profession, however, was hindered by its poor public image and its lack of statistical expertise; hence appeals by physicians for the collection of vital statistics went largely unanswered. Once Shattuck and other laymen contributed to making statistics a profession, physicians quickly began to play a prominent role in the movement. From its founding in 1847, the American Medical Association (AMA) actively worked through local and state medical societies to promote effective state registration laws. Another important factor in improving the accuracy of vital statistics that should be mentioned was the rapid growth of insurance companies around the mid-nineteenth century.[3]

Largely as a result of the activities of state medical societies, within the next fifteen years some eleven states emulated Massachusetts in enacting statewide registration laws. The drive for registration laws was least successful in the South. Although southern physicians were active in the drive for registration laws, only Kentucky, Virginia, and South Carolina passed statewide laws in the 1850s. The Virginia law, enacted in 1853, merely required the commissioners of revenue to collect statistics on births, marriages, and deaths once a year and was quite ineffective. When a registration bill was introduced in Georgia in 1849, the state legislature "fairly hooted," and the bill was viewed as another "trick of the doctors."[4] The New Orleans Board of Health repeatedly appealed for a registration law and received strong support from local medical societies. In its report for 1848 the board pointed out that 4 to 5 percent of the individuals dying in New Orleans had no death certificates. Nonetheless, despite the backing of the *New Orleans Medical and Surgical Journal* and other publications and in spite of repeated appeals from successive health boards, neither the city nor Louisiana acquired an effective registration law for many years.[5]

By 1840 the work of men such as Edwin Chadwick in England and Louis René Villermé in France was stimulating socially conscious Americans to investigate the health field. Ironically, the first significant U.S. study on health in this period was Dr. Benjamin W. McCready's work on the influence of trades and occupations on the health of workers, a long-neglected area. Two British surgeons, C. Turner Thackrah of Leeds and Philips Kay of Manchester, in 1831 and 1832 respectively, had already published studies on the health of workers, and their writings had received considerable attention in the United States. It is likely that these two books inspired the Medical Society of New York State to offer a prize for the best essay on the subject—a prize that McCready won in 1837 with his "On the Influence of Trades, Professsions, and Occupations in the United States in the Production of Disease."[6]

McCready reflected the views of many of his generation when he deplored the changes arising from industrialism and urbanism. He also shared their belief that intemperance and other moral weaknesses were responsible in part for the poor health of workers, but his studies convinced him that the greatest dangers arose from occupational hazards, poor housing, and social conditions. He appealed to the wealthy to build adequate housing for workers and their families and to enact public health measures. These actions, he wrote, would be profitable for those erecting the housing, would improve the city's health, and would be of "incalculable benefit to the laboring population."[7] McCready's work had little immediate effect, although it may have contributed to the movement for a ten-hour work day, but his essay on the general living conditions of the poor was the first of a series of writings intended to awaken the public conscience.

In 1842 Dr. John H. Griscom was appointed to the office of city inspector of New York City. This was a significant position since the inspector's duties involved reporting nuisances, inspecting buildings, and collecting mortality and business reports, among other responsibilities.

His predecessor's annual report had consisted of three pages of commentary upon the year's statistical data. Griscom greatly enlarged the number of mortality statistics and added a fifty-three-page commentary in which he presented a horrifying picture of living conditions in the city—crowded substandard housing, two-family rear dwellings containing as many as eight families, and cellars jammed with as many as forty-eight people. He described schools occupying filthy basements and criticized the city's poor food, contaminated water, filthy privies, and inadequate street cleaning. Like McCready, he believed that the construction of improved homes for the poor presented "a large field for the exercise of philanthropy, by the benevolent capitalist." To promote personal hygiene, he recommended that the city make Croton Aqueduct water freely available to the poor, construct a complete underground sewer and drain system, and establish an effective health department.[8]

Along with his contemporaries, Griscom believed that morality and poverty were closely associated, but he at least recognized that "moral degradation" was induced by a lack of privacy and by poor housing. In 1845 he expanded his 1842 report and published it under the title *The Sanitary Condition of the Laboring Population of New York*. In his introduction he mentioned that the only result of his recommendations to the mayor and council had been his dismissal from office. The aims of his present work, he wrote, were the following: first, to demonstrate the immense sickness and mortality among the poorer classes; second, to show that the causes for this were removable; third, to arouse the public and the government to take action; and fourth, to suggest courses of action. In arguing that men trained in medicine were most suitable as sanitary officers, he suggested that "a good prescribing physician" was not necessarily qualified to be a sanitary officer since sanitation "is a peculiar branch of the science . . . and as distinct as the practice of surgery."[9] Here he seemed to be suggesting that public health was a medical specialty, an idea well in advance of its time.

Griscom had started his career as a dispensary physician working with the poor, and this experience, combined with what he had seen as city inspector, turned him into a dedicated social reformer. He advocated tenement reforms, the collection of vital statistics, improved medical care for the indigent, public hygiene, temperance, and any proposal to improve the living conditions of the lower classes. His 1842 report brought him in contact with Lemuel Shattuck, and the two men corresponded, with Griscom providing information on ventilation, Shattuck supplying material relating to vital statistics, and both men exchanging their experiences in politics.[10] Griscom's inspection of tenements, schools, and public buildings led him to study ventilation and its relationship to disease, a subject that rose naturally from the miasmatic concept. In 1848 he published a 249-page treatise on ventilation in which he asserted that "vitiated air" contributed to a host of diseases and encouraged vice and "intemperance in the use of intoxicating drinks." He condemned city officials for their failure to construct a sewer system and for permitting the use of cellars for schools and homes.[11]

Griscom was an active member of medical societies, and he inevitably gravitated toward committees concerned with community health or sanitation. As chairman of the Standing Committee on Public Health and Legal Medicine of the New York Academy of Medicine, he submitted a report in 1852 on medical aid to the indigent and the need for sanitary police. He criticized the city's organization of its dispensaries (free outpatient clinics) on the grounds that there were too few of them and that they were under the control of laymen. The blame, he asserted, rested on the medical profession for its neglect of the dispensaries and on the "parsimonious spirit" of the municipal government. More significant, he argued that dispensary physicians should be better paid and that they should serve as sanitary police. He pointed out that they frequently visited the homes of the sick and were in the best position to understand the factors contributing to disease. It was only logical, he continued, to give the dispensary physicians authority to remove these causes of morbidity— obstructed drains, stagnant pools, overflowing privies, and so forth.[12]

Unlike Shattuck, Griscom's efforts bore little direct fruit, but he was a persistent gadfly, irritating municipal officials with his revelations, jarring the New York Academy of Medicine into action, nagging state officials, and, through lectures and publications, constantly seeking to awaken the public conscience. The flood of Irish and other immigrants into New York City in the late 1840s and 1850s created problems beyond the competence of the city's government to solve, and these years were ones of notorious corruption and inefficiency. Griscom's untiring efforts ultimately led to major sanitary reforms, although he was too old and sick to participate in the final struggle.

In New Orleans Edward Barton and J. C. Simonds were equally unsuccessful in achieving immediate sanitary reforms. Although New Orleans had only about one-fifth the population of New York, its warm and humid climate greatly intensified its sanitary problems. In part because a good share of the brokers, commission merchants, shippers, and other businessmen in New Orleans were a transitory population and the local citizens were relatively immune to yellow fever, there was little interest in sanitary reform. Yet although Barton and Simonds were prophets without honor in their own country, their publications were read by informed physicians and citizens throughout the United States, and they helped to shape the concepts upon which the sanitary revolution of the late nineteenth century was based.

One of the most successful reformers in the pre–Civil War era was Dr. Edwin Miller Snow of Providence, Rhode Island. During the first half of the nineteenth century, municipal authorities in Providence had taken virtually no responsibility for the health of the town's citizens. When the second cholera epidemic struck hard at Providence in 1854, Dr. Snow took it upon himself to draw up a report on it, in which he denounced the authorities for their complete neglect of sanitary affairs. Snow's report aroused the electorate, already shocked by the loss of life during the outbreak, and in 1856 the city established a health department with Snow as its head. Snow had already successfully lobbied for an effective state registration law in 1852 and promptly had been appointed city registrar for Providence. While serving in this capacity, he gave the city one of the best registration systems in the country.

As the city's health officer, he proposed an elaborate program of sanitary reform, one which included constructing sewer and water systems and building a strong professional health department. These proposals, as he must have known, were too visionary for his day. He was, however, a practical individual, and he immediately began a major, and successful, campaign to clean the city. He fought against hogs being allowed to roam free, tackled the nuisance industries and dirty streets, and sought to remedy all other sanitary problems. He instituted strict quarantine measures against cholera and smallpox and vigorously promoted smallpox vaccination. Due to his leadership, Providence became the first American city to require the compulsory vaccination of schoolchildren. The result of Snow's work was that Providence became one of the cleanest cities in America during the 1850s. Not content with his accomplishments in Providence, though, Snow soon moved on to the national scene. He took a prominent role in the national sanitary conventions of the late 1850s and in 1876 served as president of the American Public Health Association (APHA).[13]

Although Lemuel Shattuck's greatest contribution was in the area of vital statistics, he became best known for his authorship of the *Report of the Sanitary Commission of Massachusetts* (1850). Recognizing that American society was changing and that these changes were leading to higher morbidity and mortality rates, Shattuck came to believe that governmental action could improve sanitary and social conditions and thus raise the general level of health. As a statistician, he was equally sure that more accurate statistical information would reveal the causes of the rising death rate. Largely through his and Dr. Edward Jarvis's efforts, the American Statistical Society in 1848 petitioned the Massachusetts legislature to make a sanitary survey of the state. A similar petition was submitted the following year by the Massachusetts Medical Society. Shattuck was a member of the General Court himself, and, when the legislature appointed a commission to make a survey in 1849, Shattuck was the logical choice for chairman. The other two members of the Sanitary Commission, knowing little on the subject, were happy to leave the research and writing of the report to the chairman. In April 1852, Shattuck presented his celebrated report.[14]

Most well-to-do Americans in Shattuck's day still believed that poverty and immorality went hand in hand and that cleanliness was next to godliness. The laws of nature and of God were the same, and those who deviated from them paid the price in poverty, disease, and death. The wealthier classes observed that the immigrants pouring into Boston, New York, and other port cities lived crowded together in dirt and filth and were intemperate in their drinking and eating. By more than a coincidence, it seemed, they also suffered exceedingly high rates of sickness and death. To Shattuck, and most of his contemporaries, the basic problem with the poor lay, then, in their lack of moral fiber; hence a function of government was to teach them the laws of nature and to raise their moral level. Since personal hygiene was assumed to be an indication of a moral sense, another function of government was to encourage it through a program of civic cleanliness. As might be expected, Shattuck nevertheless placed great emphasis upon the gathering of statistical information to determine the exact causes of morbidity and mortality.

Shattuck's report was well received in Europe and America. The medical profession, which never doubted the lack of moral fiber among the poor, generally praised the report highly. The application of the report, however, was up to the state legislature, and by 1850 the whole tenor of Massachusetts politics was changing. The Protestant elite that had dominated the state in previous years was giving way in the face of large-scale Catholic immigration to America. The Jacksonian era had democratized government, and Massachusetts politicians, as Barbara G. Rosenkrantz has observed, were "more concerned with the voting behaviour of the immigrant and the urban poor than with their hygienic habits."[15] Following the second cholera wave, no major epidemic troubled the Northeast, and the agitation by health reformers was only beginning to filter down to the public. Until the medical profession achieved a measure of respectability and until energetic laypersons began to organize on behalf of health reform, little could be accomplished. Although most of Shattuck's recommendations eventually were accepted, his 1850 report had almost no direct impact.

In almost every American city the cholera outbreaks of the mid-nineteenth century occasioned sanitary surveys and reports. And in almost every case these reports recommended the building of water and sewer

systems, the institution of street-cleaning and garbage-collection programs, the creation of strong health departments with extensive authority,
and the passage of a whole series of sanitary measures. Carrying out these
recommendations would have required relatively huge capital expenditures and large increases in annual government budgets, but once cholera
had disappeared, the average citizen had little interest in public health.
Furthermore, the upper classes in general had no desire to tax themselves
for the welfare of the poor. In consequence, the various sanitary reports
in this period were largely ignored.

The terrible yellow fever epidemics that ravaged southern ports in the
1850s contributed little to the improvement of sanitation, but they did
lead directly to the establishment of the first permanent state board of
health. Although yellow fever had disappeared as a serious problem
north of Norfolk, Virgina, after the early 1820s, its attacks in the South
steadily intensified, reaching a peak at the mid-century. In 1853 New
Orleans experienced the worst yellow fever epidemic in its history. In
August alone the disease killed almost 5,000 people, and over 11,000
deaths were recorded in the four-month period from June through September. The exact toll from yellow fever is uncertain, but the best estimates
are around 9,000. The normal summer exodus in 1853 was increased by
the thousands who fled to escape the disease, so that the 11,000 deaths
occurred in a population numbering between 75,000 and 80,000. The
descriptions of life in New Orleans during the outbreak make grim reading: bodies piling up in the city's graveyards; entire families wiped out;
and everywhere the stench of the dead and dying. For at least two months
the entire population spent its time caring for the sick and burying
the dead.[16]

Even accustomed as they were to yellow fever, New Orleanians were
shocked by this tragedy. Motivated in part by public demand and in part
by the desire to find a rational explanation for the periodic holocausts of
fever that swept through New Orleans, in September the city's temporary
board of health appropriated $2,500 for the use of a six-man sanitary
commission to study all aspects of the epidemic. The mayor, an ex-officio
member, then appointed five physicians to serve on the commission. This
action was criticized by the editor of the New Orleans *Delta*, who wrote:
"Besides the natural tendency of doctors to disagree, this subject of yellow
fever has been peculiarly the bone of contention of the Faculty [a term
encompassing the medical profession], scarcely any two concurring in the
main points of the nature and history." He concluded that having a minority of doctors on the commission was necessary in order "to secure the
popular confidence for the report."[17]

The members of the New Orleans Sanitary Commission were all outstanding physicians. Edward H. Barton and J. C. Simonds were leading figures in the Louisiana public health movement; A. Foster Axson was a crusading medical editor; John L. Riddell was a medical professor; and S. D. McNeil, a prominent practitioner. The commission promptly sent questionnaires to the municipal governments of the major cities and to all the agencies of the federal government, as well as to selected members of the medical profession and leading citizens. It then held open hearings for three months. The commission was instructed to inquire into the etiology and mode of transmission of yellow fever; to report on sewerage and drainage problems; to study the desirability of quarantine; and, finally, to report on the city's sanitary condition. Late in 1854 the commission finished its work and issued its report. The members concluded that yellow fever was of spontaneous origin due to "peculiar meteorological conditions" and poor sanitation, and they recommended a complete sanitary program for New Orleans, one that included the construction of a sewer system. Although the entire report expressed the anticontagionist view of disease, the members, surprisingly, unanimously favored a strict quarantine.[18]

The report was generally praised, although several prominent physicians were bitterly critical of it. Shortly after it was published the Southern Commercial Convention met in New Orleans. Reflecting the rising public interest in health, the convention appointed a committee on quarantine, which urged all southern ports to institute rigid quarantines. Recognizing the need to maintain good relationships with commercial interests outside the state, some of the New Orleans newspapers joined the campaign for an effective quarantine law. Reacting to these pressures and to demands from citizens throughout the state, the Louisiana legislature, on March 15, 1855, enacted a quarantine law. An important provision of the law stated that the quarantine was to be administered by a state board of health, whose members were to be chosen for "their known zeal in favor of the quarantine system." It should be pointed out that there was a general distrust of New Orleans city officials both in Louisiana and throughout the Mississippi Valley.[19]

The law specified that three quarantine stations were to be established, and it provided $50,000 for their construction. The state board was also given authority to remove nuisances affecting health, to enact sanitary regulations subject to approval by the New Orleans City Council, and to issue warrants against sanitary offenders. While the board had quarantine authority over the entire state, its sanitary powers were restricted to New Orleans, and, obviously, even these depended upon the goodwill and support of the city government. For the next few years the board successfully exercised its quarantine authority, although not without a good deal of criticism from businessmen and commercial interests. On the score of sanitation, as was indicated earlier, little was accomplished. In 1859 the board members sadly reported that they had been unable to impress upon the city officials the need for sanitary measures or to make them realize "the utter destitution of the city in every essential of sanitary regulation necessary to health, or even to decency and public self-respect." Two years later the board conceded: "We fear the Board of Health has, from want of power, dwindled down simply into a Board of Quarantine."[20] Ironically, the 1854 report of the New Orleans Sanitary Commission had more influence nationally than it did in New Orleans.

In the meantime, despite the impact of the various sanitary reports throughout America and the increase in the number of city water and sewer systems, conditions in urban slums steadily deteriorated. The massive influx after 1845 of impoverished rural Irish immigrants unfamiliar with urban sanitary hygiene increased the crowding in the tenements and added to the worsening sanitary conditions. The nascent science of statistics was revealing an enormous number of infant deaths in the slums and a rise in the general death rate. Moreover, the filth in the slums was all too obvious to sight and smell, giving an aesthetic impulse to the rising humanitarian spirit among the middle and upper classes.

The AMA, which had conducted a sanitary survey shortly after its founding, lost interest in the subject after its first efforts came to nought. It represented only a handful of American practitioners at best, and it was too preoccupied with fighting the irregular healers to take up any other causes. Individual physicians, however, continued to play key roles in the sanitary movement. Working through local medical societies and in conjunction with health boards, they proselytized on behalf of sanitary reform. In the process they won over a number of influential laymen to their cause. By the late 1850s the ranks of the sanitary reformers were increasing rapidly, and the majority of them were zealous, dedicated individuals convinced that a complete sanitary program would solve nearly all urban health and social problems. By this date, too, the sanitary movement was in full swing in Europe, and American newspapers and medical and popular journals of the time clearly show a rising interest in the subject.

The first fruits of this growing interest were a series of national sanitary conventions held from 1857 to 1860. The occasion for calling the first convention was to standardize the widely differing local and state quarantine procedures. The precipitating factor was the series of major yellow fever epidemics mentioned earlier, which first affected southern ports and peaked in the 1850s. In 1855–56 minor outbreaks occurred on Staten

Island and Long Island, and occasional cases were reported in other northern ports.[21] At the same time, the public's memory of the cholera epidemics was still fresh. The value of quarantine had long been at issue, though, and even its advocates debated the exact form it should take. The threat of yellow fever to the North brought the whole issue to a head.

By 1857 Dr. Wilson Jewell of Philadelphia had read of the Conference Sanitaire in Paris in 1851–52 and had concluded that a meeting of representatives of the seaboard states might contribute to solving the quarantine problem. Jewell also had been an active member of the Philadelphia Board of Health for eight years, and he persuaded the board to appoint a committee of three to contact health boards in other major port cities about holding a national conference in Philadelphia. The upshot was that the Philadelphia board invited delegates from boards of health, city councils, medical societies, and boards of trade around the country to come to Philadelphia on May 13, 1857, for a quarantine convention. A total of 74 delegates representing twenty-six boards or societies attended the first meeting. Of the delegates, 22 were laymen representing state and city health boards; the rest were physicians. Philadelphia was represented by 21 delegates, Boston by 13, and Baltimore by 10. The other 30 delegates came from East Coast ports ranging from Norfolk, Virginia, to Boston. The one exception was New Orleans, which sent 5 representatives.[22]

In welcoming the delegates, Dr. Jewell stated that the paramount objective of the gathering was "to consider and recommend for adoption an improved, and as far as may be practicable, a uniform system of quarantine laws." He noted that this was the "first American congress ever convened for sanitary reform" and hailed it "as evidence of the dawn of a new era in the domain of American science." Public health has received little attention, he declared, and has lain "almost a dreary waste in our annals of progressive science." Only here and there can one find "a solitary devotee, earnestly engaged in his sanitary and statistical labors, unaided and alone."[23]

The first meeting lasted three days, a good part of which was devoted to a general discussion of quarantine and yellow fever and to setting up a temporary organization. Indicative of the strength of anticontagionist sentiment among the delegates, a motion was introduced early in the meeting stating that certain diseases could not become epidemic "unless circumstances calculated to produce diseases independent of importation exist[ed] in the community." In the ensuing discussion it was further resolved that sanitary measures could "disarm [imported diseases] of virulence, and prevent their extension, when introduced." It passed unanimously at first but was reconsidered on the final day and indefinitely postponed. Dr. James Jones, a New Orleans delegate, reported that he opposed the motion on the grounds that the convention had no authority to adopt theories about yellow fever. As a physician, he undoubtedly resented the ability of the laymen in attendance to vote on questions he considered strictly medical. Jones, however, had other reasons for opposing the motion, since he was a firm adherent of the contagionist doctrine.[24]

The second annual meeting—called by Dr. Wilson Jewell the "Great American Congress for Hygienic Reform," but officially known as the Second Annual Meeting of the Quarantine and Sanitary Convention—met in Baltimore, April 29, 1858. Some 86 delegates, of whom 44 were laymen, came from twelve states. The Northeast was best represented, but the District of Columbia, Norfolk, Alexandria, Charleston, Savannah, and New Orleans each sent one or more delegates. In his opening address Dr. William M. Kemp stated that the purpose of the meeting was to develop a code of quarantine and sanitary regulations. By this time the major issue was contagion theory versus anticontagion theory or quarantine versus sanitation. It was clear to many physicians and laypersons that yellow fever and cholera were not necessarily passed directly from one individual to another. This observation merely added another complication to explaining why these disorders became epidemic. Reflecting the swing toward the domestic causation theory, two committees were appointed to report the following year, one on "External Hygiene," or quarantine, and a second on "Internal Hygiene," or sanitation. The committee on external hygiene was instructed to survey the history of quarantine and determine whether or not it was of value. In the event quarantine was found useful, the committee was to suggest ways to make it more effective and less burdensome, and it was to recommend a uniform set of quarantine laws.[25] The delegates were unanimous in their opposition to the existing quarantine laws, and a good many favored the abolition of all quarantine measures.

The third convention took place in New York City in April 1859, with Dr. John H. Griscom presiding. As usual, the Northeast dominated the meeting. Only three southern cities sent delegates—Norfolk, Virginia, Auburn, Alabama, and Memphis, Tennessee. The delegates were welcomed to New York by Dr. Joseph M. Smith, a leader in the sanitary reform movement. Smith had served as advisor to the New York City Board of Health and as president of the New York Academy of Medicine. He was also one of the founders of the city's newly organized Sanitary Association, and he had worked closely with Griscom in mobilizing the Academy of Medicine in the fight to improve sanitary conditions in the city.[26]

The major issues at this convention were the contagiousness of yellow fever and the value of quarantine. Early in the discussion Dr. J. McNulty of New York City stated the essence of the objections to quarantine. He called it "a commercial curse" and claimed that it caused people to neglect the sanitary precautions that "could alone protect them from disease." Dr. Elisha Harris, another leader of the New York health reform movement, cited the politicalization of quarantine officers. In New York, he declared, they were usually state appointees, more concerned with "the increase of perquisites, and the increase of that personal and political power which is sure to be abused."[27]

One of the crucial issues was whether or not yellow fever could be passed from one person to another. Early in the meeting Dr. A. H. Stevens moved that personal quarantine for cases of yellow fever should be eliminated. After a heated debate he agreed to withdraw his motion until the following day. A physician from Staten Island proposed that New York City should abolish all quarantine procedures except for the detention of infected vessels during the summer months. After some discussion his motion, too, was withdrawn. On the second day Stevens's motion was reintroduced, and, after a debate (which covers over seventy-five pages in the *Proceedings*), the convention voted 85 to 6 in favor. The resolution specified that it "is the opinion of this Convention that the personal quarantine of cases of Yellow Fever may be safely abolished, provided that fomites of every kind be rigidly restricted."[28]

The debates in this meeting make it apparent that the delegates were far more concerned with sanitation than with quarantine. General P. M. Wetmore of the New York Sanitary Association made a stirring appeal for action in the field of public health, and his sentiments were echoed and reechoed by other delegates. On the final day of the convention, President John H. Griscom presented the sanitationist view of epidemic diseases. He declared that the "relative danger . . . from external causes on the one hand, and internal civic and domestic causes on the other, is about *one to one hundred*." He stressed the need to educate the public through continuous agitation, and concluded: "Let the land be covered with Sanitary Associations, and it will soon stand as much a landmark for the health, happiness and comfort of its people, as it is now a beacon-light for the politically oppressed of other lands."[29]

The proceedings of the meeting included a long report on disinfectants, which, incidentally, is a commentary on the state of medicine in 1859. Among its conclusions were that each disease required its own disinfectant, that "the poison of epidemics is not perceptible to the senses, nor, as yet, to science," and that ventilation appeared to be the best disinfectant for yellow fever.[30] Ventilation, it was thought, would disperse the particles of yellow fever contagion assumed to adhere to certain goods—the so-called fomites—such as coffee, woolens, and cotton.

The final convention met in Boston in June 1860. The rising interest in sanitary concerns is shown by the growth in the number of delegates; whereas only 73 delegates were present at the first meeting, the Fourth National Quarantine and Sanitary Convention drew 191, of whom 118 were physicians. Even more than was true of earlier meetings, the Northeast dominated the convention; Massachusetts and New York sent almost three-quarters of the delegates. The growing clash between the North and the South was made apparent by the presence of only one member from the South, Dr. Richard Arnold from Savannah. New Orleans, which had sent five representatives to the first meeting, did not send any to the last two. For the first time, however, the Midwest was represented, with Cincinnati and Columbus, Ohio, each sending one delegate.

From the beginning the tone of the speeches and addresses at the 1860 convention was optimistic and enthusiastic. Early in the meeting General Wetmore cited the accomplishments of previous conventions, chief among them the removal of the onerous and burdensome quarantine restrictions, and he urged that a permanent national sanitary organization be established. Dr. John Ordronaux in his address defined state medicine, or public health. It is, he said, "the application of the principles of medical science to the administration of justice and the preservation of the public health. It is a system of medical police, both preventive, as well as punitive and reformative." His recommendation that the convention appoint a committee on state medicine was accepted unanimously, and the new committee was instructed to report at the next meeting.[31]

The 1860 convention's papers and discussions were concentrated upon what the delegates considered "internal sanitation," that is, sewage, ventilation, street cleaning, and other matters assumed to have a relationship to disease. The younger men who were moving into leadership in the sanitary movement had little interest in quarantine. They were predominantly anticontagionists, convinced that epidemic disease was the product of dirt and filth. Dr. Jacob Bigelow of Boston spoke for all the delegates when he declared that America was standing on the "vestibule" of "one of the greatest reforms that this country has ever entered upon." Sanitary reforms, he continued, would almost eliminate the need for clinical physicians.[32] Reflecting the emphasis upon sanitary science, other speakers urged that research be done on topics such as ventilation, disinfectants, and sewage disposal. They recommended devising model laws for state and local health agencies, effective sanitary regulations, and measures to guarantee the quality of food and drugs. Recognizing the need to build public support for health reform, they advocated educating the public through local sanitary associations. The first of these had already been organized in New York, and it became a model for literally hundreds of similar associations during the next forty years.

The need to collect reliable vital statistics was taken for granted, and the discussion on this topic centered on how to accomplish this goal. The inadequate collection of birth records was attributed to the reluctance of physicians to reveal the extent of their practice and to perform a task for which they were not paid; another factor cited was the large number of births unattended by physicians. Rhode Island's registration law, which provided the town clerk with a ten-cent fee for each registration, was recommended as a model. To facilitate the collection of mortality statistics, delegates were urged to support legislation requiring a permit before a dead body could be removed or buried.[33] Unfortunately, knowing what should be done and accomplishing it were two entirely different matters, and the collection of reasonably accurate vital statistics had to await the twentieth century.

The meeting ended with expressions of goodwill and hope for the future. In response to General Wetmore's appeal, a committee was appointed to submit plans for a permanent organization at the forthcoming meeting in Cincinnati in 1861. The growing bitterness of sectional conflict, a subject preoccupying public attention at this time, amazingly did not intrude on the discussions in the convention, although the presence of only one southern delegate was significant in itself. That delegate, Dr. Richard Arnold of Savannah, while presiding over one of the last dinner sessions, praised the hospitality of Bostonians. The New England delegates responded by giving three cheers for Georgia.[34] Ten months later the outbreak of the Civil War put a stop to the national sanitary conventions and delayed the creation of a permanent national public health organization for another twelve years.

Despite the untimely demise of the national conventions, they mark the real beginning of the American sanitary revolution. The delegates included every significant figure in the prewar health movement—John H. Griscom of New York, Wilson Jewell of Philadelphia, Richard Arnold of Savannah, Edwin Miller Snow of Providence, Edward H. Barton and James Jones of New Orleans, Jacob Bigelow and Edward Jarvis of Boston, and others. Some of these men continued to work into the postwar era, but the leadership was gradually shifting to another generation, represented at the conventions by men such as Elisha Harris, E. L. Viele, and Stephen Smith of New York.

The conventions were a major force in reforming the quarantine laws, but their most significant contribution was to shift the emphasis in public health from quarantine to environmental concerns. The main function of the early health boards had been to enforce quarantine regulations, usually when epidemic disease threatened; the influence of the national sanitary conventions and the emergence of citizens' sanitary associations pressured health boards and civic authorities into facing up to the major threats to public health. Lethargy, apathy, and outright corruption still pervaded city governments, but the sanitarians, by exposing the worst conditions, periodically aroused public opinion and were able to make slow progress. Furthermore, the conventions led to a sharing of ideas and knowledge and gave moral support to those conscientious individuals who felt they were fighting lone battles in their communities. Dr. Jewell was overly optimistic in his assessment of the significance of the quarantine conventions, but he was correct in proclaiming them the dawn of a new era.

NOTES

1. Margaret H. Warner, "Public Health in the Old South," TS, pp. 10–11.

2. James H. Cassedy, *American Medicine and Statistical Thinking, 1800–1860* (Cambridge, Mass., 1984), 194–98; Dirk J. Struik, *The Origins of American Science* (New York, 1957), 229–34.

3. Howard D. Kramer, "The Beginnings of the Public Health Movement in the United States," *Bull. Hist. Med.* 21 (1947):357.

4. Richard H. Shryock, *Medicine in America: Historical Essays* (Baltimore, 1966), 131.

5. John Duffy, *The Rudolf Matas History of Medicine in Louisiana* (Baton Rouge, La., 1958–62), 1:164.

6. Benjamin W. McCready, *On the Influence of Trades, Professions, and Occupations in the United States in the Production of Disease* (Baltimore, 1943), 6–9.

7. Ibid., 41–45.

8. John Duffy, *A History of Public Health in New York City, 1625–1866* (New York, 1968), 302–5.

9. John H. Griscom, *The Sanitary Condition of the Laboring Population of New York* (New York, 1845), 2–4, 49–50.

10. James H. Cassedy, "The Roots of American Sanitary Reform 1843–47: Seven Letters from John H. Griscom to Lemuel Shattuck," *Journal of the History of Medicine and Allied Sciences* (hereafter cited as J. Hist. Med. All. Sci.) 30 (1975): 136–47.

11. John H. Griscom, *The Uses and Abuses of Air: Showing Its Influence in Sustaining Life, and Producing Disease* ... (New York, 1848), 151, 175–81.

12. [John H. Griscom], *Medical Aid to the Indigent—Sanitary Politics. Report of the Standing Committee on Public Health and Legal Medicine of the New York Academy of Medicine, Presented and Accepted July 7, 1852* (New York, 1852), 1–15.

13. James H. Cassedy, "Edwin Miller Snow: An Important American Public Health Pioneer," *Bull. Hist. Med.* 35 (1961):156–62.

14. Barbara G. Rosenkrantz, *Public Health and the State: Changing Views in Massachusetts, 1842–1936* (Cambridge, Mass., 1972), 23–24, 28–29.

15. Ibid., 34–35.

16. For a detailed account of this epidemic see John Duffy, *The Sword of Pestilence: The New Orleans Yellow Fever Epidemic of 1853* (Baton Rouge, La., 1966).

17. New Orleans *Daily Delta*, September 30, 1853.

18. Gordon E. Gillson, *The Louisiana State Board of Health: The Formative Years* (n.p., [1966]), 48, 54–57; Duffy, *Sword of Pestilence,* 130–32, 137–38.

19. "An Act to Establish Quarantine for the Protection of the State," *Acts Passed by the Second Legislature of the State of Louisiana, Session of 1855* (New Orleans, 1855), Act 336, 471–77.

20. Duffy, *Matas History of Medicine in Louisiana,* 2:190–95.

21. Duffy, *Public Health in New York City, 1625–1866,* 343–50.

22. *Minutes of the Proceedings of the Quarantine Convention, held at Philadelphia by invitation of the Philadelphia Board of Health, May 13, 1857* (Philadelphia, 1857), 3, 9, 20–23.

23. Ibid., 4–6.

24. Ibid., 28–29, 44; "Letter to Hon. Charles M. Waterman, Mayor of New Orleans from James Jones, M.D., New Orleans, Oct. 1, 1857," *New Orleans Medical and Surgical Journal* 14 (1857):326–32.

25. *Minutes of the Proceedings of the Second Annual Meeting of the Quarantine and Sanitary Convention, Convened in the City of Baltimore, April 29, 1858* (Baltimore, 1858), 3–7, 16–22.

26. *Minutes of the Third National Quarantine and Sanitary Convention held . . . New York . . . 1859* (New York, 1859), 9–16; *Proceedings and Debates of the Third National Quarantine and Sanitary Convention New York* (New York, 1859), 10–11.

27. *Proceedings and Debates of the Third National Quarantine and Sanitary Convention,* 23–24, 37–38.

28. Ibid., 43–45, 50, 201.

29. Ibid., 104; *Minutes of Third National Quarantine and Sanitary Convention,* 47–52.

30. *Proceedings and Debates of the Third National Quarantine and Sanitary Convention,* 375–78.

31. *Proceedings and Debates of the Fourth National Quarantine and Sanitary Convention . . . Boston* (Boston, 1860), 13–14, 67, 85, 278–82.

32. Rosenkrantz, *Public Health and the State,* 40.

33. *Proceedings and Debates of the Fourth National Quarantine and Sanitary Convention,* 201–5.

34. Ibid., 107–9.

8

Public Health and the Civil War

The outbreak of hostilities between the North and South in the spring of 1861 undoubtedly delayed the establishment of a national health organization, but the process of educating the public in health matters may have been stimulated by the Civil War. Wars have rarely produced major discoveries in medicine, but they have tended to speed up the application of existing medical knowledge. And public health is, to a large degree, applied medicine on the community level.

The Civil War was the bloodiest conflict in American history. The exact casualties will never be known, but approximately 600,000 men lost their lives. As was true of nearly all wars until World War II, sickness was rampant among the troops and killed twice as many men as did battle wounds. Dr. Joseph Jones, the Confederate army inspector, whose reports are among the best surviving records of Confederate losses, estimated that each soldier suffered six bouts with sickness during the course of the war. Much of the sickness was inevitable. Thousands of young men, many from isolated towns and rural areas, were brought together in crowded army camps. The result was widespread outbreaks of mumps, measles, scarlet fever, smallpox, and other highly contagious disorders. But most of the sickness, particularly after the first year of the war, could have been avoided. The soldiers' recurrent diarrheas and dysenteries, typhoid, and other enteric diseases were a direct result of the poor food and unsanitary conditions of army life.

The mobilization and mass movement of civilian and military personnel during the Civil War spread disease far and wide. Smallpox, which had been on the rise since the 1830s, once again became a serious threat. Malaria, which had retreated from New England and certain other northern areas much earlier, was reintroduced by returning troops. The civilian population was far better off, however, than the military population. The small Army Medical Corps, containing only about one hundred men, was completely overwhelmed by the enormous expansion in the armed forces. To make matters worse, it was commanded by a superannuated veteran of the War of 1812 and beset by red tape and inertia. The medical corps's problems were also compounded by the fact that, in the first flush of enthusiasm for the cause, many regiments were raised in towns and cities and sent to Washington, D.C., without surgeons or medical personnel.

In every war, at least through World War II, enteric diseases were a major problem until the troops were disciplined and until the officers learned the value of enforcing sanitary regulations. The soldiers of the Civil War, most of whom came from rural areas, were reluctant to use the latrines, particularly at night, and in short order they fouled the entire camp ground. The early latrines were often poorly constructed and dug too close to the camps, further contributing to the camps' general unsanitary conditions. Providing an ample supply of good water, always a problem for large encampments, was almost impossible under these circumstances. To add to the problems, inefficiency and chicanery often deprived the men of fresh meat and vegetables, thus inducing a great deal of acute and subacute scurvy.

Even when a full army ration was available, its benefits were largely nullified by poor cooking—beans were said to have been more deadly than bullets! In August, 1861 the *Washington Evening Star* editorialized on complaints about food by the volunteers. The fault was not the government's, the editor explained, but rather due "to the inefficiency, and sometimes, it is to be feared, to the dishonesty of regimental or brigade quartermasters and, again, the food is seldom properly cooked."[1] A treatise on military hygiene written in 1865 stated: "During the present war, in the matter of food, the great evil has been a want of variety, and especially an insufficiency of fresh vegetables." In discussing scurvy, Charles J. Stillé, in his classic *History of the United States Sanitary Commission*, stated flatly that all fresh vegetables went to the officers and virtually none to the troops.[2]

The work of the celebrated English nurse, Florence Nightingale, in the Crimean War inspired women on both sides of the American Civil War to offer their services. A few days after the opening shots, a group of prominent New York women gathered at the New York Infirmary for Women with the intent of creating a national body to coordinate all volunteer activities. Four days later, on April 29, 1861, at a meeting held at the Cooper Union, the Women's Central Relief Association was organized, with an outstanding surgeon, Dr. Valentine Mott, as president and the Rev. Dr. Henry W. Bellows as vice president. Its purpose was to determine the wants of the army, cooperate with the army's medical staff, collect medical supplies and serve as a central depot for their distribution, and recruit and train nurses. A committee was promptly appointed to arrange for liaison with the War Department and the armed forces.[3]

The committee delegation received little encouragement in Washington, D.C. The Army Medical Corps wanted nothing to do with it, and President Lincoln and Secretary of War Simon Cameron were dubious.

The delegation also found Washington in a complete state of confusion, with government bureaus in disorder and newly arrived regiments standing in the streets unfed because their officers did not know how to requisition food and quarters. Under the leadership of the Rev. Bellows and Dr. Elisha Harris, the committee formally requested Secretary of War Cameron to appoint a sanitary commission to prevent the abuses and inefficiencies that had characterized the Crimean War and to mobilize popular support for the fight to save the Union.

The proposed sanitary commission scarcely should have threatened anyone since it was to have no legal powers and sought no government money. All that was requested for the commission was that it be given office space and stationery and the right to investigate a wide range of subjects pertaining to the military. Nonetheless, President Lincoln and War Secretary Cameron first rejected the commission as a "fifth wheel." Bellows, Harris, and the others persisted in their pleading, finally winning over the government. Surgeon General Thomas Lawson had died in the meantime, and his successor, Clement A. Finley, another army surgeon in his eighties, reluctantly gave way, agreeing to the commission provided it would "never meddle with regular troops" but would restrict its activities to volunteers. On June 13, 1861, President Lincoln gave his approval to an order by Secretary Cameron creating the United States Sanitary Commission.[4]

The original Sanitary Commission consisted of twelve members—nine civilians and three army officers. The Rev. Bellows was appointed president; Professor A. D. Bache, vice president; Elisha Harris, corresponding secretary; and George T. Strong, treasurer. The civilian members, who were all prominent citizens, literally constituted the commission since the military members were too busy with their war duties. One of the commission's first acts was to appoint Frederick Law Olmsted, one of America's greatest landscape architects and an individual of unusual intelligence and energy, to the important position of executive secretary.

It is not within the purview of this study to detail the many activities of the United States Sanitary Commission, but it had a significant impact upon the Union forces and ultimately affected the entire nation. Its original purpose was to serve as an advisory body, but necessity soon turned it into a major relief agency. The commission's members discovered that thousands of sick soldiers were without food, medicine, or medical care because of transportation difficulties and a lack of hospital facilities; that thousands of discharged soldiers, many sick or wounded, were stranded in Washington because of delays in obtaining their pay or discharge papers; and that thousands more displaced soldiers were trying to locate their regiments. They also found army camps and hospitals in a dreadful state, and troops suffering from scurvy for lack of vegetables. In every case the sanitary commission swung into action, providing medical care and supplies, blankets, fresh meat and vegetables, information services, and whatever else was needed.[5] The Women's Central Relief Association, which served as the central collection agency for medical supplies for the commission, performed nobly during the war and became, in effect, the first national organization of voluntary welfare agencies.

At least as important as this direct assistance to soldiers was the success of the United States Sanitary Commission in forcing reform on the Army Medical Corps and in drawing attention to the filthy condition of so many of the army camps. The better commanders such as McClellan and Grant were concerned with the health of their troops, but many officers gave no consideration to sanitary matters—some generals in the early years of the war even looked upon the medical corps as a hindrance! The commission exerted constant pressure upon civilian and military authorities alike to improve sanitation, and at the same time it conducted large-scale educational campaigns through pamphlets and other means to teach officers and enlisted men the need for personal and communal hygiene.

The wartime experiences of the soldiers of the Civil War clearly demonstrated that the proper disposal of human wastes was essential to prevent typhoid and other enteric disorders, that fresh fruits and vegetables were necessary to prevent scurvy, and that isolation was required for contagious disease cases. These lessons were far from new, but the war—and the United States Sanitary Commission—taught them to a large segment of the American population. By the end of military action, the Sanitary Commission had affected the lives of millions of Americans and had given a strong impetus to the movement for sanitary reform.

Although the Sanitary Commission had only an indirect impact on the South, the Union army directly affected sanitary conditions in certain southern cities. New Orleans, a port with an unenviable reputation for sickness and dirt, was captured late in April 1862. As was true with many cities, New Orleans had enacted many sanitary regulations but had made little effort to enforce them. When General Benjamin Butler assumed formal military control of the city on May 1, his first general order specifically stated that all existing sanitary regulations were to be strictly enforced. To back up this order, a sanitary police force was organized.

Major yellow fever epidemics in the past had led to a periodic cleansing of New Orleans, but public enthusiasm for sanitation had never survived beyond each epidemic. Military occupation brought an unprecedented state of cleanliness to the city, one which would not be seen again until the twentieth century. Spurred on in part by the fear of yellow fever and in part by a determination to keep all sickness to a minimum, the Union commanders began a full-scale assault upon the city's accumulated filth. A labor force of two thousand men was employed to clean and drain the entire city; stables, slaughterhouses, and nuisance industries were inspected regularly; and privies and garbage collection were closely supervised.[6]

The success of the program was attested to by the chief inspector for the Sanitary Commission, who reported in January 1863 that the District of New Orleans would not be inspected in the coming weeks, explaining that "its sanitary condition has been so well maintained that the number of sick there is not very large."[7] Major General Nathaniel P. Banks, Butler's successor, was not as concerned with sanitation and was more inclined to leave it to the civilian authorities. The city council, however, impressed with the results of Butler's program and aware that its ordinances would be enforced, enacted a series of additional sanitary regulations in 1863.[8]

Along with the sanitary program, Butler and his successors maintained a strict quarantine during the summer months. From 1860 to 1867 New Orleans was relatively free of yellow fever. Since at least minor outbreaks of the disease had appeared every summer for the previous forty years, a heated debate ensued in the postwar period over the reason for this respite. A good many New Orleanians were reluctant to give Butler's measures any credit, while others attributed the absence of yellow fever either to his quarantine or to his sanitary program. In reading records of the debates, one senses that few opinions as to the cause of yellow fever epidemics were changed; and in any case, effective as the quarantine was for its day, it is doubtful that it could have kept yellow fever out of New Orleans. Clearly some other factors were involved.

Although New Orleans, by virtue of its long occupation, gained the most from the Union army's sanitary program, Memphis and other southern cities that came under federal control also benefited. Moreover, the reduction of sickness and the aesthetic improvement resulting from the military's sanitary programs encouraged southern health reformers. For example, when the army withdrew from New Orleans in 1866, the city's board of health continued to enforce health regulations. Financial difficulties, however, drastically reduced the board's budget, and the advent of Reconstruction government in 1868 compounded the board's problems. Although it functioned largely as a health board for New Orleans, it was a state office; thus the Republican governor in 1868 was able to promptly dismiss the old board and appoint a new one.

The immediate result was a bitter clash between the Democratic board, which refused to surrender its office, books, and funds, and the new board. When this issue was finally settled in favor of the Republicans, the Democratic city council refused to cooperate with the new board. This was an even more serious matter, since the council was responsible for enforcing the sanitary regulations and orders of the board. The upshot was a state legislative amendment in 1870 giving the state board authority to make and enforce sanitary regulations within New Orleans, to control the city's sanitary police, and to hold those responsible for cleaning the streets personally liable for refusing to obey the orders of the board.[9] The law should have put the board in a strong position, but the economic disruption arising from the war and the political problems brought on by Radical Reconstruction greatly limited the board's ability to function. Generally, despite considerable corruption and inefficiency, the Radical Reconstruction governments in the southern states were far more responsible to social needs than their predecessors or successors, but they were bitterly resented by the majority of whites, who successfully undermined their best efforts.

The postwar effects of the wartime sanitary programs, while generally beneficial, did vary from place to place. In 1865 Charleston created a full-time health department, with a health officer in each of the city's four health districts, and Nashville established a board of health in 1866.[10] Memphis, which had a weak board of health before the war, benefited only temporarily from the wartime cleansing. In 1866 the Memphis Board of Health advocated a strong quarantine and sanitary program to avoid the threat of cholera, but the mayor and city council refused to fund it. In 1867 no health board was appointed, and the city officials discharged the street cleaners and sanitary officers and sold the city slop carts and mule teams. The dominant commercial interests in Memphis reflected the prevailing view in the urban South that the only functions of government were to protect property and preserve the existing social order. That quarantines hindered trade and that sanitary programs cost money only reinforced this assumption. In Memphis and other southern cities, it would be some years before enlightened businessmen finally realized that a healthy population was necessary for a healthy economy.[11]

Another consequence of the war affecting the health of millions of Americans was the social disruption brought about by the end of slavery. Once the Union armies began moving into slave territory, thousands of slaves fled to them for protection. Freedom for many slaves meant the right to leave the plantation, and most of them headed in the direction of cities. In the spring of 1862 the army established the first temporary housing for freedmen in Washington, D.C. Their numbers grew, and in August they were moved into an army barracks, which became known as Camp Barker. Poor sanitary conditions and the presence of contagious disease cases forced the army to move the camp to a site in Virginia. Despite these efforts, the number of former slaves far exceeded the available accommodations, and of the estimated 40,000 who poured into Washington, many lived in miserable shacks and slums. Shortly after the first arrangements were made for them, a Freedmen's Hospital was established, but it, too, could care for only a fraction of the sick blacks.[12]

This situation was repeated wherever the Union armies moved into Confederate territory. Although many commanders did their best for the blacks, caring for them was secondary to winning the war. Also, slavery on plantations and farms had kept the blacks completely isolated, and once they began to move, they encountered a host of diseases. Smallpox may not have been the most serious of these, but it attracted the greatest attention. The use of vaccination had declined beginning in the 1830s, and smallpox among the blacks posed a threat to whites. Repeated outbreaks in Washington, D.C., were commonly blamed on the influx of freedmen and thus strained race relations; according to one historian, the outbreaks constituted more of a threat to the city's residents than the Confederate army.[13]

The precise effect of the war years on the freedmen will never be known. The evidence is clear that the majority were ravaged by diseases made more virulent by inadequate housing and food. It is equally reasonable to suppose that the freedmen also contributed to disseminating infection among the general population. A state census of blacks in Mississippi in 1866 showed a decline in population of over 56,000 compared with the federal census of 1860. Granting the inaccuracy of early statistics, these figures probably do reflect the stresses caused by the war. The descriptions of the disease, hunger, and poverty in the refugee camps in Mississippi and elsewhere leave no doubt that the black population suffered heavy losses.[14]

As the number of freedmen grew and more of the Confederacy came under Union control, in March 1865 Congress established the Freedmen's Bureau. Given a one-year life, it was intended to help the blacks make the transition from slavery to freedom. It was empowered to issue food and supplies, to develop educational facilities, and to settle the blacks on confiscated or abandoned lands. Led by an excellent director, General Oliver O. Howard, the bureau attracted a good many able and sensible individuals to its ranks. Drawing on army supplies, the bureau distributed over twenty million rations—a good many to poverty-stricken whites. The large numbers of sick blacks in all of the southern states forced the bureau to open hospitals and to provide medical care on a fairly large scale. In Washington, D.C., it took over the Freedmen's Hospital and gradually opened other hospitals and dispensaries. All told, between 1865 and 1868 the bureau operated a total of fifty-six hospitals and forty-eight dispensaries and employed about 138 physicians.[15] In Louisiana the bureau first took over the U.S. Marine Hospital in New Orleans and established another hospital in Shreveport. By October 1866, three hospitals and five dispensaries were in operation in the state.[16]

It should be borne in mind that making provisions for health care was a minor aspect of the bureau's work, since its main purpose was to educate the freedmen and help them obtain employment. In addition, the bureau was not given nearly enough funding even for this job. In 1865–66 its officials were able to call on the army for supplies, but these soon dwindled away. Many local bureau officers were conscientious individuals, but there were too few of them and too little resources. Detailed studies of blacks during Reconstruction all present the same depressing picture—one of sickness, hunger, and dire poverty. In Kentucky the bureau opened one hospital and five dispensaries. It never employed more than five physicians, although there were more than 200,000 freedmen in the state. One of the bureau's physicians estimated that only about one-fourth of the blacks could afford to pay even small medical bills. Surgeon in Chief Robert A. Bell reported in 1868 that the freedmen in Covington lived in "wretched, old dilapidated ware house[s], cellars, garrets and miserable shanties, crowded with half starved, half clad and squallid [sic] looking men, women and children with well marked disease depicted in their countenances."[17]

Similar descriptions of the freedmen can be found for other areas of the South. Chaplain John Eaton wrote of the freedmen arriving in the refugee camps as "men, women and children in every stage of disease or decrepitude . . . companions of nakedness, famine, and disease." In Vicksburg, Mississippi, the blacks occupied the caves that had been used earlier during the siege, and the Natchez Board of Health found sixteen of them occupying a cabin twelve feet square, while another family lived in a privy.[18] Some white southerners made conscientious efforts to relieve the blacks, but few sections of the South had the resources necessary for the task. With the creation of the Freedmen's Bureau, most southerners felt no further obligation to help. Moreover, many of them, embittered by the war, were not willing to give any assistance. From Owensboro, Kentucky, a bureau physician reported that the authorities were too poor to care for the needy, "even were they *willing* to do so."[19] Judging from reports, a high percentage of southern physicians refused to attend blacks unless paid in advance. Some of them justified this action on the grounds that they had to attend so many poor whites; others made no effort to disguise their anti-black attitude.

Although the Freedmen's Bureau was originally designed to last for one year, conditions among the freedmen were so bad that Congress was compelled to extend its life. It did so reluctantly, and in 1867 bureau officials in the various states were ordered to start shutting down their programs. Protests from physicians and other employees caused Congress to extend the bureau's life for yet another year, but with a greatly reduced appropriation nonetheless. In 1868 all programs except those for education were ordered discontinued, and by June 1869 the medical program came to an end. Thousands of sick, aged, and very young blacks were thrown upon local community resources. Reluctant as many were, authorities were forced to assume some responsibility for them. The recurrent smallpox epidemics, the third Asiatic cholera epidemic in 1866–67, and the return of yellow fever required some measures to help black victims and prevent the further spread of these disorders. Thus, out of sheer necessity, many towns were forced into taking public health measures. One of the duties of the bureau's physicians had been to promote health education, and, despite the political and economic difficulties of Reconstruction, some progress in public health was made in the South.

The war preoccupied the attention of most Americans, but in the major cities the accumulating filth and the inefficiency of municipal governments were reaching a crisis point. Understandably, New York City, the largest metropolis in the nation and the recipient of the greatest number of poverty-stricken immigrants, was the first major city to attempt to deal with these issues. The influx of illiterate rural newcomers not only intensified all of New York's sanitary problems but permitted the rise of political machines and broke traditional voting patterns. Appalled at what they perceived to be the ignorance, apathy, and "immorality" of the immigrants, the middle and upper classes tended to withdraw from the political scene. Health and social reformers inveighed against the prevailing social injustices and unsanitary conditions of the times, but the propertied classes had little concern for the welfare of the poor, and without their support little could be done. It was acknowledged that the city council system was an ineffective form of government; the question was what to do about it. In the 1850s, civic reform leaders decided to bypass the municipal administration by creating independent city agencies responsible to the state. Their first success came in 1857 with the establishment of a Metropolitan Board of Police for New York City, setting a pattern for health reformers to follow.[20]

Four physicians played key roles in the final drive for health reform: John H. Griscom, Elisha Harris, Joseph M. Smith, and Stephen Smith. They pushed the New York Academy of Medicine into taking a stand, worked with citizens' groups, and lobbied the New York state legislature. The first significant development in their crusade was the formation of the New York Sanitary Association in 1859. All four of the physician-reformers were active in the association, but the majority of the association's officeholders and members were laypersons. The Sanitary

Association, from the beginning, worked closely with another reform group, the New York Association for Improving the Condition of the Poor (AICP). This latter association had been working for some years to alleviate the horrible conditions in the slums. Although the AICP accepted the prevailing view of the need to improve the morals of the poor, its annual report for 1860 declared that sanitary reform "may be said, indeed, to lie at the foundation of most other reforms, and cannot be ignored without defeating the objects which the philanthropic aim to secure." Moral degradation, the report continued, is "inherent in filthy, unsanitary conditions."[21]

By 1860 the movement for health reform, solidly backed by the New York City's newspapers, was well under way. Three years earlier the New York Academy of Medicine had introduced a municipal health bill into the state legislature, but without success. In 1860 an even stronger measure to create a metropolitan board of health, with jurisdiction over Manhattan, Brooklyn, and Richmond County, was proposed. This, and a third one in 1861, also died in the legislature, and the outbreak of the Civil War temporarily set back the movement. Dr. Elisha Harris, along with many of the other reform leaders, became involved in the work of the United States Sanitary Commission, but Dr. Griscom, although not in the best of health, picked up the slack. When a fourth bill was defeated in 1862, the reformers decided to concentrate upon a campaign to educate the electorate. This campaign to create a public awareness received a major impetus from the Draft Riot of 1863. Started as a protest against the draft, the riot turned into a vicious attack on blacks. It lasted for several days, burned down a major section of Broadway, and resulted in hundreds of deaths. The bitterness and frustration demonstrated by the poorer classes brought home to the well-to-do the need for quick social action, and it may well have been decisive in convincing them of the need for reform.

Suffice to say, a group of reform-minded citizens met late in 1863 and formed the New York Citizens' Association. As might be expected, it included Harris and the physician-reformers, and it quickly absorbed the membership of the Sanitary Association. The organization grew rapidly, drawing many leading citizens into its ranks. In 1864 the association introduced a new health bill into the legislature and drafted a letter asking physicians for their support. In response, a large number of them met and organized a "Special Council of Hygiene and Public Health." The council members, familiar with the survey by Shattuck in Massachusetts and the one by the New Orleans Sanitary Commission, promptly appointed a committee under Dr. Stephen Smith to make a sanitary survey of New York City. Medical inspectors were employed at thirty dollars a month, and each was assigned to inspect one of thirty-one districts within the city. Most inspectors were dispensary physicians and thus were already familiar with the atrocious living conditions of their patients.[22]

The inspectors' reports filled seventeen volumes, but Dr. Elisha Harris condensed them into a one-volume report, which was published in June 1865. The report, as Dr. Stephen Smith subsequently acknowledged, was designed to educate the public. Aside from showing the incredible crowding and filth in the tenements, the report stressed the danger to all classes from infectious diseases. In one two-week period the inspectors found 3,200 cases of smallpox and 2,000 of typhus.[23] Even before publication of the report, the evidence of the inspectors was brought to the attention of the public through pamphlets, speeches, legislative hearings, and other methods. The entrenched political machine in the city continued to resist, but the pressure was steadily building for reform. The turning point in the battle came with the appearance of Asiatic cholera cases late in 1865. On February 26, 1866, the Metropolitan Board of Health of New York City formally came into existence.

Although physicians had initiated the health reform movement and many of them played important roles in it, the establishment of a permanent New York City health department was a broadly based joint effort by the New York Sanitary Association, the New York Citizens' Association, the United States Sanitary Commission, the New York Academy of Medicine, New York City's newspapers, and many prominent laymen. The passage of the Metropolitan Health Act of 1866 was hailed as a great victory for American democracy, yet what it did was to take away from New York voters responsibility for the city's health and turn it over to the state of New York. Under the circumstances, the reformers were probably justified, although ideally it would have been far better to have successfully educated the electorate of New York City.

The New York Metropolitan Health Act of 1866 established the first effective municipal health department in a major city and became a model for many urban health departments. It provided a single health board for New York and Brooklyn, consisting of four police commissioners, a health officer, and four other commissioners, to be appointed by the governor. Thanks to Dorman B. Eaton—a member of the Citizens' Association, but best known today for his reform of the federal civil service—specific provisions in the act transferred all existing public health authority to the new board. In addition, one section assigned to the board all powers "for the purpose of preserving or protecting life or health or preventing disease." In carrying out this mandate, the board could call on the police or could enforce orders through its own officers.[24]

The New York Metropolitan Board of Health made excellent appointments to its major bureaus. Dr. Elisha Harris, possibly the outstanding health reformer of his day, was made director of the Bureau of Registration, and Dr. E. B. Dalton was named head of the Sanitary Bureau. The latter bureau was provided with fifteen sanitary inspectors to check on streets, tenements, privies, the nuisance trades, and other sources of danger. In selecting his inspectors, Dalton relied largely on physicians, most of whom had worked in the dispensaries. The board of health promptly launched a full-scale sanitary program. At this time public opinion was highly supportive, and the appearance of Asiatic cholera in 1866–67 further strengthened the board's position. As the number of cholera cases rose, the board increased its efforts to clean the city, opened dispensaries and hospitals to care for the sick, and established a disinfectant depot and laboratory. The latter maintained disinfectant teams on a twenty-four-hour basis to clean and disinfect all premises where cholera cases were reported. By this time the connection between human wastes and cholera was well established, and the use of disinfectants probably helped to minimize the epidemic. New York was fortunate, too, in that it received a supply of relatively safe water through the Croton Aqueduct. The cholera outbreak turned out to be relatively mild, and, justifiably or not, the city's health department received the credit. The goodwill accrued by the department in the first two or three years of its existence enabled it to survive various political vicissitudes and to remain one of the best departments in the United States.[25]

It is well that New York's health department made an auspicious start. Nearly all its actions outraged some or other vested interest, and once the public's initial enthusiasm waned, its officers also had to fight public apathy and ignorance. To add to its difficulties, the board of health had been the product of a state Republican administration, and the city was generally Democratic. The first major challenge to its authority was made through the courts. At first the board lost several cases, but as the public made clear its support for the board, in the years 1866 and 1867 legal decisions increasingly favored the health officials. By 1868 the board once again began encountering serious obstacles to its sanitary program, and many old sanitary problems reappeared. Nonetheless, the health department was well organized, its personnel was generally good, and it had become a permanent part of the city administration.[26]

New York was virtually alone in having an effective health board when the 1866–67 cholera epidemic swept through the country. Elsewhere health matters were usually handled through city councils and police departments or through volunteer health officials without tangible authority.

In Chicago, where health matters had been left to the police, city residents became apprehensive in 1865 upon hearing of the threat from cholera. Responsive to public fears, the Chicago City Council appointed a committee headed by a distinguished professor of the Chicago Medical School (Northwestern University), Nathan S. Davis, to make a sanitary survey. The committee's recommendations, which included a wide range of sanitary measures, were accepted, and the boards of public works and police were instructed to put them into effect. Despite a conscientious effort by municipal officials, the epidemic proved to be serious; almost 1,000 deaths were recorded from cholera in 1867. Shaken by these events, the city council that year created a permanent board of health, consciously patterned on New York's. The seven-man board, appointed by the mayor and the judges of the Superior Court, was required by law to include three physicians.

The Chicago board, emulating the one in New York, capitalized on city residents' fear of cholera and the temporary public enthusiasm for sanitation and began a major cleanup campaign. Its sixteen sanitary inspectors, armed with police powers, began enforcing sanitary ordinances and even moved against the slaughtering and meat-packing industries. In addition to the threat of cholera, serious outbreaks of smallpox from 1865 to 1867 further convinced the public to support the board of health. The health authorities responded by vaccinating over 95 percent of the city's population of about 241,000.[27]

In quick succession other cities followed the example of New York. The 1866 Asiatic cholera epidemic struck with devastating effect in other cities, causing over 2,000 deaths in Cincinnati and over 3,500 in St. Louis. In both cities health affairs previously had been in the hands of committees appointed by boards of aldermen, but the heavy toll from the epidemic convinced citizens of the need for independent health agencies. In Cincinnati the general public suspicion of the medical profession was demonstrated by newspaper demands that physicians be excluded from the board. In consequence, the first health board consisted exclusively of laymen. The act creating the St. Louis Board of Health, however, authorized the mayor to appoint a five-man board, with three of its members to be physicians.[28] In both cities the health boards were given broad powers, including the right to promulgate sanitary regulations. These regulations, however, had to receive the assent of the city councils, which were also responsible for their enforcement.

The St. Louis Board of Health was authorized to supervise the City Health Office and Dispensary, the City Hospital, the Smallpox Hospital, the Quarantine Hospital, the Department of Sanitary Police, street cleaning, the removal of slops, and the city's scavenger boats. It was also to supervise slaughterhouses, dairies, "and every subject that can possibly affect the sanitary condition of the city." The new board met on March 15, 1867, and promptly set to work. It leased a three-story building as headquarters, appointed a staff, and began inspecting sanitary conditions. The board's expenses for the first year, exclusive of hospitals, street cleaning, and the sanitary department, amounted to $27,004.[29] Compared to other cities, this was a respectable sum, although it should be borne in mind that St. Louis had a population of over 200,000 at this time.

Pittsburgh was far more representative of American cities and towns than the foregoing cities. Its board of health, first constituted in 1851, consisted of nine members elected by the city council. It functioned only during times of emergency, and even then shared responsibility with the city's sanitary committee. From 1860 to 1869 its annual budget was only $500, although it was given additional funds during epidemics. For example, following the cholera epidemic of 1867, the board reported it was about $1,000 in debt and was granted an additional $2,000. Physicians were as little regarded in Pittsburgh as they were elsewhere in the United States. When three of them applied to fill vacancies on the board of health in 1869, the two municipal boards selected three laymen instead. This same year Dr. Crosby Gray was appointed health officer by the board. Years later he recalled that he and his assistant constituted the board's working force for a city population of 85,000, and that his supplies and furnishings consisted of one copy of the city code, two death registers, one minute book, one cesspool permit book, a variety of other blank forms, and "one antiquated desk and a half dozen chairs."[30]

In California, where malaria, cholera, and various other enteric disorders troubled the residents of the Sacramento Valley, the city and the county of Sacramento established a permanent board of health early in 1862. The five physicians who constituted the board devoted most of their energy in the board's early years to dealing with smallpox and other contagious diseases and urging the authorities to remove dead animals and other nuisances. The chief significance of this board is that it evolved into an effective health department, and that its example undoubtedly contributed to the establishment of the California State Board of Health in 1870, one of the earliest state boards.[31]

By the end of the 1860s most Americans were unaffected by public health laws and regulations. Public health, in an essentially rural society, was looked upon as an urban problem, and in most towns and cities, except when epidemic disease threatened, it was given scant consideration, or at best, it was left to the city council or the police department. Yet the sanitary movement in the United States was well under way: New York and many other cities had established reasonably effective health boards; local sanitary associations were beginning to appear; a growing awareness of the need to regulate food and water supplies was evident; and one can discern the beginnings of an interest in school and industrial health. The next thirty years were to witness the emergence of state health boards, a rapid expansion of urban health departments, and the first effort to establish a national board of health.

NOTES

1. *Washington Evening Star,* August 23, 1861.
2. Charles J. Stille, *History of the United States Sanitary Commission* (Philadelphia, 1866), 326; Frank J. Hamilton, *A Treatise on Military Surgery and Hygiene* (New York, 1865), 77.
3. Albert Deutsch, "Some Wartime Influences on Health and Welfare Institutions in the United States," *J. Hist. of Med. & All. Sci.* 1 (1946):320–23.
4. George W. Adams, *Doctors in Blue: The Medical History of the Union Army in the Civil War* (New York, 1952), 6–7.
5. Ibid.; William Y. Thompson, "The United States Sanitary Commission," *Civil War History* 2 (1956):56.
6. John Duffy, *The Rudolf Matas History of Louisiana* (Baton Rouge, La., 1958–62), 2:320–22.
7. *Documents of the United States Sanitary Commission,* vol. 2, report no. 65 (New York, 1866), 7.
8. Gordon E. Gillson, *The Louisiana State Board of Health: The Formative Years* (n.p., [1966]), 104–5.
9. Ibid., 105–8, 120; Duffy, *Matas History of Medicine in Louisiana* (1958–62), 2:323–27.
10. Joseph Ioor Waring, *A History of Medicine in South Carolina, 1825–1900* (Columbia, S.C., 1967), 161.
11. John H. Ellis, "Yellow Fever and the Origins of Modern Public Health in Memphis, Tennessee, 1870–1900" (Ph.D. diss., Tulane University, 1962), chapter 1, and "Businessmen and Public Health in the Urban South," *Bull. Hist. Med.* 44 (1970):200.
12. Betty L. Plummer, "A History of Public Health in Washington, D.C., 1800–1890" (Ph.D. diss., University of Maryland, 1984), 101–2, 189.
13. Constance M. Green, *Washington Village and Capital, 1800–1878* (Princeton, 1962), 254.
14. Marshall S. Legan, "Disease and the Freedmen in Mississippi during Reconstruction," *J. Hist. Med. & All. Sci.* 28 (1973):257–59.
15. Plummer, "Public Health in Washington, D.C.," 189.
16. Duffy, *Matas History of Medicine in Louisiana,* 2:516–17.
17. Alan Raphael, "Health and Social Welfare of Kentucky Black People, 1865–1870," *Societas: A Review of Social History* 2 (1972):145–48.
18. Legan, "Disease and the Freedmen in Mississippi," 258–59.

19. Raphael, "Health and Social Welfare of Kentucky Black People," 147.

20. John Duffy, *A History of Public Health in New York City, 1625–1866* (New York, 1968), 317. See chapter 24 for health reform efforts in the 1850s.

21. *Annual Report of the New-York Association for the Improvment of the Condition of the Poor for the Year 1860* (New York, 1860), 64–65.

22. Duffy, *Public Health in New York City, 1625–1866*, 548ff.

23. Stephen Smith, *The City that Was,* preface by John Duffy (Metuchen, N.J., 1973), 52–57, 108–13, and "The Origin and Organization of the Department of Health in the City of New York," *Medical Record* 93 (1918):115–17.

24. New York *State Laws,* 89th sess., chap. 74, February 26, 1866, pp. 114–44, and chap. 686, April 18, 1866, pp. 1462–70.

25. John Duffy, *A History of Public Health in New York City, 1866–1966* (New York, 1974), 9–19.

26. Ibid., 26–29.

27. Thomas N. Bonner, *Medicine in Chicago, 1850–1950* (Madison, Wis., 1957), 180–81; Isaac D. Rawlings, *The Rise and Fall of Disease in Illinois* (Springfield, Ill., 1927), 44.

28. Catherine V. Soraghan, "The History of St. Louis, 1865–1876" (M.A. thesis, Washington University, 1936), 31.

29. *The First Annual Report of the Board of Health of the City of Saint Louis, 1867–68* (St. Louis, 1868), 6–7, 26.

30. Pittsburgh *Evening Chronicle*, January 26, 1869; *Daily Post*, November 11, 1868; Jacqueline K. Corn, "Community Responsibility for Public Health: The Impact of Epidemic Disease and Urban Growth on Pittsburgh," *Western Pennsylvania Historical Magazine* 59 (1976):321–24.

31. Dave F. Dozier, "Beginnings of Public Health in Sacramento," *California's Health* 19 (1962):154–55.

9

The Institutionalization of Public Health

As indicated in the previous chapter, the American Civil War marked a watershed in the history of American public health. It helped usher in the sanitary revolution, and it was followed immediately by the appearance of the first effective municipal health departments and the beginning of state boards of health. More than this, the nature of public health itself was undergoing fundamental changes. In the first place, medicine, on which public health practice is based, was in the throes of a major revolution. Advances in pathology, histology, physiology, chemistry, and other fields were beginning to provide an understanding of organic and constitutional disorders, and the stage was set for the bacteriological era, which was to provide answers to the great endemic and epidemic diseases. By 1900 a good many pathogenic organisms had been identified; the role of insects and other vectors in the spread of disease had been discovered; antitoxins had been created to treat the victims of certain diseases; and vaccines were appearing on a scale large enough to protect entire populations.

New knowledge from the fields of chemistry and microbiology was also being applied in the area of public health. Laboratory testing of water, milk, and other substances of concern to public health was becoming an essential function of the better health departments, and the bacteriological revolution required them to establish laboratories for diagnostic purposes and to produce the newfound antitoxins and vaccines. The major preoccupations of public health officials were still the fight against infectious diseases and, to a much lesser degree, the inspection of food and water supplies. The increasing complexity of society and the application of science to industry in the late nineteenth century, however, were forcing health departments to broaden their concerns.

Science and technology were solving many age-old community health problems, but in the process they were creating a host of new ones. Early in the nineteenth century, John Pintard, a pioneer New York health reformer, witnessed a steam engine in operation and envisioned the day when self-propelled vehicles would eliminate horses and manure piles from urban areas, and thus put an end, he wrote, to the miasmas that were polluting the atmosphere and were so destructive to health. Pintard was correct in one respect, for the introduction of steam locomotives and railroads, electric streetcars, and the gas combustion engine in the latter half of the nineteenth century was eventually to eliminate the thousands of horses from cities. In consequence, the streets were no longer fouled with manure, and the myriads of flies and the stench from huge manure piles and stables were things of the past. Unfortunately, their place was taken by the dense clouds of smoke from the early locomotives and the more subtle pollution arising from combustion engines.

In some instances technology created problems but was later able to solve them. The advent of illuminating oil, or kerosene, shortly after the mid-century resulted in hundreds of explosions and fires. The problem arose in part from the inability of the processors to maintain quality control and in part from unscrupulous wholesalers' and retailers' adulterating kerosene with much cheaper and more volatile petroleum by-products. All too often when householders attempted to light their kerosene lamps, the volatile fuel exploded. The upshot was that health departments assigned inspectors to check on the quality of the oil. Within a few years, however, improved technology solved the problem of quality control, and the industry recognized the need to police itself.

The chemical revolution, which brought food additives to help preserve food and in some cases to improve its quality, also made possible a great many abuses. Too frequently additives were used solely for cosmetic purposes or even to disguise tainted or spoiled food; often the additives themselves were a threat to health. The same mixed blessing holds true for insecticides. They became a major factor in increasing food production and helping to eliminate or reduce diseases carried by insect vectors. Yet the excessive application of these powerful chemical weapons proved a major danger to public health and the environment. Likewise, the same chemistry that brought new and effective therapeutics was also used to produce an even greater number of proprietary drugs. Many of these patent medicines disguised symptoms and caused patients to delay proper treatment; others contained harmful and dangerous ingredients.

In other cases technology proved immensely beneficial. The rise of the textile industry and the invention of the sewing machine made possible the mass production of cheap cotton clothes, a development that was a major factor in promoting personal cleanliness. The transportation revolution not only solved the problem of horses and stables in urban areas, but also enabled cities to receive their milk and dairy supplies from distant milk sheds, thus eliminating the need for dairies, another source of flies and foul odors. An incidental result of this change in dairy production was improved health conditions in rural areas. In order to guarantee the quality of its milk supply, New York City civic authorities began a rigorous inspection of dairies in Upstate New York and other areas shipping milk to the city. The same situation held true for New York's water supply. As the city was forced to draw water from more distant rivers, lakes, and reservoirs, it was compelled to prevent or minimize pollution from sewage and other sources. The net result was to carry the benefits of public health developments to areas well beyond the boundaries of major cities.

A fundamental role of public health departments has always been to recognize community and individual health problems, find a way to solve them, and then, where feasible, turn the problem over to some other agency or body. For example, the quantity and quality of the water supply was a major concern of health officials in the nineteenth century. By the twentieth century technology and bacteriology had made possible an ample supply of safe water, and the responsibility for safe water supplies now rests largely in the hands of separate water boards or departments. The same is true of sewer systems. Inspection of privies and cesspools was a perennial source of difficulty for health boards until the advent of effective sanitary engineering and the construction of comprehensive sewer systems. Here again, health departments were able to spin off the responsibility to sewerage boards or combined water and sewerage boards. In other instances health departments have worked with private industries or trade associations to promote self-policing of products or services vital to health. Health officials have not surrendered all responsibility in cases such as these, but their supervision is usually nominal.

The late nineteenth century was a period when health departments were rapidly broadening their concerns. In so doing they were reflecting the changing views of American society. Whereas sinfulness and lack of moral character were held to be largely responsible for poverty and disease early in the first half of the nineteenth century, increasingly the middle and upper classes began to recognize the role of environment in shaping people's lives. Moreover, whereas formerly epidemics had been attributed to God's displeasure, scientific knowledge was now providing a more logical explanation. The success of the New York Metropolitan Board of Health in minimizing the 1866–67 Asiatic cholera outbreak seemed proof that science held the possibility for solving all health problems. Rather than eliminating social problems by concentrating on improving the moral character of the poor, now it seemed the solution lay in improving the environment of the poor. Cleanliness, long associated with godliness, now became an end in itself as the equation of disease with dirt became more firmly entrenched. The Christian humanitarians of earlier years now turned sanitation and cleanliness into a moral cause.

In the drive to improve the environment, health reformers took up the cause of school health, tenement reform, ventilation in public buildings, air pollution, and a host of other matters affecting health. The new emphasis on scientific public health did not allay the bitter arguments between the sanitationists and the contagionists, but the public, showing little concern for the subtle variations in the many medical theories presented on both sides of the debate, required public health officials to enforce both quarantine and sanitary regulations. Even with the discoveries in bacteriology, the miasmatic thesis still remained basic to the sanitary movement and continued to play a role in public health thinking until the early years of the twentieth century. For example, in the spring of 1885 the New York City Board of Health resolved that the "laying of all telegraph wires underground in one season . . . would prove highly detrimental to the health of the City in that portion densely populated through the exposure to the atmosphere of so much subsoil, saturated, as most is, with noxious gases."[1] Even as late as 1900 health departments were still preventing gas and water companies from digging up the streets during the warm season for fear that disturbing the soil would release a potentially dangerous miasma, and until World War I sewer gas was considered by most Americans to be a source of disease.

The late nineteenth century also witnessed the rise of professions and of specialization within them. Despite strong opposition from the American Medical Association, the expansion of medical knowledge literally forced physicians and surgeons to concentrate in specific areas. Physicians working with health boards and health departments soon recognized that dealing with community health problems differed greatly from private practice, and the organization of the American Public Health Association in 1872 clearly indicated the emergence of a new medical specialty. By this date dozens of new professions were beginning to appear on the scene. The public health field contributed to their growth by creating a demand for professionals such as sanitary engineers, chemists, microbiologists, and statisticians. Whereas formerly the vast majority of members and employees of health boards had been laymen, supplemented by physicians, the late nineteenth century witnessed the professionalization of health departments. This is not to say that as of 1900 a complete transformation had been made, but in major cities the process was well under way.

The shift toward professionalization reflected a major change in the public's view of government. In the early national period Americans followed the English tradition of placing government in the hands of men of learning and intelligence. The Jacksonian era replaced this with an egalitarian philosophy that any good American could handle any government position—or any other job, for that matter. The middle years of the century saw a massive influx of illiterate Irish, most of whom settled in eastern port cities and helped pave the way for political machines. Native Americans, and particularly the Protestant middle class, despairing of corrupt politicians and distrusting the average voter, sought to place government in the hands of appointed professionals based on merit. The Pendleton Act of 1883, which established the civil service system, was part of an effort to create a corps of professional federal employees. This attempt to distance government workers and officeholders from politics belonged to the wider movement in this period to bring greater efficiency into government and business affairs. Professionalization and efficiency were the key methods by which the Progressive Movement, in full swing by 1900, hoped to create a brave new society. Health departments helped lead the way toward professionalization, and their successes undoubtedly reinforced the optimism of the Progressive reformers.

If a date can be assigned to the professionalization of public health it would be the appearance in 1872 of the American Public Health Association. The New York Metropolitan Board of Health had attracted widespread attention, and, as noted earlier, had become a model for other municipal health agencies. It received a good many inquiries from other cities, and the upshot of this extensive correspondence was a recognition of the need for a national organization. In April 1872 ten health reformers from New York and other cities held a preliminary meeting. Among those present were Drs. Stephen Smith and Elisha Harris of New York, Edwin Snow of Providence, J. H. Rauch of Chicago, and C. C. Cox of Washington, D.C. At this meeting a decision was taken to create a permanent organization, and Dr. Smith was elected chairman of a committee to draw up a tentative constitution. Circulars were sent to cities and states announcing a meeting to be held in Long Branch, New Jersey, September 12. As of this date only four states and the District of Columbia had established boards of health, although some form of health agency existed in well over one hundred cities.[2]

The September gathering included representatives from New York, Pennsylvania, Louisiana, Rhode Island, Connecticut, Ohio, Illinois, and Washington, D.C. A constitution was adopted stating that the goal of the association "was to be the advancement of sanitary science and the promotion of organizations and measures for the practical application of public hygiene." The first secretary, Dr. Elisha Harris, stressed that the association was a voluntary one in order to bring together a wide range of individuals concerned with public health. At this meeting Dr. Smith was elected president, and a call was issued for the first annual meeting, to be held in Cincinnati in May 1873. The original constitution required a quorum of twenty-five, and when the members assembled in May, they were compelled to adjourn the meeting for lack of a quorum. Undeterred, those present determined to call for a second meeting in New York the following November. At this gathering the original constitution was revised slightly, reducing the quorum to nine, and the APHA officially began.

New members were to be elected to the association through nomination by its executive committee and a vote of two-thirds of the members present. Dues were set at five dollars, and new members were to be chosen on the basis of "their acknowledged interest in, or devotion to, sanitary studies and allied sciences, and to the practical application of the same." Despite a slow start, the association grew rapidly. The 1880 meeting in New Orleans drew some four hundred members, and about seven hundred attended the annual meeting held in Savannah the following year. Recognizing that disease knew no boundaries and that public health problems were universal, in 1884 Canada was invited to become a constituent member of the association. Five years later approaches were made to Mexico, Cuba, and the Central American countries. Mexico accepted the invitation in 1892, and the other countries followed.[3]

Founding members such as Drs. Stephen Smith, Elisha Harris, Edwin Snow, and A. N. Bell, who had attended the sanitary conventions in the 1850s, must have been delighted with the surging interest in sanitary reform in this period. Newspapers in every major city, medical journals, and popular magazines all welcomed the new organization. Health and hygiene were popular topics, and citizens' sanitary associations were springing up throughout the country. The rapid growth of the APHA was further aided by the equally rapid development of local and state health agencies—a development in which the APHA itself played a role. In 1872 only six states had health boards; six years later Elisha Harris proudly noted that, at the beginning of the association's seventh year, nearly fifty cities had reasonably efficient health departments and sixteen states had boards of health.[4]

One of the association's first actions was to send a questionnaire to every town of over 5,000 inhabitants. The questionnaires covered virtually every subject of concern to community health—even including the town's altitude, the amount of paved streets, and the ventilation of public buildings. Detailed answers were requested in connection with the water supply, sewer systems, vital statistics, and the community's health agency, if it had one. In reporting the results of the survey, Dr. John M. Toner noted "how grudgingly legislatures invest Boards of Health with sufficient power to properly perform their important trust" and how the courts are reluctant to support health laws "lest they seem to abridge the rights of property and individual freedom." Thousands of dollars, he said, are spent to apprehend those who violate the laws of property, but legislatures refuse to spend fifty or one hundred dollars for removing nuisances that may be "slowly destroying scores of valuable lives."

The survey was not as complete as had been hoped, Dr. Toner explained, since those who received the questionnaires either did not understand the inquiries or else were indifferent to them. He commented, too, that the least understood and most backward branch of sanitary science was sanitary engineering. Health boards too frequently authorized the construction of sewer systems while giving little attention to the system's size or the need for a comprehensive system. Every health board, he added, needed the services of "a competent sanitary engineer." Although Toner was appalled at the inadequacy of the reported methods for handling sewage, the most revealing information from the survey was the lack of vital statistics and the want of paid health officials in America.[5]

From the beginning, the papers read at the annual meetings covered a wide range of topics, but they still reflected the old major concern with epidemic disease. Asiatic cholera reappeared in 1866–67 and then again on a smaller scale in the early 1870s, while yellow fever struck New Orleans and the coastal cities in 1867, flared up occasionally in the intervening years, and then became epidemic again in 1873. Of the papers delivered at the two meetings in 1873, fifteen were on Asiatic cholera, five on yellow fever, five more on quarantine, one on an epizootic among horses, and several others on a variety of topics. Significantly, the secretary of the association commented at the 1880 meeting in New Orleans that this was the first time in four years that yellow fever had not absorbed the main interest of the session.[6]

As the nineteenth century advanced, the emphasis on epidemic disease declined and the range of subjects at the APHA meetings widened. In addition to sewage and garbage disposal, the subject of ventilation became of major interest. In view of the widespread fear of miasma, it was only logical that sanitarians would worry about the concentration of fetid odors indoors. The result was a host of articles dealing with ventilation in schools, tenements, factories, and public buildings. But ventilation was only one of the problems found in these places, and the number of articles dealing in general with the health of schoolchildren, workers, and tenement dwellers shows a steady increase. Indicative of the new emphasis upon medical sociology, a Mr. Henry Lomb of Rochester, New York, gave $2,000 to be awarded for prize essays on four topics, which he selected. Of the winning essays announced at the 1885 association meeting, one dealt with the homes and food of workers, a second with the sanitary condition of schools, and a third with disease and injuries in factories and workshops.[7]

Even the forbidden topic of venereal disease received some notice. In 1870 St. Louis experimented with the medical inspection of prostitutes—an experiment that touched off a heated debate in newspapers and medical journals. Some years later the medical director of the navy, Dr. Albert G. Gihon, delivered a paper on venereal disease before the APHA, in which he stressed the need to protect innocent women and children and urged the establishment of a well-organized sanitary service to track down and isolate all venereal disease cases. He mentioned that he had broached the subject three years earlier but nothing had been done. Ironically, the curtain of silence on the subject was just falling; in 1882 a proposal to require the reporting of venereal disease was rejected on the grounds that it would bring public disapprobation on the association.[8] In this matter, too, the APHA reflected the spirit of the times.

Another evidence of growing professionalism was the multiplication of books relating to public health and the appearance of professional journals. Nearly all the health periodicals published in America in the pre–Civil War period were popular magazines—and these continued to increase in the postwar period. The first significant American public health journal was the brainchild of Dr. A. N. Bell of New York, one of the founders of the APHA. In 1873 under his editorship, volume one of *The Sanitarian* was published. In his foreword to the first issue, Dr. Bell announced his intention to make "the results of the various inquiries . . . for the preservation of health and the expectation of human life" available to the public and the medical profession. After noting that the "resources of sanitary science are inexhaustible," he stated that in addition to pure medical subjects, he proposed to discuss the "practical questions of State Medicine"—the health of the armed forces, marine health, quarantine, civic cleanliness, the food supply, occupational health, and other topics. He added, too, that no advertisements "of even questionable character" would be accepted.[9] He was an inveterate reformer, and for the next thirty years he published articles covering almost every social issue of consequence. In addition to purely sanitary topics, he published articles on such subjects as venereal disease (a problem the APHA and the AMA refused to touch), sweatshops employing women, the health of blacks, and child labor.

Beginning with the first annual meeting, the APHA published an annual volume entitled *Public Health: Reports and Papers of the American Public Health Association*. Many of the articles were picked up and reprinted in medical journals or summarized in newspapers and magazines. By the 1880s many health departments were publishing their own annual reports along with pamphlets, broadsides, and other publications designed to educate the public and the medical profession. The appearance of *The Sanitary Messenger* (Baltimore, 1878), *The Sanitary Engineer* (1880), and

The Sanitary News (1882) showed that specialization was developing within the public health field. Even a cursory examination of the *Index-Catalogue of the Library of the Surgeon-General's Office* of the 1870s and 1880s indicates the rapid growth of health publications. The rising public interest in the subject can also be seen by glancing through the *Guide to Periodical Literature* for these years. *Harper's, The Atlantic, Scientific American*, and other popular magazines all carried articles on community health topics.

One great contribution of the APHA was the inclusion of laypersons in its membership. In the post–Civil War period business and civic organizations began to take an active interest in public health. In part it reflected a growing awareness of the deplorable conditions in urban areas coupled with the rising social consciousness of the middle class. By the 1870s a host of sanitary associations and other volunteer groups began emerging. The movement was strongly supported by responsible business leaders who recognized that a reputation for an unhealthy environment hindered community growth. This was particularly true in the South, where many major cities were notorious for their unsanitary conditions and pestilences such as yellow fever.

For Americans today, who tend to view the American medical profession as extremely conservative, it may come as a surprise to realize that in the nineteenth century it strongly supported all public health measures. Individual physicians were in the forefront of the early health and social reform movements. They initiated the sanitary movement, and, while the movement gathered strength with the recruitment of leading lay reformers, physicians continued to play a significant role. In the latter part of the nineteenth century they helped organize and lead most of the citizens' sanitary associations.

Medical societies, too, actively sought to educate their members on public health matters. Local medical societies constantly agitated for municipal health boards, and state societies led the battle for state boards. The New York Academy of Medicine was one of the better organizations in this respect. Its Committee on Public Health took the early initiative in the fight to establish the New York Metropolitan Board of Health, and its members included some of the leading health reformers in New York City. Over the years the committee investigated a wide range of public health issues, took an active role in city and state politics, and constantly prodded the membership of the academy into taking a stand on social issues.

The American Medical Association, from its founding in 1847, devoted most of its efforts toward improving medical education and requiring licensure laws—efforts that were aimed, at least in part, at eliminating competition from homeopaths and other irregular practitioners. But it also strongly supported health reforms in general and the development of public health boards at all levels of government. In response to the enormous death toll on ships bringing Irish immigrants to America, in 1852 the AMA petitioned Congress to require all vessels carrying steerage passengers to have a surgeon aboard. The AMA Committee on a National Health Council reported to the association in 1872 that it had contacted thirty states, urging their officials to establish state health departments. The committee also defined state medicine "as the application of medical knowledge and skill to the benefit of communities," adding, "which is obviously a very different thing from their application to the benefit of individuals in private or curative medicine."[10]

Year after year the AMA actively pushed for a national health agency, and its section on state medicine reported annually on the number of states with boards of health. The annual addresses by the association's presidents almost invariably mentioned the need for state health boards and a national health agency. Significantly, virtually all of the early presidents of the APHA were also prominent members of the AMA. In 1883 an article in the *Journal of the AMA (JAMA)* proclaimed: "Public health ever goes hand in hand with true liberty, and is the companion of orderly habits and pure morals." After discussing various health problems, the author declared: "Sanitary Science, therefore, is a segment of political economy, and should receive encouragement by the State as a wealth-creating factor—riches, indeed, to the whole people far above that of any other earthly value."[11]

One of the explanations for the progressive attitude of the medical profession lies in the division within its ranks. As was true of all professions in America for most of the nineteenth century, physicians collectively were not held in high regard. In the first place, medicine had lagged behind the advancing front of science and technology, and there was little that physicians could do for most patients. Second, medical education was woefully limited. The majority of physicians had acquired their knowledge through a limited apprenticeship and one or two short annual courses in a medical school. Most of these schools had minimal, if any, requirements for entrance, and few students who could afford to pay their fees failed to obtain a degree. Since all licensure laws had been repealed by the 1850s, anyone could practice medicine. The result was a flood of practitioners, and in the ensuing competition for patients, the average physician eked out a bare existence.

In contrast to these struggling doctors were the professional elites. Generally they came from the middle and upper classes, received a college or university education, acquired a medical degree at one of the better

American schools, and then completed their education by studying in medical centers in Britain and the Continent. These were the individuals who edited the medical journals, dominated the AMA and local medical societies, taught at the best medical schools, led the fight to reform medical education, and were active in social and health reform. They were also the leaders in the sanitary reform movement and the APHA. Financially secure by virtue of their social position and relatively high income, they saw no threat to their economic position in espousing public health and other reforms. Average practitioners, struggling to make a living, were far more concerned with improving their own economic status than with the welfare of society, and, when revisions in the AMA's constitution at the beginning of the twentiethth century gave them a greater voice, the AMA began taking a more conservative stance. Nonetheless, the old guard of elite physicians continued to control the AMA until the battle over national health insurance in the World War I period. Henceforth all proposals for government action were judged on the basis of whether or not they threatened the private practice of medicine.

While there can be little doubt that the majority of physician leaders of the sanitary movement were sincere in their belief that public health should be in the hands of the medical profession, consciously or not, many physicians recognized that laying claim to a growing area of general concern would raise the professional status and social prestige of their profession. In earlier years the inability of doctors to deal with major diseases and sicknesses had compelled them to emphasize their moral leadership. This same attitude was expressed in a different form by Dr. Samuel Osgood in a paper before the APHA in 1874: "Once the priests were physicians, now the physicians are becoming, in their way, priests, and giving laws not only to their own patients, but to society. . . ."[12]

Addressing the 1878 Buffalo meeting of the AMA, Dr. T. G. Richardson, dean of the University of Louisiana Medical School (presently Tulane University), in urging the association to encourage the creation of state health boards, declared that state medical societies should insist on "the right of nomination for appointment to such boards" lest the positions fall into the hands of mere office hunters.[13] In his inaugural address as president of the New York Academy of Medicine in 1885, Dr. Abraham Jacobi declared that physicians were the "natural advisors in all matters concerning sanitation and health," adding that the two medical societies in New York City ought to be the authorities on all matters of health. He foresaw the day when presidents of health boards would be either nominated or appointed by the medical profession, and he predicted "that no Board of Education, no Board of Charities [would] be complete without a prominent medical member."[14] Expanding this thesis further, in 1894 the editor of the *Cincinnati Lancet-Clinic* proclaimed: "In the settlement of great sociological questions affecting the masses of people . . . none are so well prepared to cope as the learned physicians of the country."[15] Several factors contributed to the raising of the medical profession's status toward the end of the nineteenth century, and the role of physicians in the public health movement certainly ranks among them.

NOTES

1. New York City, Minutes of the Board of Health, April 3, 1885, New York City Health Department MS, p. 390.

2. Mazÿck P. Ravenel, ed., *A Half Century of Public Health* (New York, 1921), 13–14.

3. Ibid., 17–18; *Selections from Public Health Reports and Papers Presented at the Meetings of the American Public Health Association (1873–1883)*, Public Health in America Series (New York, 1977), ix, xiii–xv (hereafter cited as *Selections from Public Health Reports of the APHA (1873–1883)*. For good short accounts of the early meetings see Harold M. Cavins, "The National Quarantine and Sanitary Conventions of 1857–1858 and the Beginnings of the American Public Health Association," *Bull. Hist. Med.* 13 (1943):419–25, and Howard D. Kramer, "Agitation for Public Health Reform in the 1870's," *J. Hist. Med. & All. Sci.* 3 (1948):473–88.

4. Elisha Harris, "Significance of the Recent Epidemic—Duties of the American Public Health Association," in *Selections from Public Health Reports of the APHA (1873–1883)*, 163.

5. John M. Toner, "Boards of Health in the United States," in *Selections from Public Health Reports of the APHA (1873–1883)*, 499–501.

6. Cavins, "The National Quarantine and Sanitary Conventions," 419–20.

7. Ravenel, *A Half Century of Public Health*, 23.

8. John Duffy, "The Physician as a Moral Force in American History," in *New Knowledge in the Biomedical Sciences*, W. B. Bondeson et al., eds. (Dordrecht, 1982), 11–12; Albert G. Gihon, "On the Protection of the Innocent and Helpless Members of the Community from Venereal Diseases and their Consequences," in *Selections from Public Health Reports of the APHA (1873–1883)*, 57–58.

9. A. N. Bell, *The Sanitarian* 1 (1873), foreword.

10. Morris Fishbein, *A History of the American Medical Association, 1847 to 1947* (Philadelphia, 1947), 55, 83–84.

11. James E. Reeves, "The Eminent Domain of Sanitary Science, and the Usefulness of Boards of Health in Guarding the Public Welfare," *Journal of the American Medical Association* (hereafter cited as *JAMA*) 1 (1883):612.

12. Burton J. Bledstein, *The Culture of Professionalism: The Middle Class and the Development of Higher Education in America* (New York, 1976), 94–95.

13. Fishbein, *A History of the American Medical Association*, 97–98.

14. Abraham Jacobi, *Inaugural Address*, New York Academy of Medicine pamphlets, (New York, 1885), 10.

15. Editorial, "Medical Politics," *Cincinnati Lancet-Clinic* 72 (1894):308–9.

10

The Growth of Municipal and State Boards of Health

As noted earlier, the American public health movement was based largely upon the European experience. The Paris Clinical School, which dominated medicine in the early nineteenth century, enabled France to take the initiative in public health, but by the 1840s and 1850s Great Britain had assumed leadership. The public health movement received a further impetus from the emergence of a united Germany in the latter part of the century. Germans were already making strides in science and technology, and under Bismarck the German government fostered public health as a means of strengthening the state.

In consequence, in attempting to deal with the whole range of sanitary issues, American health reformers were able to draw on the experiences, knowledge, and literature of Britain and other countries. Dr. John H. Griscom modeled his work, *The Sanitary Condition of the Laboring Population of New York,* on Edwin Chadwick's 1842 classic study, and American reformers frequently cited British and European public health works. In the first series of the *Index-Catalogue of the Surgeon-General's Library,* far more British and European publications were cited than American ones.

The major differences between the United States and Western Europe, however, ensured that the evolution of American public health agencies would follow a somewhat different path than those of Europe. While early events in history had led Britain to place a considerable emphasis upon the role of local government because the English people were homogenous and their country was small, the sanitary movement in England led directly to the formation of a national health agency. The French government, and the German government established under Bismarck in the later nineteenth century, were highly centralized, with the result that in France and Germany, too, public health reforms tended to come from the top. Moreover, in all three countries the population was more docile and obedient to authority than that of the United States—the British, through the class system; the French and Germans, by long tradition of authoritarian government.

In America the British emphasis upon local government continued throughout the nineteenth century, aided in part by the sheer size of

America. Local and state government took precedence over the national government in most matters of direct concern to the people. The United States was founded as a federation of separate colonies, and, as the complexity of society required action on a scale beyond the local level, the people looked to state government rather than to federal government. Moreover, the settlers and immigrants who braved the New World tended to be more individualistic, and the American frontier experience accentuated their dislike for authority. Public health measures could be imposed upon them only with difficulty; consequently, as health reformers discovered by the late nineteenth century, education had to be a main function of health agencies.

One other factor of considerable importance in the institutionalization of public health in America was the effect of regionalism. Sectional variations in climate, terrain, economic systems, and cultural patterns greatly affected the nature of diseases and health problems. The predominantly rural South, with its malaria, hookworm, and pellagra and its slave plantation system, clearly differed from other sections of the United States; and the health problems of New England varied considerably from those of the Gulf Coast states, the Midwest, and the West.

The phenomenon of major urban growth, which made possible the start of the sanitary movement in America, began in the early nineteenth century on the East Coast, then spread to the Midwest and, to a lesser degree, to the South in the second half of the century, and finally reached the West Coast by the beginning of the twentieth century. Consequently, the Midwest and, in particular, the West Coast were able to benefit from the experience of the older cities in the East. This ability is clearly illustrated in the development of sanitary engineering.

The piecemeal and haphazard construction of sewers and drains in eastern cities created inadequate systems that could be replaced only at a huge cost. Some years ago, for example, it was estimated that two billion dollars would be needed to replace the New York City sewer system with a dual one separating rainfall drainage from sewerage. Even today a heavy rain in New York, as well as a number of other cities, can overwhelm the sewer plants and cause the discharge of improperly processed sewage into harbors and streams. The development of sanitary engineering in the 1870s and 1880s enabled more recent towns and cities to incorporate newly developed technology into their sewer systems and building codes at minimum cost. They could draw on the experience of the older cities and towns when they established municipal health agencies and health codes.

The New York City Health Department, which largely established the pattern for health departments in Chicago and a good many other cities, has a history that illustrates the problems besetting municipal health agencies in the later nineteenth century. After an auspicious start aided by the threat of Asiatic cholera, the department began to languish in the 1870s. The Depression of 1873 and a long period of inefficiency and corruption in government reduced the department's budget and its capacity to operate effectively. Then, as now, health departments had to depend to some extent upon the cooperation of other municipal departments such as the police and building departments, and in New York City this cooperation was given grudgingly. To illustrate the problem, in 1878 Mayor Smith Ely, Jr., declared that in order to dispose of street dirt it was necessary to gain the assent of three city departments and two state ones, not one of whom "seemed to be in sympathy with any of the others."[1]

In the 1880s the widespread corruption in New York's city government permeated the health department. Increasingly, accusations of negligence were made as political appointees replaced experienced health workers, and in 1885 General Alexander Shaler, president of the New York Board of Health, was accused of taking bribes. Although Shaler's two trials resulted in hung juries, he was removed from office. The publicity, fortunately, focused attention on the health department and led to a major overhaul. By the 1890s the health department, under new leadership, was once again one of the best in the country.[2]

Despite its political problems, the department steadily widened its activities. Smallpox, which had once again become a major threat in America, peaked in New York in 1875, when its death toll reached 1,280. The health department, as early as 1867, had resolved that schoolteachers and students must have vaccination certificates. A more serious smallpox outbreak in 1868–69 led the department to appoint sixty health inspectors to make a house-to-house check in tenement areas to see that all residents were vaccinated. As smallpox continued to flare up, in 1874 a permanent vaccination force was established. Spurred on by the 1875 epidemic, in 1876 the department began producing its own vaccine on a farm in Lakeview, New Jersey. These measures should have enabled New York to vanquish smallpox, but such was not the case. In the first place, the department never had enough funds for the inspection services; in the second place, many citizens objected to free vaccinations for the poor; third, the antivaccination movement was just getting under way. In addition to all these problems, the flood of immigrants into the city, most of whom objected strongly to being vaccinated, supplied a constant pool of nonimmunes. Nonetheless, smallpox was more or less under control by 1900.[3]

Dr. Charles F. Chandler, a chemist who took over the health department in 1873, deserves credit for two developments that contributed notably to improving infant and child health. The first of these was the start of laboratory testing of the city's milk supply, which had been a source of complaint for many years. The second, a far greater contribution, was the establishment of what was called the Summer Corps. Beginning in 1876, Chandler obtained a special appropriation of five thousand dollars to employ about fifty physicians during the month of August. Each physician was assigned a specific tenement district and was to visit every household in it. The Summer Corps was to treat sick children, advise mothers on child care, investigate sanitary conditions, and report any violations of the sanitary or health laws. Although the corps physicians' intrusions were at first resented, the tenement dwellers soon welcomed them, and in succeeding years the corps performed a notable job of providing medical care and health education for the poor. When newspaper reporters accompanied some of the physicians in 1882, their accounts of the deplorable tenement conditions stimulated demands for reform. The success of the program led the New York state legislature in 1890 to provide a special appropriation, known as the Tenement House Fund, to employ the Summer Corps for the months of July and August. By this time, a number of private organizations and newspapers also had organized summer programs to help tenement mothers and children.[4]

One other area into which the New York City Health Department ventured, but with only limited success, was that of school health. A limited inspection of schoolchildren for vaccination had been made during the smallpox epidemics from 1867 to 1875, but the city's board of education—which in New York, as in most other cities, was highly politicized—wanted no interference from other city agencies. In 1872–73 two health inspectors made a sanitary survey of the schools and found nearly all of them to be in a deplorable condition. The board of education quietly pigeonholed the report. In 1877 the *Medical Record* declared that the board of education had defied all attempts by health inspectors to examine schools on the grounds that it could handle its own affairs. Periodically health inspectors did check on schools, but the health department was reluctant to tangle with the board of education, and no effort was made to enforce the sanitary regulations.

While working for the department in 1869, Dr. Chandler was assigned the task of safety-testing kerosene (known as illuminating oil) because of a series of recent explosions caused by kerosene. He reported that of seventy-eight samples tested, all contained a high percentage of naptha, and many were pure naptha. Apparently unscrupulous dealers were adulterating kerosene with naptha, a volatile substance, which at that time was considered relatively worthless.[5] When the board of health passed an ordinance against the sale of unsafe oil, it was thrown out by the New York courts on the grounds that illuminating oil came under the jurisdiction of the city's fire department. A number of other city health departments also began testing kerosene; fortunately, a few years later the industry solved the problem by instituting a policy of self-regulation.

By the 1890s other city and state health departments were establishing vaccination programs, checking on milk and meat, occasionally venturing into the schools, and originating or supplementing programs comparable to that of New York City's Summer Corps. As municipalities grew in size and living standards improved, most of them expanded their health departments. New York City began in 1866, with a sanitary bureau consisting of a superintendent and fifteen inspectors. This bureau was responsible for the surveillance and control of communicable diseases, as well as all matters relating to sanitation. By the 1880s it had expanded to include four divisions: sanitary inspections, contagious diseases, plumbing and drainage, and food inspections and offensive trades. A tenement house law in the 1890s led to its further expansion. This same period also witnessed the establishment of laboratories in health departments at both local and state levels.[6]

The growth of other health departments in the East was similar to, if somewhat slower than, that of the department in New York City. Baltimore appointed a building inspector in early 1871, empowered its health commissioner to require vaccination in 1882, appointed its first plumbing inspector in 1883, began regulating tenements in 1886, and appointed three food inspectors in 1894. Yet Baltimore generally followed a laissez-faire policy toward contagious diseases, with the exception of smallpox, and the city provided only a few hospital beds for the poor.[7]

Newark and Camden, New Jersey, are probably representative of moderate-sized cities and towns in the East. Newark established a board of health in 1857, but the board apparently did nothing for the next twenty years. Between 1870 and 1880 Newark's spending for public health amounted to only seven cents per person. In 1892 two able health officials were appointed, and, with strong support from the local medical society, they made the Newark Health Department into a much more effective agency.[8] Camden, which grew from 20,045 in 1870 to 41,659 in 1880 to become the forty-fourth largest city in the country, had only one mile of properly paved streets as of 1886. The city council had established a sanitary committee in 1872, but the committee was reluctant to take any but the most primitive sanitary measures. An independent board of health under the direction of a physician was not established until 1886—and this development came several years after a state public health law had made the appointment of a board mandatory.[9]

Midwestern cities were generally smaller and of more recent origin than those of the East. Partly for these reasons, their overall death rates tended to be lower, although there were exceptions. The St. Louis Board of Health, established in 1867, consisted of the mayor, the police commissioner, the health officer, and two physicians. In 1871 the sanitary police, formerly part of the regular police force, were incorporated into the city's health department. The department at this time was responsible for investigating contagious diseases, sanitary matters, and the quality of milk and was also in charge of the city's poorhouse, its quarantine and smallpox hospitals, and the city's insane asylum. In 1871 the department's expenses, exclusive of those for the hospitals, were $17,056. Of this sum, almost $6,000 was paid for the removal of offal from the city's sewers and for the scavenger boats which dumped the city's wastes into the Mississippi River. By 1880 the total budget of the health department, including the costs of the city hospitals and related institutions, was $272,801. This included $16,400 for the board of health and another $5,000 for the "abatement of nuisances."[10]

St. Louis was the first city in the United States to attempt to deal with the problem of prostitution and venereal disease. In 1870 the city council passed what was termed the Social Evil Ordinance, a law providing for the licensing and medical inspection of prostitutes. A physician was assigned to each of the city's six districts. Women found to be infected with venereal disease were sent to a special Social Evil Hospital financed by license fees levied on brothels and individual prostitutes. The local medical society was somewhat ambivalent at first toward this reform, but in 1871 gave its tentative support. The ordinance created a stir throughout the United States and led medical journals for the first time to discuss the subject at length. Church members and other groups in St. Louis were outraged, and in 1874 they pressured the state legislature into repealing the clause in the city's charter allowing it to regulate bawdy houses.[11]

The St. Louis Board of Health, which fully supported the law, deplored its repeal in its annual report for 1874, calling the repeal "a hasty and inconsiderate action" taken before the value of the law could be clearly established. It pointed out that under the ordinance the number of prostitutes and the incidence of venereal disease had greatly diminished, and that one-third of the women entering the Social Evil Hospital had been reformed. Four years later the health department published statistics showing that the number of prostitutes found diseased had been far lower under the inspection system than without it, and once again the health officials regretted that the law had been repealed. By this date, however, the "purity movement" was in full swing, and little would be done about venereal disease until well into the twentieth century.[12]

Chicago, which was emerging as a major industrial city, suffered all the health problems of rapid urbanization, but unfortunately it did not have the reform tradition of cities such as New York and Boston. Although it had established a good health department under the impetus of a strong health reform movement in the late 1860s, the city government proved unable to handle the city's growing problems. In 1894 the United States Commissioner of Labor asserted that sanitary conditions in Chicago were worse than those in the major eastern cities.[13] Louisville, Kentucky, and Cleveland, Ohio, were far more representative of midwestern cities. In Louisville, where the population increased from 100,000 in 1871 to 150,000 in 1874, the board of health reported a decline in overall mortality from 23.0 per 1,000 in 1871 to 16.5 in 1874. Cleveland, which was about the same size as Louisville in 1874 but grew much faster, estimated its annual death rate from 1873 to 1886 at between 18 to 19 per 1,000.[14] New York City's death rate in these same years declined from about 30 per 1,000 to 26.

Midwestern urban areas, like their counterparts in the East, were subject to the vicissitudes of politics. Cincinnati established a fairly effective health department shortly after the Civil War, and the health of its residents ranked with that of the inhabitants of Cleveland and Louisville. Yet in 1883 a *JAMA* correspondent reported that political maneuvering in the city had resulted in the replacement of an excellent health board with one made up "of five saloon-keepers and an advertising, so-called, doctor." The writer added that the new board had selected "an oldtime politician, a chronic place-seeker, who at one time was in the lumber business, as the Health Officer." The correspondent finally noted that there was little sickness in the town and that the state legislature was expected to remove the new board.[15]

The South was slow to recover from the Civil War and Reconstruction, and few advances were made in public health there until the closing years of the nineteenth century. The Louisiana State Board of Health, which was essentially a New Orleans board, devoted its main energy to dealing with repeated smallpox and yellow fever epidemics. Since yellow fever was the major threat, most of the board's efforts were directed toward enforcing the quarantine regulations designed to keep this pestilence at bay, a statement which holds true for most of the health boards in the Gulf Coast and southeastern port cities. The Louisiana board did make occasional inspections and published a number of studies, and it may have helped reduce the number of yellow fever outbreaks in New Orleans, but it did little else to improve the health of the state's citizens. The limited sanitary measures taken in the 1880s and 1890s in New Orleans were largely the work of citizens' sanitary groups, but private funds alone could scarcely support a sanitary program for a city its size.

Memphis, one of the larger interior cities in the South, was an exception to the general picture of slow progress in southern public health. Along with New Orleans, Memphis shared an unenviable reputation for being one of the filthiest places in the United States. To make matters worse, in 1872 its annual death rate of 46.6 per 1,000 was the highest of any major city in the country. In theory Memphis had a board of health, but neither it nor the mayor and council felt any real sense of responsibility for community health. It took two major yellow fever epidemics, one in 1873 and another in 1878, to shake the city officials out of their lethargy. By the time of the second outbreak, the city's population had been reduced to about 48,000. On this occasion the fever sickened half the population and killed over 5,000. As the terrified inhabitants fled the city, they carried yellow fever up the Mississippi as far north as Louisville and Cincinnati. The Memphis municipal government collapsed completely, and in January 1879 the governor of Tennessee replaced the mayor and council with a commission form of government.

Horrified by the inordinate loss of life and aware that Memphis steadily had been losing population, the city's business and professional men decided that something had to be done. Fortunately, in response to the 1878 yellow fever epidemic, which had ravaged almost every southern port and spread far up the Mississippi Valley, a national board of health had been established, and Memphis promptly appealed to the board for help. Headed by Dr. John S. Billings, a group of health and sanitary experts from the national board met in Memphis on November 22, 1879. Among their immediate recommendations was the construction of a sewer system. Within a matter of weeks the governor had convened the state legislature and provided the new city government with the authority to move ahead with a sewer program. In the meantime, eight physician medical inspectors and twenty-six subinspectors began a house-to-house sanitary survey of Memphis.[16]

The survey presented a devastating picture of sanitary conditions in Memphis. Most dwelling places were described as being in poor condition; the basements in over 21 percent of the city's buildings were ill-ventilated or damp or else had water standing in them; foul and overflowing privies were found in 6,000 homes; and only 215 buildings were connected to the privately owned sewers of Memphis. The city's entire sanitary force consisted of nine carts, thirteen mules, and sixteen men who were expected to collect garbage and street refuse once a week. In fact, only half the work reported was done, and four of the city's ten wards received virtually no service. The small and inadequate private water works had gone into bankruptcy in 1879, although its demise had had little impact, since the majority of citizens relied on cisterns and shallow wells— most of which were adjacent to privies.

Determined to improve the reputation of Memphis, the city's businessmen and leading citizens employed the nation's chief sanitary expert, Colonel George E. Waring, to plan and construct a sewer system.

The work began under Waring in 1880 and was taken over by the city engineer in 1883. By 1886 all but the two poorest wards had sewers. In the meantime a citizens' group, the Auxiliary Sanitary Association, had promoted a public latrine, and, as the sewer lines were extended, most of the privies were replaced with water closets. After a long struggle with the private water company, a new private company took over, and by 1887 it was able to provide Memphis with an ample supply of good water from artesian wells. In the meantime an effective garbage system was organized, streets were paved, and hogs and cattle were driven from public thoroughfares. Under a strong board of health with full authority, nuisances were removed and health and sanitary laws strictly enforced. By 1890 Memphis had been transformed from one of the dirtiest cities into one of the cleanest. Before the bacteriological revolution had affected the nation, an effective sanitary program had reduced the mortality rate in Memphis from 46.6 per 1,000 in 1872 to 21.5 in 1889.

Atlanta, the city which best represents the rise of the New South after Reconstruction, was affected only indirectly by the 1878 yellow fever epidemic, but its businessmen learned a lesson from it. They came to realize that health and prosperity were intimately related, and they, too, embarked on a sanitary program. Without the shock of a major epidemic, sanitary progress was slower, but by the 1890s Atlanta had an ample supply of water and most of the city was supplied with sewers. The Atlanta Board of Health, while not quite as effective as the one in Memphis, functioned reasonably well for its day. It must be remembered, however, that even in Atlanta and Memphis, two of the most progressive southern cities, the sanitary reforms largely excluded those sections of the city occupied by blacks.[17]

In the prebacterial era, the age of a city and the density of its population clearly affected general health. This fact becomes clear as one examines the cities of the Midwest and West. Urban death rates in the Midwest were well below those in most eastern cities, and the lowest rates were found on the West Coast. For example, the San Francisco health officer reported in 1877 that epidemics of smallpox and diphtheria in the past year had raised the annual death rate from 17.6 to 20.6 per 1,000. He blamed the epidemics on the 30,000 Chinese living in the city, "who disregard our sanitary laws." At that time the city had a population of 300,000.[18] Newark, with about half that population, in this same year had a death rate of almost 30 per 1,000. For the fiscal year 1887–88, when San Francisco had grown larger, the mortality rate was 18.27 per 1,000. Seattle, a much smaller city, had an annual rate of 12.47 in 1884 and 11.5 in 1891.[19]

Both of these West Coast cities enjoyed equable climates and occupied areas that had not been subjected to generations of pollution. They also had relatively good health departments, and San Francisco had the advice and support of one of the better state health boards. San Francisco's health problems were complicated, like those of the major East Coast cities, by a large influx of illiterate immigrants from rural areas. The wide cultural gap between the sanitary practices of the Chinese immigrants and the other Californians made the work of the city health department more difficult, and undoubtedly contributed to increasing the city's death rate.

As California's first major city, San Francisco began constructing its sewer system before engineers had begun to apply their knowledge to sanitary problems. By 1876 the city had over 74 miles of brick sewers—far more than most eastern cities of the same size. In that year a survey by William Humphreys showed that the sewer lines did not conform to the natural terrain and were too large for proper drainage. His recommendations to unify the system, install smaller sewer pipes, and extend the outflow into San Francisco Bay were accepted. The major criticism of Humphrey's sewer system was that during the dry season there was not enough rainfall to clear the sewers.[20]

San Francisco's health department, as established in 1870, consisted of a five-man board, a health officer, a deputy health officer, a secretary, and three inspectors. The duties of the health inspectors were to recommend sewers where needed and to check on nuisances, contagious diseases, and citizens' complaints. One inspector was assigned to supervise the city's markets and food supply. In succeeding years the number of the department's health inspectors and other employees steadily increased.[21]

In overview, one of the most striking features of the 1870–90 period was the growth in the number and effectiveness of municipal health departments. The sanitary revolution in America was in full swing, and health and sanitation were virtually synonymous. Sanitary engineering came into its own, and many large and medium cities and towns expanded their old sewer and water systems or else built new ones. Even in those municipalities where little progress was made, citizens' sanitary associations were demanding action. The collection of garbage and refuse was systematized, and health departments began to broaden their activities.

Possibly the key factor in all this was a rising standard of living, without which municipalities could not have afforded the enormous capital costs of the sewer and water systems nor the steadily increasing operating costs of health and sanitary programs. The constant fall in urban mortality rates beginning in the 1870s, well before advances in bacteriology and other areas of medicine could be applied on a broad scale, attests in part to the efficacy of the sanitary movement. The improvement in health, however, also rested on rising living standards, which meant better food, housing, and working conditions for urban workers. These improvements, of course, were purely relative, since living conditions in city tenements, when compared with those of today, were still exceedingly grim, and life expectancy was short.

One of the obvious lessons of this period, drawn from experiences with contagious diseases, was that no community was an island. With yellow fever striking the southern coastal states and spreading up the Mississippi Valley, and with recurrent outbreaks of smallpox and Asiatic cholera plaguing the entire country, state officials took it upon themselves to proclaim statewide quarantines. The sanitary movement also demonstrated the interdependence of communities. Water pollution, for example, affected not only the community responsible for the pollution but also other communities dependent upon the polluted water source. In addition, sanitation was a moral cause for most of the early reformers, and they envisioned state action as a means of spreading the good word. Not surprisingly, the emergence of municipal health boards in the immediate post–Civil War years led to demands for state boards.

Most of the early health agencies at the local level functioned primarily as advisory bodies. The New York City Metropolitan Board was the first to be given wide authority and to use this authority with effect, but most other city health boards were dependent upon the cooperation of municipal councils or other city departments to enforce their regulations. Too often this cooperation was virtually nonexistent, and health officials in frustration began demanding the right to enforce their own rules and regulations. This experience led many health reformers to insist that the proposed state health boards be given wide authority over local communities. In a report to the first session of the American Public Health Association in 1873 Dr. Stephen Smith of the New York City Health Department insisted that state boards must be given the power "to compel execution of sanitary works in towns where they are neglected." The rights of the individual should be subordinated to the welfare of society, he declared, adding, "Private rights should not be allowed to create or maintain public wrongs."[22] On the other hand, Dr. Elisha Harris, also of the New York City Health Department, warned that a state board would need to move cautiously because of the public prejudice against stringent regulations and the jealousy with which local units guarded their autonomy. The prime need for all health agencies, he said, was to educate the public.[23]

The APHA, from the beginning, was a staunch advocate of state boards. At one of its early meetings a standing committee was appointed on state and local sanitary organizations. In 1875 this committee submitted a model act for a state board of health, which the APHA promptly sent to all state governments. The proposed legislative bill recommended that the members of this model board, half of whom were to be physicians, should receive expenses but no compensation. The board would have some limited powers but was essentially intended to gather and disseminate information on health and sanitary matters.[24] Despite strong support from the APHA and the AMA, state and local medical societies, municipal health agencies, and citizens' health and sanitary associations, in most states health boards came into existence only after years of struggle.

The Louisiana State Board of Health, technically the first state board, was established in 1855 as the result of a series of major yellow fever epidemics. For the rest of the century, however, its jurisdiction rarely extended beyond New Orleans, and its main function was to serve as a quarantine agency. The second state board, and the first effective one, was established in Massachusetts in 1869. Dr. Henry I. Bowditch, a dedicated reformer who became chairman of the first board, told AMA delegates in 1874 that the creation of the Massachusetts Board of Health was the conclusion of a thirty-year war with politicians.[25] While it was true that he and others had been advocating a board for many years, the law providing for it passed almost without debate as part of a reorganization of the state's administrative apparatus. The legislative committee proposing a "State Board of Health and Vital Statistics" said it should have the power to investigate and advise on matters pertaining to public health, "but without any authoritative control or right of active interference." Other than an amendment authorizing the board to investigate the use and effects of liquor, the original bill was quickly enacted into law.[26]

Massachusetts was fortunate in the choice of members for its first state health board. Three of them were well-educated physicians, and the other four were a historian, a lawyer, a civil engineer, and a businessman, respectively. Dr. Henry I. Bowditch, a leading physician-reformer, was chosen as chairman, and Dr. George Derby, lecturer on hygiene at Harvard and editor of the state's registration reports, was made secretary. One of the first decisions of the board was to move against the slaughterhouses, one of the most obnoxious of the so-called "noxious trades." By attempting to remove a glaring public nuisance, the board won widespread public support and was able to persuade the Massachusetts legislature in 1871 to pass an offensive trades act. This measure gave the board authority to enforce its recommendations, even to the point of closing slaughterhouses if it deemed this action necessary. In these early years it conducted a series of investigations into tenement conditions, smallpox and vaccination (subjects discussed in every early report), food adulteration, water pollution, ventilation, and sewerage.[27]

While tackling the slaughterhouse problem, the state health board also began sending circulars to prominent physicians in Massachusetts towns without health boards, requesting information and urging them to push for a local board. By 1869 most of the larger cities in Massachusetts already had health boards, and the state had one of the best records for collecting vital statistics. Under the active leadership of Bowditch and Derby, the number of local health boards rose steadily in ensuing years. In 1878 the state board was given general supervision over water supplies and authorized to issue orders to prevent pollution. The first period of major activity ended in 1879, when, for a combination of political reasons and from financial stringency, the state board of health was merged into a "Board of Health, Lunacy, and Charity." Although Bowditch was appointed to the new board, he resigned shortly thereafter, convinced that health affairs would suffer from political interference.

As Bowditch had feared, the new board ran into problems, although the board's health committee functioned relatively untouched by the scandals that plagued the Massachusetts state administration in the 1880s. It continued to gather information and give assistance to local boards. In 1882 a pure food and drug act conferred additional power on the state's health officials. By the 1880s water pollution and sewage disposal were becoming major problems, ones that had become of increasing concern to the board. In 1886 the board was given a liberal appropriation to investigate and conduct experiments with water purification and the processing of sewage. In addition, towns and cities contructing new water or sewer systems were required to consult with the state board. The net effect was that by the 1890s Massachusetts was leading the way in the area of sanitary engineering.

In 1886 the Massachusetts Board of Health was reconstituted as a separate unit, and, under the leadership of Henry Pickering Walcott from 1886 to 1914, it continued as a model for other state boards. As Barbara G. Rosenkrantz points out, although the new board established in 1886 was given additional legal powers, it relied largely upon persuasion and education to enforce its decrees. The high quality of its leadership and its obvious concern for community welfare had created such strong support for the board that opposing interests were reluctant to clash with it.[28]

The state of Michigan modeled its board of health on that of Massachusetts. Michigan did not have as many colleges and universities as Massachusetts, nor did it have the long tradition of reform that characterized the New England area, but in some respects Michigan was more progressive than Massachusetts. The founder of the Michigan board was Dr. Henry B. Baker, who had been involved in army hygiene and sanitation during the Civil War and subsequently served on the state board of agriculture. He was already convinced of the need for a state board of health, and, after reading a copy of the first report of the Massachusetts Board of Health, he persuaded the Michigan State Medical Society to help promote a similar agency for Michigan. In the meantime he was appointed to help the secretary of state compile vital statistics. His medical partner, Dr. Ira H. Bartholomew, was president of the state medical society and won election to the state legislature. The fight for a state health agency was already gaining public support because of the frequency with which illuminating oil was exploding and a national scare about the use of arsenic in wallpaper and other products. Suffice to say, with Bartholomew leading the fight in the legislature, in 1873 the Michigan State Board of Health was established.[29]

The first members appointed to the Michigan board by the governor were four physicians and two ministers. Dr. Baker was chosen secretary, a position he held from 1873 to 1905. The choice of secretary could hardly have been better since Baker was a dedicated public health worker and the state's leading advocate of vital statistics. Due to Baker's influence, from the beginning the Michigan board was given responsibility for gathering vital statistics. It was also to conduct sanitary investigations and to draw up sanitary laws and regulations. Reflecting public concerns, the first three papers published by the board dealt with illuminating oil, poisonous papers, and the hygiene of school buildings.[30] The Michigan board members, as was the case in Massachusetts, were consistently capable and distinguished men. The first president was a socially conscious physician; the second, a professor of chemistry interested in school health; the third, a lawyer and member of the legislature, helped to strengthen state health laws; and the fourth, who held membership on a school board and on a county board of supervisors, promoted state sanitary conventions.[31]

Following the example of Massachusetts, the Michigan board promptly began contacting all cities, townships, and villages asking for reports on health and sanitary conditions. In the early years less than one-third of the localities responded to the board's queries, but in 1877 the legislature enacted a law requiring each township to appoint a health officer, leading to a rapid increase in the number of reports.[32] The law created a need for qualified health officers and led the board in 1878 to conduct examinations in "Sanitary Science." Candidates were subjected to rigorous testing in biology, diseases, physical science, sanitary engineering, sanitary inspection, and sanitary law. Eight candidates were examined in 1879, but Michigan was too far ahead of its time, and within two years a lack of interest forced the state board to give up the program.[33]

Although the Michigan board had a limited budget of only about four thousand dollars annually for the first few years, it conducted a wide range of investigations, published many pamphlets and monographs, and conducted an effective health education campaign. Baker was convinced, as were many contemporary physicians, that meteorology lay at the basis of many epidemics, and the Michigan board, which was far from alone in taking this tack, gathered detailed statistics attempting to correlate meteorological data with disease. Fortunately this work did not interfere with the far more productive task of gathering vital statistics and promoting sanitation.

As the state law requiring all Michigan communities to establish health boards gradually took effect, the state board, after considerable preliminary work, held two sanitary conventions early in 1880, one in Detroit and a second one in Grand Rapids. They were designed to inform and encourage local health officials and to educate the public. These proved so successful that over the next eighteen years some forty-five of these conventions were held.[34] As of 1883, the Michigan board had sixteen standing committees dealing with a wide range of health and sanitation topics and was in regular contact with nearly 1,400 local health boards. Local health work was further strengthened in this year by a law requiring a minimum compensation of two dollars per day for local health officers.[35]

As the Michigan board moved more and more into the regulation of food and water, a special committee of board members conferred with the regents of the University of Michigan about establishing a state laboratory. A joint petition to the state legislature resulted in an appropriation in 1887, and Dr. Victor C. Vaughan, who was to become an outstanding public health figure, was appointed director of the first Michigan "State Laboratory of Hygiene." Although the laboratory did not open officially until 1888, as early as October 1886 Dr. Vaughan began studies on cases of milk poisoning, and in 1887 started work on typhoid.[36] Like its counterpart in Massachusetts, the Michigan state board began auspiciously and capitalized on this felicitous beginning to maintain a leading rank among state health boards.

On the West Coast the California public health program got off to an excellent start with the establishment of a state board of health in 1870. The members of the board, all physicians, were instructed to collect vital statistics (the permanent secretary assumed the duty of registrar), to consider legislation respecting liquor, and to investigate the subject of ventilation and other sanitary questions. At its first meeting, the board established standing committees on schools and public institutions, vital statistics, and intoxicating liquors. In its first two years reports were prepared on school diseases, consumption, female hygiene, burial grounds, the water quality of Lake Tahoe, and the "Social Evil" problem among the Chinese. In the succeeding years the board recommended the establishment of a national sanitary bureau, the creation of chairs of hygiene in all medical schools, and the organization of a national health council for state boards of health.[37]

Despite the California board's initial success, it was not able to mobilize public support as was the case in some other states. Its urgent appeals for improved registration laws and a measure requiring all towns and cities to appoint a health board went unheeded until the closing years of the century. The board's biennial report for 1890–92 complained that the board's duties were too general and its functions purely advisory, and as late as 1896 only 25 of the 57 counties in California were reporting vital statistics.[38]

In addition to the foregoing states, a number of others established relatively effective health boards. Minnesota's board of health, created in 1872, followed the Michigan pattern of promoting local health boards and keeping in contact with them, and the Illinois board in 1885 conducted a statewide survey of sanitary conditions.[39] A good many state boards undertook vaccination programs against smallpox and investigated consumption (pulmonary tuberculosis), malaria, and other diseases— including those of cattle. They also studied food adulteration, immigrant diseases, and climatology.

By 1900 most states had established health boards, but the majority of these boards were powerless and ineffective. The chief function of a good many of them was simply to license physicians. Even the best of them rarely had an annual budget of as much as $5,000 before 1900, and few had any authority. In North Carolina the state legislature designated the entire state medical society as its board of health and appropriated a board budget of $100. Although the board was established in 1877, it was 1909 before it had a budget large enough to employ a full-time health officer.[40] When the Kentucky State Board of Health in 1883 called a meeting of county and local health officers to organize a sanitary convention, only four of the seven state board members and twelve local officials attended. Dr. A. T. McCormack wrote in 1918 that his father, as health officer, and his mother, as clerk, constituted the entire Kentucky Board of Health from 1878 to 1910.[41]

The Kansas board complained in 1891 that it was purely advisory and had no authority over sanitary affairs. Two years later, when, under the threat of a cholera outbreak, the board spent $2,200 for sanitary work, the state refused to pay the board's expenses, causing the entire board to resign.[42] In 1885 and 1887 the Missouri legislature failed to appropriate any funds for its board of health, and the governor did not bother to replace board members whose term of office had expired. Seven years later the Missouri Board of Health reported that the state still had no local health boards nor any reports of vital statistics.[43] If state health board members generally commanded little respect, the situation was even worse for local health officials. A statement in a late nineteenth-century board of health report best characterizes the local health officer's status:

"As a general rule he labors without funds, without legal powers, without aid, and without sympathy."[44] Despite this discouraging picture, good progress was made in several states, and nearly all of them at least recognized the need for a state health board.

NOTES

1. John Duffy, *A History of Public Health in New York City, 1866–1966* (New York, 1974), 73.

2. Ibid., 77–82.

3. For this and much of the succeeding material on New York City I have drawn on my history of public health in New York City.

4. These private agencies included such organizations as the Tribune Fresh Air Fund, the Evening World Summer Camps, St. John's Guild, and the Hebrew Sanitarium.

5. *President Chandler and the New York City Health Department, 1866–1883* (New York, 1883), 2–3.

6. For a quick survey of the origins of the sanitary bureau see A. E. Abrahmson, The Sanitary Bureau—a Pioneer Unit in Public Health, New York City Health Department MS.

7. William T. Howard, *Public Health Administration and the Natural History of Diseases in Baltimore, Maryland, 1797–1920* (Washington, D.C., 1924), 55–58, 70–72, 152.

8. Stuart Galishoff, *Safeguarding the Public Health: Newark, 1895–1918* (Westport, Conn., 1975), 10–16.

9. Sam Alewitz, "The Life and Times of Camden," *Journal of the Medical Society of New Jersey* 81 (1984):741–42.

10. *Fourth Annual Report of the Board of Health of the City of St. Louis* (St. Louis, 1871), 4; *The Mayor's Message, with Accompanying Documents to the City . . . of St. Louis, 1871* (St. Louis, 1871), 21; *Annual Report of the Health Commissioner of . . . St. Louis . . . 1879–80* (St. Louis, 1880), 6.

11. For the best account see John C. Burnham, "Medical Inspection of Prostitutes in America in the Nineteenth Century: The St. Louis Experiment and Its Sequel," *Bull. Hist. Med.* 45 (1971):203–18.

12. *Seventh Annual Report . . . Board of Health . . . St. Louis* (St. Louis, 1874), 28–29; *First Annual Report, Health Department of . . . St. Louis Under the Provisions of the New Charter . . . 1878* (St. Louis, 1878), 20.

13. Thomas N. Bonner, *Medicine in Chicago, 1850–1950* (Madison, Wis., 1957), 20.

14. Annual Report of the Louisville Board of Health for the Year Ending February 24, 1871, and Annual Report . . . December 31, 1874, Microfilm Records of the WPA Kentucky Medical History Project, reel 25, University of Louisville Kornhauser Health Sciences Library (hereafter cited as Microfilm Records of the WPA Ky. Med. Hist. Research Project); *First Annual Report of the State Board of Health . . . Ohio . . . October 31, 1886*, 158, 161.

15. "Cincinnati Letter," *JAMA* 1 (1883):149.

16. John H. Ellis, "Memphis' Sanitary Revolution, 1880–1890," *Tennessee Historical Quarterly* 23 (1964):59–72; Thomas H. Baker, "The Yellow Fever Epidemic of 1878 in Memphis, Tennessee," *Bull. Hist. Med.* 42 (1968):241–64.

17. John H. Ellis, "Businessmen and Public Health in the Urban South during the Nineteenth Century: New Orleans, Memphis, and Atlanta," *Bull. Hist. Med.* 44 (1970):199–212, 346–71.

18. *Report of the Health Officer of the City and County of San Francisco for the Year Ending June 30, 1877* (San Francisco, 1877), 3, 13.

19. Reports of the Seattle Health Department prior to 1900, Report of City Health Officer for 1884, University of Washington Library TSS; *Report of the Board of Health, City of Seattle for the Year Ending December 31, 1891* (Seattle, 1892), 3.

20. William P. Humphreys, *Report on a System of Sewerage for the City of San Francisco* (San Francisco, 1876), in Pamphlets on San Francisco, vol. 8, no. 5, Bancroft Library; I. H. Stallard, *The Problem of the Sewerage of San Francisco: A Polyclinic Lecture* (San Francisco, 1892), 14–15.

21. *An Act to Establish a Quarantine and Sanitary Laws for the City and County of San Francisco, and Orders and Regulations Adopted by the Board of Health,* pp. 3–4, in Pamphlets on San Francisco, vol. 8, no. 1 (San Francisco, 1870), Bancroft Library.

22. Stephen Smith, "Reports upon Physiological Subjects Relating to Hygiene," in *Selections from Public Health Reports . . . of the APHA (1873–1883),* 15.

23. Elisha Harris, *General Health Laws and Local Ordinances, Considered with Reference to State and Local Sanitary Organization* (Cambridge, Mass., 1874).

24. Harold M. Cavins, "The National Quarantine and Sanitary Conventions of 1857 to 1860 and the Beginnings of the APHA," *Bull. Hist. Med.* 13 (1943):423.

25. Howard D. Kramer, "History of the Public Health Movement in the United States, 1850 to 1900" (Ph.D. diss., University of Iowa, 1942), 99.

26. Barbara G. Rosenkrantz, *Public Health and the State: Changing Views in Massachusetts, 1842–1936* (Cambridge, Mass., 1972), 52–53.

27. George C. Whipple, *State Sanitation: A Review of the Work of the Massachusetts State Board of Health* (rpt., New York, 1977), 1:41–53.

28. Rosenkrantz, *Public Health and the State,* 87–88.

29. Theodore R. MacClure, "The State Board of Health and a Quarter Century of Public Health Work in Michigan," *Teachers' Sanitary Bulletin* 1 (1898):51–53.

30. *First Annual Report of the Secretary of the State Board of Health of the State of Michigan . . . September 30, 1873* (Lansing, 1874), 2–3, 7, 31.

31. Ola G. Hylton, "A History of the Public Health Movement in Michigan, 1888–1913" (Ph.D. diss., University of Michigan, 1943), 5–8.

32. *Fifth Annual Report of the Secretary of the State Board of Health of the State of Michigan . . . September 30, 1877* (Lansing, 1878), xiv–xix.

33. *Seventh Annual Report . . . Board of Health . . . Michigan . . . 1879* (Lansing, 1880), 511–12; MacClure, "The State Board of Health in Michigan," 61.

34. *Eighth Annual Report . . . Board of Health . . . Michigan . . . 1880* (Lansing, 1881), 184ff.; MacClure, "The State Board of Health in Michigan," 68.

35. Foster Pratt, "Address of the Chairman . . . ," *JAMA* 1 (1883):163; MacClure, "The State Board of Health in Michigan," 57.

36. *Fifteenth Annual Report . . . Board of Health . . . Michigan . . . 1887* (Lansing, 1888), xxxix–xlv, 1.

37. *First Biennial Report of the State Board of Health of California for the Years 1870 and 1871* (Sacramento, 1871), 1, 3–10, 15, 20–21, 32–33, 43–46; *Second Biennial Report . . . 1871, 1872, and 1873* (Sacramento, 1873), 8, 21–23.

38. *Twelfth Biennial Report . . . Board of Health . . . California . . . 1890 to 1892* (Sacramento, 1892), 5; *Fourteenth Biennial Report . . . 1894 to 1896* (Sacramento, 1896), 5–6.

39. Philip D. Jordan, *The People's Health: A History of Public Health in Minnesota to 1948* (St. Paul, 1953), 73; *Eighth Annual Report of the State Board of Health of Illinois, 1885* (Springfield, 1886), ix–xv.

40. Benjamin E. Washburn, *A History of the North Carolina State Board of Health, 1877–1925* (Raleigh, 1966), 1, 10.

41. Editorial, *Louisville Medical News* 15 (1883):167; Dr. A.T. McCormack, untitled, *Southern Medical Journal* 11 (1918):624–29. Both of these citations are from the Microfilm Records of the WPA Ky. Med. Hist. Research Project.

42. *Seventh Annual Report of the State Board of Health of the State of Kansas, 1891* (Topeka, 1892), ix.

43. *Annual Report of the State Board of Health of Missouri . . . for 1888* (Jefferson City, 1890), 7; *Annual Report . . . for 1893,* 6–7; *Annual Report . . . for 1894,* 1ff.

44. Harriet S. Pfister, *Kansas State Board of Health* (Lawrence, 1955), 35.

11

Hospitals and the Federal Government's Role in Public Health

The hospital—as a place to undergo surgical procedures or receive treatment for major illnesses—is essentially a twentieth-century development. For most of American history hospitals were designed to care for the sick poor or for ill and destitute strangers. Respectable citizens, until the early twentieth century, expected to be born, treated, nursed, and allowed to die in their own homes. Even aside from the stigma of charity associated with them, hospitals generally had an exceedingly poor reputation, looked upon by rich and poor alike as a place where the sick poor were sent to die.

The forerunners of today's hospitals were the almshouses and pesthouses of the eighteenth century. Out of necessity the almshouses had to provide some medical care for sick inmates. The early pesthouses, on the other hand, rarely provided anything but custodial care, since their main purpose was to protect the community by isolating those sick with infectious diseases. Exactly when the first American institution designed exclusively to cure the sick was founded is a subject of considerable debate among historians, as was noted in chapter 2. The two main claimants to the title of oldest hospital in the United States are Charity Hospital in New Orleans, founded in 1736, and the Pennsylvania Hospital, which dates back to 1752. Both were charitable institutions, but they were established to provide medical treatment for the sick rather than to care for the indigent, aged, and chronically ill.

Regardless of which hospital is the oldest—and there are other claimants—by the end of the eighteenth century nearly all towns of any size had an almshouse, usually occupied by the aged and chronically sick poor, and a pesthouse. As of 1795 only two hospitals were functioning in the original thirteen colonies: the Pennsylvania Hospital, already mentioned, and the New York Hospital, which opened its doors in 1791. Both institutions were private but received state assistance. The next thirty years saw the development of several municipal and many private hospitals. Massachusetts General in Boston, Bellevue in New York City, the Philadelphia Hospital, and Charity in New Orleans were typical of muncipal institutions, although Charity was taken over by the Louisiana territorial government in 1811. Most of the private hospitals were charitable institutions, but a few accepted private patients—primarily travelers, businessmen, and other well-to-do individuals away from home.

In the eighteenth and nineteenth centuries the state of medical knowledge precluded hospitals from doing much more than providing nursing care, and most of this care was of a low order. Except for those who belonged to religious orders, nurses tended to belong to the worst elements in society. Descriptions of many nineteenth-century hospitals almost defy credulity. Patients of all ages and disorders were often jammed together in crowded wards, and the air was thick with the smell of putrefying wounds, dirty linen, and all of the other odors associated with unwashed humanity. Small wonder that down to the end of the nineteenth century the poor often hid their sick to prevent them from being sent to hospitals.

Until the Civil War hospitals were restricted largely to the major cities. For example, neither New Jersey nor Indiana had a single hospital in the antebellum years. In 1857, Newark, New Jersey, with a population of 60,000, had forty churches but not one hospital. Milwaukee in 1848 had one hospital operated by the Sisters of Charity.[1] The Civil War, which coincided with the advent of anesthesia and antiseptic surgery, gave a sharp impetus to the growth of both private and public hospitals.

From the standpoint of medical care for the urban poor, a more significant development was the rapid growth of dispensaries. Many of these were founded by philanthropic individuals, while others were established by medical schools and groups of physicians. A dispensary offered physicians a chance to hone their skills in a particular medical specialty and to give their apprentices and students opportunities for clinical experience. Whatever the motives of the founders, by the end of the nineteenth century dispensaries provided a major share of medical care for the urban lower-income groups.

Since the majority of hospitals and dispensaries were founded by philanthropic laypersons, these institutions tended to be managed by lay boards. In addition, it was customary to allow donors or patrons to designate which patients should be admitted. As the state of medicine improved and physicians achieved a more professional status, they clashed with the lay administrators, and in the early twentieth century they gained control of the hospitals. Over and above the problem of lay control, the dispensaries constituted what the medical profession felt was a grave threat to their economic well-being. Estimates vary, but by the 1890s dispensaries in New York City alone were providing free medical care to almost a quarter of the city's population.[2] Physicians, whose average income was low at this time, accused the dispensaries of treating patients who could afford private fees. In the 1890s the AMA and local medical societies launched an all-out assault on the dispensaries, and this attack, combined with changes in medicine that outdated much of dispensary practice, led to their virtual elimination by World War I.

Hospitals provided the opening wedge by which the national government entered the field of community health care, starting with the colonial era. The life of seamen in the colonial days was dangerous and hard, and the British practice dating back to the sixteenth century of making some provision for sick and injured seamen was introduced into the American colonies in the eighteenth century. In 1708 the Virginia Council ordered that a house be made available for the use of sick seamen, the expenses to be paid from the King's revenues. In 1780 the Virginia legislature passed a law requiring that nine pence a month "hospital money" be collected from all seamen and marines in the state. A similar law was enacted by South Carolina in 1785 and by North Carolina in 1789.[3] Massachusetts, Pennsylvania, and other colonies also made some provision for sick and disabled seamen.

One of the first measures introduced into Congress was one to provide medical care for seamen, proposed in 1789. Although nine years elapsed before effective action was taken, in 1790 Congress did pass a law requiring all merchant vessels with ten or more crewmen to carry a medicine chest complete with instructions. Partly as a result of political infighting, it was not until 1798 that Congress enacted a law creating the United States Marine Hospital Service. It required ship captains arriving in port to deduct twenty cents a month from the pay of every crewman aboard their ships, the money to be paid to the collector of the port. These funds were to be used for the care of sick and disabled seamen in existing hospitals or other institutions. If any surplus money was accumulated, the President was given discretion to use it to build hospitals. A year later an amendment extended the Hospital Service Act to include the officers and men of the United States Navy.[4] The navy soon discovered that allowing naval personnel to be treated along with civilians was not satisfactory. Aside from the problem of the dubious character of some hospitals, the naval officers lost control over their men; a good many naval patients lingered in the civilian hospitals, and many of them simply disappeared. On the insistence of the navy, Congress in 1811 enacted a law authorizing the creation of separate naval hospitals.[5]

The first medical officer of the Marine Hospital Service, Dr. Thomas Welsh, was appointed to the Boston district by President Adams in 1799. He had charge of a temporary hospital for several years until a new building was erected in 1804. In the meantime, in 1801 the federal government purchased a hospital that the Commonwealth of Virginia had provided for seamen in Norfolk. Another hospital was erected in Newport, Rhode Island, and a fourth was authorized for Charleston, South Carolina. The Charleston situation illustrates much of what was wrong with the hospital service in the early years. The United States Treasury Department did not pay the city the $15,000 authorized for the building of the hospital. Charleston officials repeatedly protested, but it was not until 1830 that Congress recompensed the city for construction costs and $12,050 in interest.[6]

For over forty years the Marine Hospital Service relied largely on private and municipal hospitals. The case of New Orleans was fairly typical of the way in which the hospital service operated. On learning in 1801 that many seamen and Mississippi River boatmen were sick and dying in New Orleans, at that time still under Spanish control, President Jefferson requested Congress to extend the Marine Hospital Act to New Orleans. Congress complied with his request and provided an annual appropriation of $3,000 to supplement the 20 cents collected from each seaman and boatman. The medical officer of the service was left free to make his own arrangements—either to contract with an existing hospital or else to set up his own institution. He was given a salary of $1,000 and funds for a staff. In addition he was given a daily hospital allowance of 75 cents per patient for maintenance. Since the Marine Hospital Service was a source of political patronage for many years, marine patients were shunted around between private institutions and Charity Hospital with every shift in the political wind.[7]

As the midcontinent developed, the Mississippi River became the major transportation route for grain, lumber, and other products for the entire area. In consequence, New Orleans and other Lower Mississippi towns and cities had a large transient population of raftmen, bargemen, seamen, brokers, and businessmen. For most of the century the majority of patients in New Orleans Charity Hospital were from out of state. The governors of both Louisiana and Mississippi circulated the northern states requesting financial help for their hospitals. Charity Hospital was in desperate straits in 1817, and only a gift of $5,000 from the Pennsylvania legislature temporarily tided it over.[8] By 1830 the towns and cities along the entire Mississippi River began petitioning Congress for Marine hospitals to relieve them of the care of sick rivermen. The 1832 Asiatic cholera epidemic, which spread far up the Mississippi Valley, greatly intensified the demands for federal action, and Congress responded in March 1837 with an act authorizing the secretary of war to purchase sites for Marine hospitals on Lake Erie and the Ohio and Mississippi Rivers.

This act inaugurated an era of hospital building, much of it pure pork-barrel politics. Between 1840 and 1861 some twenty-seven hospitals were erected, most of them on the Great Lakes and the Mississippi and Ohio Rivers. A commission report on the state of Marine hospitals submitted in 1851 noted delicately that the condition and expense of hospitals varied widely, that there was no uniformity in their operations, and that no system of inspection existed. The 1837 legislation extending the Marine Hospital Service to inland waterways led New Orleans, along with every other city with any claim at all, to request a Marine hospital. Work began on the New Orleans hospital in 1838, but in 1841, after $38,000 had been spent, the unfinished building was temporarily abandoned. In 1845 a small appropriation was made to preserve the dilapidated structure from the weather, and finally in 1848 the hospital was completed, at a total cost of $122,772.70.

In 1854, probably under pressure from the Louisiana delegation, Congress appropriated $248,000 for an even larger hospital. Construction began in late 1856 on a three-story building with a cast-iron framework. Despite a foundation based on many pilings, the building sank two feet before it was finished. In the meantime Congress appropriated an additional $151,659 in 1856 and another $85,000 in 1858. With the outbreak of the Civil War, the hospital was used successively as the Confederate Arsenal and Hospital, the Union Hospital, and the Freedmen's Bureau Hospital. It was never satisfactory as a Marine hospital, and in the postbellum years marine patients continued to be shifted around from hospital to hospital. In 1882 it was estimated that $100,000 was necessary to make it habitable. In part because of the hospital's poor location, the Marine Hospital Service decided it was totally unsuitable, and in 1896 the building, which had cost the federal government about half a million dollars and had stood empty for most of its life, was sold to the city for $25,000.[9]

In 1869 Treasury Secretary George S. Boutwell decided that the hospital service needed reorganizing and directed a leading hospital expert, Dr. John Shaw Billings, and Dr. W. D. Stewart to report on the service's hospitals. Their report presented a discouraging picture of waste and mismanagement. It noted that several hospitals were located in places where they were not needed; that the leading ports of New York, Philadelphia, and Baltimore had no hospitals; and that the one in New Orleans was completely unsuitable. The upshot was a congressional act reorganizing the Marine Hospital Service and placing it under the control of a medical director. Dr. John M. Woodworth, a distinguished Civil War surgeon, was chosen as the first supervising surgeon, and under his administration the service steadily improved. He required examinations for surgeons, established an administrative system along military lines, weeded out unnecessary and inadequate hospitals, and gradually built an effective organization.[10]

The history of the United States Marine Hospital Service is inextricably intertwined with the history of the first national quarantine law and the first federal health agency, the National Board of Health. As early as 1796 Congress had enacted a law authorizing federal agents to cooperate with state authorities on quarantine matters. Then, in response to the yellow fever epidemics at the end of the eighteenth century, a series of petitions requesting a national quarantine law was sent to Congress, but to no avail. For much of the nineteenth century quarantine control in the Northeast rested primarily in the hands of towns and cities, while in the South it remained largely under state control. During these years the danger from Asiatic cholera led to the introduction of several bills into Congress, but these, too, proved abortive.

By the 1870s health reform was in the air, and the emergence of the American Public Health Association, along with a more effective AMA and a revived Marine Hospital Service, helped make possible a national quarantine act and the first national board of health. An additional stimulus to congressional action was provided by outbreaks of cholera and yellow fever in 1873 and a major yellow fever epidemic in 1878. Yet despite this strong pressure for national action on the health front, only limited progress was made. The issue of states' rights was undoubtedly a major factor in this, but a series of personality clashes also contributed to delaying action at the national level.

Drs. Billings and Woodworth were strong individuals who jointly made significant contributions to strengthening the Marine Hospital Service. Billings, a major figure in the APHA, favored a national health board. Woodworth, an exceedingly capable administrator and empire builder, was equally determined that the Marine Hospital Service should assume responsibility for the nation's health. His first aim was to expand the service into a national quarantine agency that would supervise quarantines and gather information about the spread of contagious diseases throughout the world.

Beginning in 1873 several bills were introduced into Congress to establish a national sanitary bureau and a national quarantine system. The first of these was drawn up by Dr. Christopher Cox, president of the Washington, D.C., Board of Health. His bill, introduced by Senator James Patterson in December 1873, proposed a sanitary bureau under the aegis of the Interior Department to gather information on public health matters and to help state and local quarantine authorities. About the same time, another bill was introduced into the House of Representatives to create a national board of health consisting of the surgeon generals of the army and navy and the supervising surgeon of the Marine Hospital Service. This board would have the authority to establish and enforce a national quarantine system. Both of these bills, and subsequent bills, received short shrift in Congress. Significantly, one national quarantine bill did manage to pass the House, but only after a clause had been eliminated from it that gave the national board control over state and local quarantine officials.[11]

Ironically, the southern states, the leading exponents of states' rights, favored a national quarantine, while the northern states, where yellow fever was no longer a serious threat, generally were in opposition. Dr. John Woodworth, undeterred by the failure of the early national quarantine bills, maintained steady pressure on Congress with strong support from southerners. Aroused to action by a severe yellow fever outbreak in Savannah, delegates from nearly all the southeastern ports of the Atlantic Coast met in Jacksonville, Florida, in the spring of 1878. Not content with merely petitioning Congress for a national quarantine system, they worked closely with Dr. Woodworth and introduced a bill to create such a system. The opponents of the measure used a variety of arguments. Quarantine, they said, was a police power, and as such belonged to the states. They argued, too, that a uniform quarantine law could not meet the needs of special local circumstances. Whatever the logic of the opponents' arguments, a major reason for their opposition lay in the fact that local quarantine systems were a lucrative source of income for cities and states and an equally valuable source of political patronage.

The bill passed the House, but not before its opponents had effectively gutted it by two amendments. The first specified that any quarantine regulations of the federal government could not impair or conflict with the laws or regulations of states or municipalities; the second stated that the federal government could not interfere with any state or local quarantine agencies. The debate in the Senate took place in April 1878, when yellow fever was ravaging Havana and the West Indies. The threat of yellow fever to the South, an impassioned plea by Senator John G. Gordon of Georgia, and the knowledge that the bill was innocuous enabled it to pass easily on April 29. For Dr. Woodworth the law was a dubious victory. The Marine Hospital Service was responsible for administering the law, and the law did provide that the service was to gather worldwide information on contagious diseases. On the other hand, the law gave the federal government no real authority over quarantine, and the House had further weakened the measure by failing to appropriate funds for its implementation.[12]

During the 1870s the American Public Health Association staunchly supported the movement for a national sanitary bureau. The AMA favored one, too, but a measure of ambivalence characterized its support. Dr. Bowditch, a leading member, in 1874 declared that it would be premature to establish a national health board until effective health boards had been created at the state level.[13] Two basic problems confronted the health reformers. In the first place, the issue of states' rights was bound to cause objections to any grant of authority to the federal government. In the second, the concept of governmental responsibility for health and welfare was only beginning to gain ground. Alleviating ravaging epidemics or major calamities was seen as a matter for individual philanthropy rather than government action. These two factors guaranteed that any federal health measures taken in the nineteenth century would be of an exceedingly limited nature.

As has been the general rule respecting community action on behalf of public health, it took a major crisis to push through the law that established the first national health board. Although repeated cholera scares, largely unjustified, swept the country in the latter part of the nineteenth century, it was yellow fever, a disease of the South, which precipitated congressional action. Whenever yellow fever raged in the Caribbean area, it was almost certain to spread to southern ports, the most important of which was New Orleans because of its role as entrepôt for much of the Mississippi Valley. After a major epidemic in 1867 which killed over three thousand people in New Orleans and hundreds of others elsewhere, yellow fever continued to break out every summer, but in succeeding years it seemed to be tapering off, and New Orleans newspapers confidently began asserting that the disease would soon disappear.

In 1878, however, the pestilence struck with devastating force. The first case in New Orleans was diagnosed at the end of May, and other cases began appearing in June. The board of health, knowing that an official announcement of the presence of yellow fever would virtually isolate New Orleans and disastrously affect its economy, hesitated until July 12 before conceding the existence of the disease. By the end of July full-scale epidemics were under way in New Orleans, Natchez, Memphis, and other towns on the lower Mississippi River. New Orleans suffered over four thousand deaths; Memphis, as mentioned in chapter 10, was devastated; and epidemics occurred in every Gulf Coast state from Florida to Texas. More significant because of its impact on the nation, the disease swept up the Mississippi River as far as Cairo, St. Louis, and Cincinnati, and cases were quarantined in New York and other northern cities. Rapid and detailed newspaper reports of the ravages of the fever, made possible by technological developments, created apprehension and outright panic throughout the South and the entire Mississippi Valley.[14]

As the horrifying conditions in the plague-stricken cities became known, Americans in all parts of the country rallied to help—churches, benevolent groups, and individuals contributed money, food, and clothing. The most effective of the relief agencies were the Howard Associations, groups of young businessmen in southern cities who dedicated themselves to the sick and dying in times of yellow fever epidemics. The federal government did very little. Dr. Woodworth of the Marine Hospital Service announced that he was unable to take action against the pestilence since Congress had provided no money. Secretary of War McCreary, late in August, informed reporters that although no law authorized him to distribute army supplies, he would give what could be spared.[15]

As yellow fever became a matter of national concern, all the old arguments about the disease's cause and its means of spread were revived and embellished with new theories and hypotheses. The South, which had always been dubious of the Louisiana quarantine system and had frequently accused the New Orleans' health authorities of concealing the existence of the disease, demanded a national quarantine law—a demand with which many health leaders in New Orleans concurred. For once the South had strong allies in the North, for the presence of yellow fever far up the Mississippi Valley mobilized widespread support for a national quarantine system.

By the fall of 1878 newspapers and medical journals throughout the country were joining in the call for federal action. Reflecting this widespread sentiment, on December 2, 1878, President Rutherford B. Hayes began his second annual message to Congress by speaking of the recent "fatal pestilence" that had disrupted the nation's health. In a commentary upon the inaction of the federal government, he proudly mentioned that it had supplied 1,800 tents and $25,000 worth of food and medicines—this in the face of an epidemic that had cost the Mississippi Valley alone some 20,000 lives and economic losses estimated at between $100 to $200 million. "The fearful spread of this pestilence," President Hayes continued, "has awakened a very general public sentiment in favor of national sanitary administration, which shall not only control quarantine, but have the sanitary supervision of internal commerce in times of epidemics. . . ." He then urged Congress to give the whole subject "early and careful consideration."[16]

With the Forty-fifth Congress in recess during the epidemic and no extra funds in his agency, in September 1878 Surgeon General Woodworth obtained private money, part of it from a New York philanthropist, Mrs. Elizabeth Thompson, for a yellow fever commission to investigate the disease and report to the APHA at its convention in Richmond on November 20. At this meeting the commission members pointed out that they had been given too little time for a proper investigation. Nonetheless, they concluded in their report that the disease was imported and was transmitted solely by human intercourse. The members also agreed that disinfectants and the existing therapeutics were useless, and that only a "rigorous quarantine to the extent of total non-intercourse had proven effective."[17]

The gathering of the APHA members in November was notable for its tension. The nature of yellow fever was the dominant issue, and, as had been true of the early sanitary conventions, the delegates were sharply divided between the contagionists, who believed in the importation thesis, and the sanitarians, who were firmly convinced that the disease originated in dirt and filth. While most delegates adhered to one or the other of these basic concepts, they were also prepared to present a great many variations on the two themes. Surgeon General Woodworth played a rather dubious role at the meeting. Disregarding the suggestions of the APHA's executive committee at the opening executive session devoted to the order of business, he issued a printed program which proposed to give every yellow fever theorist a full hearing. Had this program been accepted, it would have led to endless arguments and discredited the association, thereby strengthening Woodworth's position as a leading public health expert. Although his program was rejected and he was personally criticized, Woodworth continued to play a significant role at the convention.[18]

In the lengthy discussions on yellow fever at the APHA meetings, Dr. John Billings, showing a very early appreciation of developments in bacteriology, suggested that arguments and theories about the cause and spread of the disease were useless until what he termed the "yellow fever poison" could be identified. In any event, the convention agreed that yellow fever was imported and that quarantine was essential, although the members stressed the need for state and local authorities to undertake sanitary programs. The convention also resolved to appoint a special legislative committee to draw up bills and lobby for a national health service. Newspapers and medical journals throughout the country reacted favorably to the decisions of the APHA and added their voices to the call for national action.

The Senate and House, responding to President Hayes's appeal in his annual address, and also to public pressure, each appointed committees to examine the question of how contagious diseases could be prevented. The two committees met jointly on December 16 and agreed to establish a board of experts to study the issue. Congress concurred and appropriated $50,000 for this purpose. The board reported to Congress on January 30, 1879, but by this date several bills had already been introduced into the House and Senate.

On December 10, Senator L. Q. C. Lamar of Mississippi proposed to establish a department of health that would have supervised the Marine Hospital Service, administered a national quarantine system, gathered public health information, and directed a corps of sanitary engineers. Its head would have had cabinet status and assumed all functions of the surgeon general. This bill, which had strong support from Dr. Wood-worth, in effect would have transformed the Marine Hospital Service into a bureau of health, with Dr. Woodworth in charge. Many of the leaders in the APHA had qualms about giving too much authority to the head of a national agency, particularly since it appeared that Woodworth was the intended director. Congress, always conscious of states' rights and reluctant to act on any health measure, did not permit the bill to come out of committee.

The APHA—recognizing the need to move slowly and, for the most part, believing that health matters were best left to state and local authorities—pushed for a much milder bill, but this, too, failed. After discussing and rejecting these and other proposals, on the last day of the session, March 3, 1879, the House and the Senate passed a bill that had been introduced by Representative Jonas McGowan of Michigan a few days earlier. It had been strongly supported by the APHA, largely because it proposed a national board of health consisting of seven civilians and certain national officers. The bill originally included a clause for an appropriation of $500,000, but this was deleted. The "Board of Health" created by this bill was without funds and virtually powerless. Its main functions were to gather information and advise government departments on health matters. It was also to work with the National Academy of Science in planning for a permanent health department to be presented at the next Congress.[19]

It is clear that Congress, reluctant to create a strong federal agency—and feeling that health was not its concern—simply evaded the issue. The clash between the APHA and Woodworth of the Marine Hospital Service also helped reduce any chance for an effective law. John S. Billings and other leaders in the APHA opposed the bills that would have transformed the Marine Hospital Service into a health department, and Supervising Surgeon General Woodworth used his political strength to undermine any measures to create a separate health agency.

When the forty-sixth Congress met later, in March, bills were introduced immediately to expand the authority of the national board. Senator Isham Harris of Tennessee consulted with the national board members before introducing his bill to require certificates of health on ships arriving from infected ports and to give the board control over a national quarantine system. The board was hesitant about assuming responsibility for quarantine, believing that its chief role was to help state and local health agencies. It did, however, suggest that an appropriation of $650,000 be added to the bill.

After various political maneuvers, the Harris bill passed both houses of Congress on June 2, 1879. By this time amendments had specified that the national board could not make its own rules and regulations but had to follow those of the states. Other amendments reduced the appropriation to $500,000 and limited the life of the board to four years. The national board, however, now had both funds and some authority. It could make regulations pertaining to vessels coming from infected ports, but it was required to cooperate with local agencies in administering quarantine laws. If local regulations were lacking or inadequate, the board was then authorized to assume responsibility. The major effect of the law was to make the National Board of Health responsible for quarantine and to restrict the Marine Hospital Service to its original function.

The final step in the creation of the National Board of Health came with the enactment of a law on July 1, 1879, which authorized the board to rent office space, employ clerical help, and use the government printing office. It was also empowered to construct temporary quarantine hospitals and other buildings in times of emergency. Without the vivid recollections of the 1878 yellow fever epidemics and the threat of cholera, it is doubtful that Congress would have created this first federal health agency. The fears and doubts expressed by many congressmen about this "experiment" in public health, however, did not bode well for its future.[20]

The eleven-member National Board of Health, which included some of the most prominent names in sanitation and health, was dominated by leaders of the APHA. One member, Stephen Smith, was a founder and former president of the APHA; James Cabell of Charlottesville, Virginia, was then serving as the APHA's president; and John S. Billings of the U.S. Army and Hosmer Johnson of Chicago would later become presidents of the association. On April 2, 1879, the national board elected James Cabell as its president, John S. Billings as vice president, and T. J. Turner of the U.S. Navy as secretary. These three men, along with Drs. Stephen Smith of New York and Preston Bailhache of the Marine Hospital Service, formed the national board's executive committee. Since Cabell and Smith frequently could not attend the executive committee meetings, the other three members, with Billings taking a decisive role, largely determined policy.[21]

The board promptly organized a number of standing committees to deal with matters such as contagious diseases, food adulteration, and sanitary legislation. Its instructions had been to conduct scientific investigations, but the board decided it would be better to give grants for this purpose to sanitarians, engineers, and scientists. The board's duties also included submitting a plan for a permanent national health agency. After a number of studies and meetings, no consensus could be reached, and the question was simply dropped. The two areas where the board proved most successful were in establishing and improving local and state health boards and in helping to develop more effective quarantine measures.

In connection with the national effort to improve the quarantine system, the Tennessee State Board of Health called for a meeting, in the early spring of 1879, of all state health boards in the Mississippi Valley to plan joint action in the event of another yellow fever outbreak. The national board was more than happy to cooperate and sent observers to the first meeting, which was held on April 30. Seven state boards and six cities were represented at this meeting in Memphis. The group first decided to constitute itself as the Sanitary Council of the Mississippi Valley and, second, decided to fully endorse the concept of a national health agency. It also decided to meet the following week with the National Board of Health, which was holding a session in Atlanta, Georgia. The national board had chosen Atlanta because the Association of Medical Colleges and other medical groups were meeting there at the same time. Working in conjunction with the Mississippi Valley Sanitary Council, the national board worked up a set of rules and regulations pertaining to maritime quarantine and then formulated another code for dealing with inland quarantine (waterways and railroads).[22]

If the National Board of Health was to have any success with quarantine, it was essential that it secure the cooperation of state and local officials. While the board was assumed to have responsibility for a national quarantine system, the law creating it was vague and poorly defined—a situation that ultimately contributed to the board's demise. In any event, the Atlanta meeting—in which the board consolidated its position with AMA and the Mississippi Valley Sanitary Council—gave it a good start. In preparation for the anticipated yellow fever attacks, the national board divided the Atlantic and Gulf Coasts into eight districts, assigning an inspector to each one. The inspectors were qualified physicians, familiar with the board's quarantine regulations and with the latest knowledge of sanitation. Their instructions were to report on sanitary conditions, inform the board immediately of any contagious disease cases, and aid and assist local health officers. In addition, temporary inspectors were appointed who were to swing into action at the appearance of yellow fever, applying isolation and disinfection measures where necessary and educating local officials in threatened areas. Since disease prevention in New Orleans was critical in holding yellow fever at bay, in May the board sent Dr. John Rauch of Chicago, a founding member of the Mississippi Valley Sanitary Association, to inspect the quarantine system. He reported some weaknesses and recommended that the board grant funds to upgrade the city's quarantine station and enlarge its inspection staff.[23]

In July 1879 the national board was given its first test when yellow fever was reported in Memphis. The board promptly sent additional inspectors, recommended a mass evacuation of the city, and notified all states up the Mississippi River of the danger. A grant of $10,000 was made available to help enforce water and railway quarantine measures and to restrict the spread of infection. Despite its efforts, the board received limited praise. Cotton brokers and other businessmen objected to the strictness of the quarantine; many citizens criticized the mass evacuation; and the state of Tennessee was unhappy over what it felt was the refusal of the board to help support the refugees camped outside Memphis. The board was not at fault in this instance since its funds were restricted.

At about the same time, Dr. Samuel M. Bemiss, the board's representative in New Orleans, reported several cases of yellow fever and declared the city infected. The New Orleans medical profession and businessmen, who tended to assume that a few cases of yellow fever were a normal summer occurrence, were outraged. On August 1 the board granted $10,000 to New Orleans to help with isolation, fumigation, and quarantine measures, but fortunately the outbreak was minor.[24] Although the board acted decisively on the news of yellow fever in Memphis and New Orleans, and although its measures probably contributed to restricting the fever's spread, it won few friends. Where local officials were cooperative, matters went smoothly, but too often this was not the case. Moreover, its grants involved considerable red tape and required strict accounting from the recipients, further irritating state and local officials. The Louisiana Board of Health, as was true of nearly all health boards, was highly sensitive to the reactions of the business community, and it resented the intrusion of the national board into what it considered local matters.

Following the 1879 epidemic, the national board, at the request of the Tennessee Board of Health, send a three-man delegation to make a sanitary survey of Memphis. The notable work of the board in connection with the complete sanitary reform of Memphis has already been recounted in chapter 10. In July it sent a delegation to study yellow fever in Havana. Other than recognizing the endemicity of the disease in Cuba and noting Memphis's unsanitary conditions, the commission learned little about the cause of yellow fever.

Meanwhile the board was encouraging cities and states to undertake sanitary surveys, providing limited funds to stimulate the formation of better health departments and sanitary programs, promoting an interest in more accurate vital statistics, and subsidizing research and studies on such topics as food and drug adulteration, air and water pollution, the engineering of sewer systems, and soils and drainage. Among the leading sanitarians and scientists conducting these studies were professors from Harvard, Johns Hopkins, the University of Virginia, and other leading schools.[25]

Considering the amorphous nature of the law creating the National Board of Health and the general suspicion with which it and other federal agencies were viewed, it is not surprising that it was short-lived. One of the key factors in its demise was the active opposition of Dr. Joseph Jones, who in 1880 became president of the Louisiana State Board of Health. Jones was a strong irascible individual and a firm believer in states' rights. He had no love for Dr. James Cabell, president of the national board, and he clashed with the board's representatives in New Orleans, Drs. Bemiss and Stanford E. Chaillé. Jones's refusal to work with the national board aroused opposition even in New Orleans, where the New Orleans Auxiliary Sanitary Association and the Medical and Surgical Association both passed resolutions supporting the efforts of the national authorities. Jones dismissed these criticisms in his board of health report for 1881, asserting that the "true and only guide" for public officials were *"the organic laws of the States."*[26] Jones was an intelligent and able individual who contributed to medicine and public health, but insofar as yellow fever was concerned, New Orleans was the key to the Mississippi Valley. By flatly rejecting the authority of the national board, Jones helped to undermine its position in both the South and the entire Mississippi Valley.

Anxious to strengthen local quarantine systems and develop effective local health departments, Billings and his associates repeatedly petitioned Congress for additional funds. Congress, which had had reservations about the original appropriation of $500,000, insisted that this amount was intended to be spent over the four-year life of the board. Fortunately for the United States, if not for the national board, no major epidemics of yellow fever or Asiatic cholera occurred during the next few years, and, as memories of the 1878 outbreaks receded, so did enthusiasm for a national public health board. The vested interests of politicians in state and local quarantine agencies in the Northeast, the doctrine of states' rights in the South, opposition from the Marine Hospital Service, and public apathy were all contributing factors in its decline. Part of the problem was that the public perceived the board as having full authority over the quarantine system and access to unlimited funds. By expecting too much, the public came to believe that the board was weak and ineffective.

Dr. John B. Hamilton, who succeeded Woodworth as surgeon general and as director of the Marine Hospital Service, was an intelligent individual well versed in the politics of Washington. His maneuvering was largely responsible for the virtual end of the national board. In the summer of 1882 he persuaded the House to take the $100,000 annual appropriation to prevent the importation and spread of contagious diseases away from the national board and give it to the Marine Hospital Service.

At the same time, the national board was given a small appropriation but found its activities restricted to investigating cholera, smallpox, and yellow fever. The following March 2, the law under which the national board operated expired, and the Marine Hospital Service took over all national responsibility for quarantine and public health.[27] The board continued in nominal existence until 1893 when a new quarantine act specifically repealed the law creating the board.

Dr. Billings continued to fight for a national bureau of health, but Dr. Hamilton outmaneuvered him at every turn, while continuing to expand his own agency. When Billings and his supporters arranged for the Congressional Committee on Commerce to report favorably on a bill to set up a bureau of health, Hamilton mobilized opposition to the bill. A main purpose of the proposed bureau was to study Asiatic cholera. Hamilton in his testimony pointed out that the Marine Hospital Service had already established a laboratory in 1887 in charge of one of his officers, who had studied bacteriology for five years. Having eliminated all competition, the hospital service under Hamilton and his successor, Dr. Walter Wyman, succeeded in becoming the major federal health agency. It steadily assumed more control over quarantine affairs, and, as the new wave of immigrants flooded into the United States in the 1880s and 1890s, the Marine Hospital Service began taking responsibility for examining them for contagious diseases.[28]

The massive influx of immigrants in the late nineteenth century coincided with a series of outbreaks of cholera in Russia and Eastern Europe, creating widespread fears of cholera in America. The repercussions of a particularly serious epidemic in Russia in 1892 were largely responsible for the first effective national quarantine law. Signed by President Benjamin Harrison on February 15, 1893, the law required all vessels bound for the United States to have a certificate of health from the American consul and assigned medical officers of the Marine Hospital Service to foreign ports to make the necessary inspections. Furthermore, their captains were to submit the certificate to the federal quarantine officer at the port of debarkation before landing cargo or passengers. In addition, the Marine Hospital Service was given responsibility for examining all state and local quarantine facilities to determine whether or not they measured up to the federal standards. The hospital service already had nine quarantine stations, and the law provided that any state or municipality wishing to surrender its facilities to the federal government would be recompensed. In consequence, several states immediately complied and gradually the service assumed control over the rest of them.[29] Thus by the end of the century the Marine Hospital Service had become the chief health agency of the United States.

NOTES

1. David L. Cowen, *Medicine and Health in New Jersey: A History* (Princeton, N. J., 1964), 91; Dotaline E. Allen, "History of Nursing in Indiana" (M.S. thesis, University of Indiana, 1948), 8–9; Stuart Galishoff, *Safeguarding the Public Health: Newark, 1895–1918* (Westport, Conn., 1975), 7–8; Peter Harstad, "Health in the Upper Mississippi Valley, 1820–1861" (Ph.D. diss., University of Wisconsin, 1963), 177.

2. New York Academy of Medicine, Minutes of the Section on Public Health, November 30, 1893, New York Academy of Medicine MS, p. 83.

3. Wyndham B. Blanton, *Medicine in Virginia in the Eighteenth Century* (Richmond, Va., 1931), 270, 289; Joseph Ioor Waring, *A History of Medicine in South Carolina, 1670–1825* (Columbia, S.C., 1964), 109.

4. Ralph C. Williams, *The United States Public Health Service, 1798–1950* (Washington, D.C., 1951), 28–32.

5. F. L. Pleadwell and W. M. Kerr, "Lewis Heermann, Surgeon in the United States Navy," *Annals of Medical History* 5 (1923):124–25.

6. Harry S. Mustard, *Government in Public Health* (New York, 1945), 35; Williams, *The United States Public Health Service*, 35–36.

7. John Duffy, *The Rudolph Matas History of Medicine in Louisiana* (New Orleans, La., 1958–62), 1:449–56; William E. Rooney, "The New Orleans Marine Hospital, 1802–1861" (M.A. thesis, Tulane University, 1950), 34–35.

8. Duffy, *Matas History of Medicine in Louisiana*, 1:432; *Pennsylvania Archives*, 4th ser., 5 (Harrisburg, Pa., 1900), 122–23.

9. Rooney, "New Orleans Marine Hospital," 54–57, 86–99; Duffy, *Matas History of Medicine in Louisiana* (1958–62), 2:215–18, 513.

10. Bess Furman, *A Profile of the United States Public Health Service, 1798–1948* (Washington, D.C., n.d.), 114–16, 121ff.

11. Christopher C. Cox, "A Report Upon the Necessity for a National Sanitary Bureau," in *Selections from Public Health Reports of the APHA (1873–1893)*, 522–32; Peter W. Bruton, "The National Board of Health" (Ph.D. diss., University of Maryland, 1974), 51–53.

12. Bruton, "The National Board of Health," 54–60.

13. Howard D. Kramer, "A History of the Public Health Movement in the United States, 1850–1900" (Ph.D. diss., University of Iowa, 1942), 161–62.

14. Jo Ann Carrigan, "The Saffron Scourge: A History of Yellow Fever in Louisiana, 1796–1905" (Ph.D. diss., Louisiana State University, 1961), 179–86.

15. Bruton, "The National Board of Health," 87.

16. James D. Richardson, *A Compilation of the Messages and Papers of the Presidents, 1789–1907* (n.p., 1908), 7:492.

17. John H. Ellis, The New Orleans Yellow Fever Epidemic in 1878: A Note on the Affective History of Societies and Communities, TS, pp. 13–15.

18. Bruton, "The National Board of Health," 120–22.

19. Ibid., 125–29, 133–54.

20. Ibid., 154–65.

21. Ibid., 166–70; Williams, *The United States Public Health Service*, 77–78.

22. Bruton, "The National Board of Health," 170–76; Jo Ann Carrigan, "The National Board of Health, 1879–1883," TS, pp. 18–22.

23. Dr. J. H. Rauch, "Report on Quarantine in New Orleans," in *Annual Report of the National Board of Health, 1879* (Washington, D.C., 1879), 458–60.

24. Bruton, "The National Board of Health," 206–210.

25. Carrigan, "The National Board of Health," 22–28.

26. Duffy, *Matas History of Medicine in Louisiana*, 2:471–76; *Annual Report of the Louisiana State Board of Health for 1880* (New Orleans, 1880), 46–123. The latter contains a long discussion of the problems between the Louisiana and national health boards along with transcriptions of all correspondence. For another version, see *Annual Report of the Board of Health, 1883* (Washington, D.C., 1884), 42–55.

27. Furman, *Profile of the United States Public Health Service*, 184–88.

28. Ibid., 194–96, 199ff; Williams, *The United States Public Health Service*, 82–84, 103, 176–78.

29. Furman, *Profile of the United States Public Health Service*, 211–12.

12

Health and Sanitation at the Close of the Nineteenth Century

The last twenty years of the nineteenth century saw the sanitary revolution in full swing. Towns and cities were establishing water and sewer systems; garbage collection and the removal of nuisances were improving; and health departments were expanding and moving into other areas of health concern. Commendable as this progress was, rapid increases in urban populations nullified many of the gains being made. By the time a water or sewer system was completed, it was already inadequate. Housing seldom kept up with the population increase, with the result that more and more people were jammed into aging, shoddily built, filthy tenements. The introduction of steam and electric cars at the end of nineteenth century was a tremendous step forward, but horses were still the main source of urban transportation. This meant the continuing presence of stables, manure piles, manure in the streets, and the omnipresence of myriads of flies.

In most cities dairy stables, too, contributed to the flies and noisome atmosphere. Even though municipal systems for collecting garbage were improving, they were always subject to the vicissitudes of politics. A New York citizens' association reported that from 1881 to 1895 total corruption prevailed in the street-cleaning department and that the streets were so filthy it was impossible to tell whether the surface was asphalt or stone.[1] Periodically a reform government would overhaul the city's street department and temporarily clean the streets. New York, which had experienced a number of these temporary reforms, in 1895 selected a nationally known sanitationist, George E. Waring, as its street commissioner. Waring, who provided his men with white uniforms and gave the name "White Wings" to street cleaners, for a few years made New York an example for the nation.[2] Generally, accumulated piles of garbage and refuse characterized most urban areas. The one exception was the neighborhoods occupied by the well-to-do, which usually received special attention from the city authorities.

The larger cities by 1900 had banned hogs and large domestic animals from roaming the streets, but since the authorities were usually slow in removing carrion, the odor from dead horses, dogs, and cats constantly assailed residents' nostrils. Keep in mind that dead horses, like abandoned automobiles today, were simply left in the streets. In the 1890s the offal contractors removed an average of eight thousand dead horses a year from the streets of New York.[3] And New York differed in this respect from other cities only in matter of degree.

Descriptions of other towns and cities make it clear that conditions there closely resembled those of New York City. An observer in Milwaukee in 1889 commented that the garbage remained so long in the streets that it eventually attempted to remove itself "by crawling away, in the shape of active little worms." There, too, dead animals, debris, and horse manure, compounded with the odors from slaughterhouses and unflushed sewers, gave the town a distinctive atmosphere.[4] Chicago, with its vast stockyards and slaughterhouses, must have been unbearable in summer; and New Orleans, with an inefficient government and a moist, hot atmosphere, must have tested the nostrils of even the hardiest residents in the warm months.

In the post–Civil War years the development of sewer systems that poured human wastes directly into adjacent lakes and rivers—the usual source of the local water supply—made water pollution a major problem by the 1880s and 1890s. Along with being a collecting point for sewage, these same water bodies were convenient receptacles for industrial wastes, garbage, dead animals, and any other refuse. As early as 1864 Pittsburgh and its surrounding towns petitioned the Pennsylvania legislature to make it "a penal act to empty the chemicals and residium from the distillation of carbon oil into the Allegheny River."[5] Despite years of agitation by medical societies and health officials, little was accomplished. In 1897 Governor Daniel H. Hastings of Pennsylvania complained to the legislature that the water pollution situation in the state was more acute than when the state board of health had begun its work. The trouble lay, he continued, in the assumption that property owners had the right to dump anything they wished in water bodies fronted by their property.[6]

As the Midwest developed, the pollution of the Ohio River—the water source for most of the towns and cities on its banks and tributaries—became a major problem. The Ohio State Board of Health reported in 1891 that nearly all towns on the Ohio River discharged their sewage into the river and drew their water supply from it as well. It also noted that in many cases the sewage outlet and the water intake were close together. In the town of Bellaire the water intake was located immediately downriver from the sewage discharge. A legislative study of water pollution on the Ohio River confirmed the worst fears that the Ohio was literally becoming an open sewer. Fear of cholera and a steady rise in the rate of typhoid fever gave further impetus to the movement to improve water supplies. A report in 1888 by an APHA committee on water pollution, which argued that the introduction of wholesome water was the key factor in reducing the rate of typhoid, was widely reprinted in state health board reports.[7]

By 1890 the pollution of water supplies was affecting nearly every major city. In Chicago most sewage was poured into the Chicago River, which flowed directly into Lake Michigan. Not only did the river function as an offensive open sewer running through the city but the city's water supply was drawn from waters polluted by the river. To improve the quality of the lake water, in 1892 construction of a drainage canal was started, which, when finished in 1900, reversed the flow of the Chicago River away from the lake. Baltimore and New York were fortunate in having adequate supplies of good water, but the discharge of raw sewage and every other type of waste into their harbors created an incredible stench. In Baltimore the foul odors from the harbor and local rivers and streams reached every part of the city by 1890, but it took three sewerage commissions and twenty-five years before Baltimore had a complete sewer system.[8]

New York City in these years not only provided its citizens with an ample supply of good water but was also a leader in protecting its upstate watershed from pollution. Its sewage, however, was simply discharged into the adjacent rivers and harbor. As early as 1871 a law was passed that prohibited the dumping of carrion, offal, and other objects into the harbor, and the office of shore inspector was created to enforce the law. While this law was a step in the direction of eliminating gross pollution, nothing was done about the growing flood of industrial, commercial, and human wastes that were turning the harbor into a virtual cesspool. No further action was taken by New York until the Passaic River became so badly polluted that a group of New Jersey communities formed the Passaic Valley Sewerage Commission and established a system to discharge all the sewage from a population of about 500,000 people into upper New York Harbor. Belatedly New York City and state authorities appointed a series of sewerage commissions, but it was well into the twentieth century before anything was done. As late as 1914 the raw sewage from some six million people was still being discharged into the harbor.[9]

Insofar as improving the quality of America's drinking water goes, some progress had been made in protecting water sources and in developing filtration systems, but as of 1900 the pollution of the nation's rivers, lakes, and harbors continued almost unabated. An encouraging sign was that commissions appointed by state legislatures and municipal councils were studying the problem, and in a few places projects were under way to reduce pollution. The reasons for this slow progress were twofold: first, filtration systems and sewage treatment plants were expensive; second, pollution of water bodies was only rarely a local problem. In most instances any solution required the cooperation of many communities and, not infrequently, as in the case of the Ohio Valley system, the cooperation of several states. One other factor deserves mention: the technology involved in water filtration and sewage treatment was still developing, and debates over the merits of the various treatment methods further delayed action.

The deplorable condition of housing for the poor was a problem that increasingly occupied the attention of reformers in these years. As cities developed, the lower economic groups tended to occupy older housing in the central city. As these buildings decayed, they were gradually torn down to make way for tenements. Long after indoor plumbing was made possible through the advent of sewer systems, the older housing units and many of the poorly constructed tenements continued to rely on privies. When water was introduced into tenement housing, it often was not available above the first floor. The thousands of poverty-stricken immigrants who poured into the major Eastern cities in the 1880s and 1890s, primarily Eastern Europeans, had no choice but to jam themselves into the cheapest housing, often an entire family to a room. Lacking adequate toilet and washing facilties, the tenement dwellers' homes were notorious for their filth and odors.

New York City, the home of the largest tenement population, was a leader in tenement reform. Beginning in 1867 the city promulgated a series of ordinances that regulated the construction of, and conditions within, tenements. One of the early laws required landlords to provide one privy for every twenty inhabitants. In 1887 amendments to the law increased the required number of privies or water closets to one for every fifteen residents and also prohibited the location of privy vaults or cesspools under tenements without a special permit.[10] In these same years a drive was made to eliminate the many damp basement apartments of the city.

The general interest in sanitation in the 1880s led many cities to attempt to control plumbing, but the regulations were difficult to enforce since so much of plumbing is hidden. A New York City inspector reported in 1890 that every "ruse was employed to deceive." One contractor, he declared, opened up an entire street and closed it without laying a single pipe.[11] Another major problem that discouraged and undermined tenement regulations was that many tenements were owned by wealthy and influential individuals who were far more concerned with their income than with the welfare of their tenants. Nonetheless, although tenement housing was still poor as of 1900, the urban slums were generally improved over what had been the case in the pre–Civil War period.

While the urban poor in other cities and towns did not live in the six-story walk-ups that were coming to characterize New York City, living conditions for them were equally grim. An observer in Pittsburgh in 1906 declared that a significant part of the city's population was herded into cellars unfit for human habitation, dilapidated old shacks, and housing units with inadequate toilet facilities and insufficient water supplies. The author cited cases of entire blocks relying upon one outside hydrant for water and asserted that 19,000 families were still dependent upon privy vaults.[12] Since most major cities had inadequate sewer systems and many large towns had no systems at all, it is safe to say that as of 1900 the majority of Americans living in towns were still relying on privies, many of which were infrequently emptied. In almost every city and town piles of refuse, garbage, and debris cluttered the areas occupied by the lower economic groups, and crowded housing was the norm.

As might be expected, health conditions throughout America were poor. Infant mortality was high, and infectious diseases such as diphtheria, scarlet fever, and typhoid annually exacted an enormous toll. The disease that may have been responsible for the highest number of deaths was tuberculosis, but in 1890 even many physicians did not consider it contagious. All these disorders, however, were familiar ones and occasioned little public concern. Between 1880 and 1896 the annual deaths from diphtheria in New York City never fell below 1,000, and for three of these years it was in excess of 2,000. Yet even when the number of deaths rose above 2,000, newspapers, not considering the disease epidemic, paid only limited attention to it. Meanwhile, the press and the public worried about Asiatic cholera, which was of no consequence after 1873, and smallpox, which was relatively minor compared to the other epidemic disorders.[13]

The incidence of smallpox had steadily increased after 1830, but then had declined somewhat as a result of vaccination programs in the postbellum years. Smallpox flared up again in the early 1890s. It may have been a horrible and fatal disorder, but so was diphtheria, which caused many, many more deaths. Smallpox, however, was not restricted largely to children, unlike diphtheria, scarlet fever, and measles; and it was the one disease for which a preventive was available. It was also associated with immigrants, few of whom had been vaccinated, who occasionally brought the disease with them. Ironically, the large-scale use of vaccination in the late nineteenth century was responsible for a vociferous antivaccination movement, one that found strong support among Germans, Poles, and the newer immigrant groups.

The significance of the movement is shown by its effect on the Milwaukee Health Department. A series of smallpox outbreaks in the postwar years had led Milwaukee to build a relatively effective health agency, but an epidemic in 1894 had the reverse effect. As the number of smallpox cases increased, parents in the city's German and Polish neighborhoods refused to allow their children to be vaccinated and hid those sick with the disease, and mobs occasionally prevented ambulances from carrying smallpox patients to the Isolation Hospital and sometimes even attacked officials guarding quarantined premises. Egged on by the German-language press and the Anti-Vaccination Society, the city council dismissed the health commissioner and greatly reduced the powers of the health department.[14] The Milwaukee case, which weakened the power of the health authorities, was unusual, but in other cities, too, rioting occasionally resulted from efforts to enforce vaccination and quarantine regulations.

While infant mortality and deaths related to contagious diseases were undoubtedly higher in the urban slums than in smaller towns and rural areas, and higher among the lower classes than among the middle and upper classes, the ravages of disease seemed to spare no one, and losing an infant or child was common to almost all families. Respiratory and enteric infections winnowed the entire population, and malaria prevailed generally in the South as well as in other areas ranging from the East Coast to California. A higher living standard and the application of sanitary measures were reducing the incidence of the major killer diseases, but their virtual elimination awaited the application of new understandings of disease causation in the twentieth century.

Since blacks, with a few exceptions, were generally poor, their morbidity and mortality rates were considerably higher than those of whites. An article entitled "The Health of Negroes in the South," published in 1887, estimated the black death rate at almost double that of whites. One of the several southern health officers cited by the article's author stated that in Savannah, Georgia, 7 whites and 114 blacks died in 1885 without medical attention.[15] The rise of Jim Crow legislation in the 1880s and 1890s did nothing to improve black health.

As might be expected, the highest infant mortality rates were associated with the urban slums. Particularly problematic for major cities were the large numbers of foundlings—babies simply left in the streets. Jacob Riis asserts that in one year 170 live and 72 dead babies were picked up off the streets of New York. In New York City these foundlings were turned over to the female inmates of the almshouse, where they "seldom survived a year." A special infant asylum was built in 1866, but it, too, had a mortality rate of about 70 percent. To make matters worse, for those who wished to get rid of babies, infant boarding houses or baby farms existed where the mortality was almost 100 percent.

Newspapers occasionally denounced the city's infant care program, but they had little success in improving it. The *New York Times* in 1883 described the babies in New York's Infant Hospital as "mere skeletons with a bit of blue-black skin drawn over them." Despite this publicity, the death rate in that institution during the 1880s continued to average around 60 to 70 percent. When 96 percent of the infants turned over to the institution in 1896 died, the commissioner of charities blandly explained that the figure was not as bad as it appeared since many of the babies were ill on arrival and others had been sent by their parents to avoid funeral expenses. Fortunately, a new health commissioner with an interest in infant health remedied the situation shortly after.[16]

The life expectancy of tenement babies was far better than that of foundlings, but it was still exceptionally low. An unsanitary environment, poor food, and a lack of knowledge by mothers of how to care for their babies all contributed to the infant death toll. Fortunately, beginning in the 1870s the work of the New York City Health Department's Summer Corps and a number of private organizations slowly helped to improve infant and child well-being. Fresh-air camps, educational programs, free milk stations, and medical advice all contributed to reducing the deaths of children under five from 48.35 percent of the city's total annual deaths in 1875 to 40.66 percent in 1890.[17] In other cities, too, health departments and philanthropic organizations were promoting maternal and child welfare. A rising social consciousness among upper economic groups in the late nineteenth century brought forth a host of voluntary associations motivated by a desire to improve the health and welfare of the poor. They pressured city officials into supporting sanitary programs, fought to improve tenements, demanded regulation of milk and foods, and sought to help infants and children in the slum areas.

Another area of child welfare that needed attention was education. The idea that all children should be educated originated with the New Englanders in the early colonial period, but the beginnings of public school systems date back to about the 1820s and 1830s. Since education was essentially a local responsibility and seldom had a high priority, schools received minimal funding, and the majority of public schoolhouses were filthy, dilapidated buildings. They were described by state school officials in the pre–Civil War years as dirty, rundown, gloomy, fetid, crowded, and lacking in toilet facilities. Few school boards erected schoolhouses, and most schooling was conducted in old residences, stores, barns, warehouses, and empty structures. In the 1830s and 1840s the reports of state school superintendents repeatedly describe children crowded together in miserable, filthy school buildings, devoid even of privies. As late as the Civil War, in almost half of the public schools, boys relieved themselves on one side of the building and girls on the other. In 1848 the Connecticut school superintendent suggested that the small proportion of girls attending public schools was due to the reluctance of mothers to subject their daughters to the exposure this entailed. Virtually all observers agreed, too, that the deplorable school environment contributed to the excessive amount of disease and sickness among the children.[18]

Some improvement came in the latter part of the century, but except in a few of the major cities, the sanitary conditions in schools remained incredibly bad. It was not until 1887 that New York—one of the early states to show concern for its schoolchildren—passed the first state law requiring separate privies or water closets for boys and girls. By this date other states, too, were beginning to take an interest in school conditions. As might be expected, the New England states, with their tradition of education and sanitary reform, were among the leaders in improving school health. Following a number of piecemeal reforms, in 1888 Massachusetts passed a comprehensive sanitary code for school buildings, and other states rapidly followed suit.[19]

Well before this time, health boards had recognized the value of using schools as bases for mass vaccination. In 1850 Massachusetts enacted a statewide compulsory vaccination law. Stimulated by a series of widespread smallpox outbreaks, by the 1880s most city health departments were either supervising the vaccination of schoolchildren or urging school boards to do it. The movement for the compulsory vaccination of schoolchildren and general vaccination of the public was slowed by public apathy, the rise of the antivaccination movement mentioned earlier, and by sharp jurisdictional clashes between school boards and health officials. Nonetheless, working through school systems, health officials were successful in seeing that the majority of Americans were vaccinated by 1900.[20]

As the sanitary movement blossomed in the 1870s, it was only natural that the subject of the health of schoolchildren would arouse reformers' attention. In 1875 the American Social Science Association heard several of its members speak on the need for medical inspection in schools. The emergence of state boards of health in these years provided a strong impetus to the school health movement. In 1881, for example, the Illinois Board of Health, in making a sanitary survey of the state, specifically instructed its medical inspectors to investigate school conditions.[21] In New York, Boston, and other cities, health officials and reformers continued to agitate for the appointment of school physicians, but success was not achieved until public apathy was shaken by widespread epidemics of smallpox, diphtheria, and scarlet fever in the 1890s.

A major diphtheria outbreak in Boston in 1894 was responsible for the establishment of the first permanent system of school medical inspection. In November of that year the Boston Board of Health appointed fifty physicians, one for each school district, to visit all schools and examine any students appearing ill or complaining of illness. In the course of examining approximately 5,000 children over a period of four months, the inspectors uncovered 58 cases of diphtheria, 19 of scarlet fever, 42 of measles, 17 of whooping cough, 55 of mumps, and 7 cases of congenital syphilis.[22]

The success of these programs in Boston and other New England towns led the Chicago Board of Health to assign eight of its physicians to the schools. Since Chicago had some 273,000 children in school, these medical inspectors made no attempt to make regular school inspections but concentrated on identifying children with the more obvious contagious disorders. Despite this early start in school inspection, it was 1907 before Chicago had a relatively effective system. New York City, with a strong health department, was next to swing into action. In 1897 the city's health department established a Division of Medical School Inspection and systematically began to check the schools for cases of contagious diseases.[23]

Other cities, too, moved into the area of school inspection. As of 1902 some twenty-three cities claimed to have systems for inspecting the health of schoolchildren, but most of these were limited in scope, designed only to meet emergency situations. For example, Brookline, Massachusetts, one of the pioneers in the field, reported in 1898 that since neither diphtheria nor scarlet fever had been epidemic, it was not considered necessary to inspect the schoolchildren.[24] Fortunately for the cause of school health, in the process of checking for contagious diseases, school inspectors uncovered a host of other medical problems among the children, and their reports were ultimately responsible for moving the focus of school health programs well beyond the sanitary condition of school buildings and contagious diseases.

The late nineteenth century saw a revived interest in the regulation of food, a subject of concern to governing authorities from earliest times. As detailed earlier in chapters 1–3, in the American colonies some of the earliest ordinances and laws dealt with the quality of flour, the size of loaves of bread, and the condition of food markets. These regulations were eliminated in the early nineteenth century, and it was toward the end of the century before state and municipal authorities again attempted to guarantee the quality of certain foods.

The first item to arouse concern was milk. Large distilleries had early discovered that the residues from producing alcohol could be used to feed cows. There would have been nothing wrong with feeding this so-called swill to cows if the animals had been given supplementary feed. Unfortunately swill was their sole food supply, and the cows were routinely jammed together in conditions of almost indescribable filth. The milk, generally known as swill milk, was a thin bluish liquid nearly devoid of fat. Enterprising dairymen were able to turn this liquid into a rich creamy mixture by generous additions of magnesia, chalk, and plaster of paris.

Beginning in the 1820s and 1830s protests against swill milk began to appear in city newspapers. By the 1840s physicians were urging their medical societies in New York, Boston, and other cities to take up the fight against swill milk. They were joined by local health boards, but such boards as existed in the pre–Civil War years had little authority or influence. Medical societies tended to be somewhat ambivalent, and civic authorities had little interest in the subject. They recognized that swill milk was consumed largely by the poor, a group whose political influence has always been negligible. In addition to the problem of swill milk, adulteration of regular milk by water, chalk, and other substances was also becoming a major problem.[25]

Massachusetts and the city of Boston were the first to take action against milk adulteration. A state law in 1856 prohibited any form of adulteration, and in 1859 Boston appointed a milk inspector to enforce the law against feeding distillery wastes to dairy cattle. An equally important ordinance in Boston in 1864 prohibited the use of milk from diseased cows.[26]

In New York a series of newspaper campaigns, culminating in a full-scale exposé by Leslie's *Illustrated Weekly* beginning in 1858, finally led to success. By 1860 the milk reformers had gained powerful allies in the New York Academy of Medicine, the Association for Improving the Condition of the Poor, and the New York Sanitary Association. Unable to force action from the city government, at that time subservient to distillery and dairy interests, they turned to the state legislature, and in June 1862 secured an act that levied a fifty-dollar fine on anyone selling impure or adulterated milk, prohibited the keeping of cows in crowded and unhealthy conditions, and required milk-wagon drivers to show the source of their milk.[27] Washington, D.C., in 1863 passed a law against unsanitary cow yards, and in 1871 enacted another one against milk adulteration. Gradually in the succeeding years other cities began to regulate milk supplies, but progress was slow. As late as 1904 only six cities used dairy inspectors.[28] It should be borne in mind that enacting laws to ensure the quality of milk was not easy, but it was still much easier than enforcing them.

By the 1870s state legislatures—under pressure from honest dairy farmers and processors fearful of competition from unscrupulous processors and from producers of dairy substitutes such as oleomargarine—began to pass a number of laws regulating the dairy business at all levels. In cities such as New York, milk inspectors were appointed, dairy cows were examined for diseases, and licenses were required from individuals and companies handling milk. It is safe to say that most of the state laws in the late nineteenth century were intended to eliminate the sale of oleomargarine and other dairy substitutes, but their indirect effect was to improve the quality of dairy products in general.

Scientific developments in these years, most notably in chemistry and bacteriology, led to laboratory testing of milk. In 1870 the New York Health Department appointed a chemist, Dr. Charles F. Chandler, and instructed him to investigate the city's milk, food, and water. Chemical analysis at this time was limited, and Chandler and the other early municipal chemists concentrated largely on determining the amount of excess water in the milk supply. As bacteriology developed, it became possible by the 1890s to determine the extent of pathogenic organisms in milk, and the first result of this was the rise of the certified milk movement.

The founder of the certified milk movement, Dr. Henry L. Coit of Newark, New Jersey, had fought for a state milk law in 1890. When this effort failed, he persuaded the Essex County Medical Association of New Jersey to establish a Medical Milk Commission. This commission then contracted with dairies to produce milk under close supervision. This product, called "certified milk," was guaranteed to be fresh, wholesome, and free of pathogenic organisms. Coit's idea proved so successful that by 1906 milk commissions had been established in some twenty-seven cities.[29] The next step in producing safe milk was the introduction of pasteurization. Nathan Straus, a New York philanthropist, in 1893 opened milk stations where the poor could obtain good milk either free or for a nominal sum. In 1894 he began pasteurizing the milk.[30] Pasteurization at this time, however, was a highly debatable issue, and the large-scale pasteurization of milk did not come until well into the twentieth century.

Although the adulteration of milk attracted public attention in the early nineteenth century, the major drive for pure food and drug regulation began in the 1870s. Health officials and medical societies helped spearhead the movement, but its success was due in part to the efforts of a number of influential businessmen. It was also helped by lurid tales in newspapers and magazines, some of which were true, of poisonous adulterants. The basic reasons behind the growing public apprehension about food were the loss of contact between producers and consumers and the sense of unease that rapid change brings in any society. The introduction of canned goods in the 1870s, for example, undoubtedly contributed to suspicions about food in general. It was widely believed in the latter part of the century that food adulteration was both common and dangerous to health. Recent historical studies tend to minimize its threat to health, claiming that most adulteration in the nineteenth century was fraudulent but not poisonous. A proponent of this thesis, Michael Okun, recently argued that reputable businessmen and trade associations joined with health reformers in promoting food regulations in order to protect themselves from dishonest competition.[31]

Whatever the motivation, beginning in the 1870s states and municipalities began passing laws relating to specific foods or drugs. The first state law applying generally to food was passed by Illinois in 1874, but little more was accomplished for a few years. In 1879 Congressman Hendrick B. Wright of Pennsylvania introduced the first federal bill to prevent food adulteration, but it was too far in advance of its time. By this date public health leaders, medical societies, and business and trade associations in New York and New Jersey were joining forces to push food adulteration laws through their state legislatures. After considerable political maneuvering, in 1881 almost identical bills were enacted in New Jersey and New York. The legislation prohibited the sale of adulterated food and drugs, specified what the term "adulterated drug" meant, assigned responsibility for the law's enforcement to the state board of health, and set fines for violations of the law.[32]

This same year Michigan and Illinois passed comparable laws, and in 1883 Massachusetts passed an even stronger law against food adulteration. By 1895 twenty-seven states had enacted some type of food adulteration measures. Although some of them were modeled on the New York law, the laws varied widely, ranging from comprehensive statutes to very limited ones. Several minor pieces of legislation wended their way through Congress, but they were largely concerned with trade. The first one, in 1886, taxed and regulated the sale of oleomargarine, undoubtedly reflecting the influence of the dominant agricultural interests of legislators.[33] The others were of little significance, and federal action awaited the Pure Food and Drug Act of 1906.

Another subject that troubled virtually all health reformers and worried the public in the latter part of the nineteenth century was air pollution. Unlike the present-day concern with air pollution, the public's fears were related to the miasmatic doctrine of disease causation. Typhus, for example, was assumed to be caused by a combination of filth, crowding, and poor ventilation; and sanitationists in general assumed that malodorous smells, whether from sewers, unclean and unventilated buildings, or other sources, were in themselves the cause of fevers and other diseases. By the 1830s and 1840s physicians and health reformers were discussing the danger arising from crowded unventilated schools, tenements, and public buildings.

By the 1870s medical and sanitary journals, popular magazines, newspapers, and public health reformers all joined in warning about the danger from poor ventilation and sewer gas. In 1874 Dr. Edward H. Janes, addressing the APHA on health conditions in the tenements, spoke of the foul odors that accumulated in them and declared: "It is this odor which indicates the commencement of that condition known as crowd-poisoned atmosphere, and which, if allowed to increase, furnishes the specific germs which develop typhus, ship or jail fever."[34] Two years later Professor William H. Brewer informed the association that chemists were unable to explain why, or if, gases of decay had deleterious effects, but that the fact that typhoid had been caused by the escape of sewer gas seemed to have been proven "beyond a reasonable doubt."[35] Dr. Richard McSherry informed the Baltimore Academy of Medicine in 1882 that the city desperately needed pure air. Baltimore's air is so polluted, he declared, "that adults grow ill and children die of it by thousands, especially during the summer heats, with each recurring year." The air was poisoned by the "vast collection of decomposable refuse" and the city's thousands of privy pits and cesspools.[36]

Ironically, in 1886 an article on house sanitation in the *Journal of the American Medical Association* suggested that the space under the floors, which seldom receives "pure air," might be the source of germs, and the author suggested that this space be filled with asbestos or other material.[37] The construction of sewer systems and water closets increased the specter of sewer gas and was undoubtedly responsible for the enactment of plumbing codes toward the end of the century. Many early water closets were located outside the main building as a safety measure. By 1900 bacteriologists had laid to rest the sewer gas thesis, but it was well into the twentieth century before many health workers and the public accepted their findings.

The public demand for fresh air and the ventilation of buildings and homes gained strength with the discovery of the airborne transmission of respiratory and other disorders. The drive against tuberculosis, which began in the 1890s, was particularly effective in this respect. As of 1900, however, there was little concern for industrial air pollution. A number of laws were passed against smoke pollution, but smoke was considered more of a nuisance than a danger to health. Until the virtual elimination of the great killer diseases in the early years of the twentieth century and the development of more sophisticated methods for analyzing air, few individuals gave much thought to the more subtle forms of air pollution.

The late nineteenth century, which saw the United States emerge as a major industrial power, also witnessed the appearance of the first significant labor laws. Before the large influx of immigrants in the 1880s and 1890s little concern had been shown for industrial health. The expanding

American economy created a perennial labor shortage; thus many of the worst abuses that characterized the early industrial revolution elsewhere did not appear here. Moreover, most employers shared the moral values of their colonial forefathers who emphasized social responsibility and moral discipline. It was assumed, too, that the wealth created by a market free of government control would benefit the workers as well as the capitalists. Even before the Civil War, however, health reformers were beginning to point out that health was the sole property of the wage earner, and that, as property, it required a measure of government protection.

The Civil War, by giving a major impetus to American industry, created a class of urban industrial workers whose background and skills no longer fitted them to take advantage of the free land in the West; it also raised the prestige of the political economists who were seeking to devise means for evaluating the nation's wealth and productive capacity. Political economists recognized from the start that the health of a country's people was a major factor in determining that country's strength, and by the 1870s they were joining with health reformers in arguing for state responsibility for the health of workers. As was the case in Britain, the first American labor regulations were designed to remedy abuses in factories and pertained largely to women and children. The deplorable conditions under which home workers and those in small sweatshops labored received little attention until much later.[38]

Massachusetts led the way in regulating child labor, enacting laws in 1824, 1836–37, and 1842. Other states were slow to follow, and as of 1879 only two other states, Rhode Island and Pennsylvania, had any restrictions on child labor. The first action on behalf of labor came as a result of the Depression of 1837, when President Martin Van Buren decreed a ten-hour day for all federal workers. By 1853 five states had enacted ten-hour laws, but they applied largely to state employees. Although the immediate postwar years saw a rising interest in occupational health, the result, in terms of legislation, was minimal. Dr. George Derby of the Massachusetts Board of Health wrote that the health of workers was of primary concern to the board but that health statistics on them were difficult to obtain. He recognized, as did other reformers, that the unsanitary living conditions of most workers made it difficult to differentiate between medical problems arising from occupational hazards and those arising from other sources.[39]

In addition to taking the initiative in limiting child labor, Massachusetts made a significant contribution to occupational health by appointing the first factory inspectors and establishing a State Bureau of Labor Statistics in 1870. In this same year the state legislature required the state board of health to report annually the number of minors employed in factories, to ascertain the causes of death among factory children, and to compare their rate of mortality with that of other minors.[40] Some years elapsed before the factory inspectors' reports of the grim conditions under which men, women, and children labored brought legislative action, but the accumulated evidence in these reports helped reformers in Massachusetts and elsewhere to overcome the argument that labor laws infringed on the right of personal property and the sanctity of individual contracts (the right of adults to contract their own labor and that of their children).

In the nineteenth century employers had little responsibility for hazards in the workplace. Although Pennsylvania was one of the more progressive states with respect to occupational health, the Pittsburgh *Daily Post* could report in 1867 that a meeting was to be held to devise means "for the relief of destitute families" arising from a boiler explosion at the "Iron Works in Pitt Township." The explosion had killed seventeen men and injured more than twenty. The same paper reported two months later that a "boiler ordinance" was pending before the Philadelphia City Council and called on the Pittsburgh authorities to enact a similar measure to protect lives and property.[41] Yet it was 1886 before the first law in the nation requiring the reporting of industrial accidents was passed by Massachusetts, and only three other states had enacted comparable laws by 1900.

Most of the laws passed in the 1880s and 1890s related to women and children. New York State made a stab at protecting female employees in 1881 with an amorphous law requiring employers to provide them with seats. A much more comprehensive law was enacted in 1886. It limited the working hours of women under 21 and minors under 18 to sixty hours per week "unless for the purpose of making necessary repairs." Children below the age of 13 could not be employed in manufacturing, and those between the ages of 13 and 16 were required to have a certificate signed by their parent or guardian. The law's most important feature was a clause authorizing the governor to appoint two officers, a factory inspector and an assistant, to enforce the law.[42] In succeeding years New York's laws regulating labor were steadily strengthened. In 1892 the working age was raised to 14, and several safety and health measures, such as proper guards on machines and exhaust fans for ventilation, were required. Four years later an important amendment to the 1886 law broadened it to include retail stores, one of the chief places of female employment. It also required minors between the ages of 14 and 16 to obtain a certificate from the local health board or department.[43]

Probably more typical of the labor laws were those of Maryland. In 1888 a maximum ten-hour day was established for children under 16, and in 1896 industrial plants were forbidden to employ children under the age of 12. Significantly, the law did not apply to 16 counties in the state, including Baltimore, the chief industrial center.[44] By 1900 a start had been made toward eliminating the medical problems arising from the workplace, but concrete action was limited to only a few states. Even in the states where factory inspectors had been appointed, there were too few inspectors for the task assigned to them. Labor unions, which might have been expected to push for improved occupational health conditions, were too busy fighting for mere survival and for the eight-hour day to have any other concerns.

As the nineteenth century drew to a close, the sanitary movement was beginning to improve the quality of urban life. In the major cities morbidity and mortality rates were declining, and life expectancy, which had started to fall in the 1830s and 1840s, was on the rise. The incidence of the great killer diseases was still high, but improved sanitation and a higher standard of living were improving the general health. Sanitary science, or public health, was becoming both institutionalized and professionalized, and in the urban centers, health departments were contributing notably to educating the public and to eliminating or reducing the worst threats to community health.

For the great majority of Americans, who lived in rural areas or in towns with populations of less than 2,500, community health had little meaning. With a few exceptions, health departments were restricted to the larger cities; and state health boards, whose annual budgets seldom exceeded $5,000, were for the most part ineffective. Happily, by this time the bacteriological revolution, probably the most significant development in the history of medicine, was changing the entire focus of the public health field—a change that would profoundly affect life in the twentieth century.

NOTES

1. *Campaign Book of the Citizens' Union, September-October, 1897* (New York, 1897), 54–55.

2. Martin V. Melosi, *Pragmatic Environmentalist: Sanitary Engineer George E. Waring, Jr.* (Washington, D.C., 1977), 12–16.

3. John Duffy, *A History of Public Health in New York City, 1866–1966* (New York, 1974), 126.

4. Ronald L. Numbers and Judith W. Leavitt, *Wisconsin Medicine: Historical Perspectives* (Madison, Wis., 1981), 157.

5. *Daily Pittsburgh Gazette,* January 8, 20, 1864.

6. *Pennsylvania Archives,* 4th ser., 11, 759–61.

7. *Sixth Annual Report of the State Board of Health of ... Ohio ... October, 1890* (Columbus, 1890), 6–9.

8. William T. Howard, *Public Health Administration and the Natural History of Diseases in Baltimore, Maryland, 1797–1920* (Washington, D.C., 1924), 120–21.

9. Duffy, *Public Health in New York City, 1866–1966,* 118, 519–20.

10. Ibid., 230–35.

11. *Annual Report of the Health Department of the City of New York, 1890* (New York, 1891), 51–52.

12. Roy Lubove, ed., *Pittsburgh* (New York, 1976), 87ff.

13. John Duffy, "Social Impact of Disease in the Late Nineteenth Century," *Bulletin of the New York Academy of Medicine* 43 (1971):798–99.

14. Judith W. Leavitt, "Politics and Public Health: Smallpox in Milwaukee, 1894–1895," *Bull. Hist. Med.* 50 (1976):553–68.

15. Horace W. Conrad, "The Health of Negroes in the South . . . ," *The Sanitarian* 18 (1887):502, 505.

16. Duffy, *Public Health in New York City, 1866–1966,* 208–11.

17. Ibid., 211–13.

18. John Duffy, "Early Days of the School Health Movement," *Conspectus of History* 1, no. 7 (Cambridge, 1981):46–47; Duffy, "School Buildings and the Health of American School Children in the Nineteenth Century," in *Healing and History: Essays for George Rosen,* Charles E. Rosenberg, ed. (New York, 1979), 164–65.

19. Duffy, "School Buildings and Health in the Nineteenth Century," 169, 175.

20. John Duffy, "School Vaccination: The Precursor to School Medical Inspection," *J. Hist. Med. & All. Sci.* 33 (1978):344–55.

21. Duffy, "Early Days of the School Health Movement," 54–55.

22. Ibid., 56–57.

23. Ibid., 58–61.

24. Ibid., 61.

25. For a discussion of the early swill milk problem, see John Duffy, *A History of Public Health in New York City, 1625–1866* (New York, 1968), 427–37.

26. Mazÿck P. Ravenel, ed., *A Half Century of Public Health* (New York, 1921), 285–86.

27. Duffy, *Public Health in New York City, 1625–1866,* 431–36.

28. Ravenel, *A Half Century of Public Health,* 286.

29. Ibid., 267.

30. Gordon Atkins, "Health, Housing, and Poverty in New York City, 1865–1898" (Ph.D. diss., Columbia University, 1947), 243ff.

31. Michael Okun, *Fair Play in the Marketplace: The First Battle for Pure Food and Drugs* (DeKalb, Ill., 1986), 128, 136, 159–61, 287–95; see also Howard D. Kramer, "Agitation for Public Health Reform in the 1870s," *J. Hist. Med. & All. Sci.* 3 (1948):481.

32. Okun, *Fair Play in the Marketplace,* 116, 149, 158–68.

33. Ravenel, *A Half Century of Public Health,* 214–15.

34. Edward H. Janes, "Health of Tenement Populations and the Sanitary Requirements of Their Dwellings," in *Selections from Reports and Papers of the APHA (1873–1883),* 118.

35. William H. Brewer, "The Gases of Decay and the Harm They Cause . . . ," in ibid., 118.

36. Richard McSherry, "The City Needs a Change of Air," *The Sanitarian* 10 (1882):385.

37. "A Danger in House Sanitation," *JAMA* 6 (1886):264.

38. For an excellent account of the early occupational health movement in America see Craig Donegan, "For the Good of Us All: Early Attitudes toward Occupational Health with Emphasis on the Northern United States from 1787 to 1870" (Ph.D. diss., University of Maryland, 1984).

39. Ibid., 339; George Derby, "Health of Minors Employed . . . ," *Second Annual Report of the State Board of Health of Massachusetts* (Boston, 1871), 409–23.

40. Donegan, "For the Good of Us All," 342–43.

41. Pittsburgh *Daily Post*, November 11, 1867, January 4, 1868.

42. *New York State Laws*, 104th sess., chap. 298, May 18, 1881, vol. 1:402; 109th sess., chap. 409, May 18, 1886, vol. 1:629–30.

43. Ibid., 115th sess., chap. 673, May 18, 1892, vol. 1:1372–79; 119th sess., chap. 991, May 29, 1896, vol. 1:1135–42.

44. Howard, *Public Health Administration in Baltimore,* 80–81.

13

Bacteriology Revolutionizes Public Health

Based on the valid assumption that cleanliness, fresh air, and pure water were essential to community health, and on the less valid assumption that epidemic diseases were caused by an indefinable substance known as miasma, the sanitary movement made a major contribution to community health in the nineteenth century. But even as sanitation, in conjunction with a rising standard of living, was raising the health and life expectancy of urban populations at the end of the nineteenth century—and, to a much lesser extent, that of the majority of Americans, who still lived in rural areas and small towns—developments in bacteriology were in the process of revolutionizing both medicine and public health.

The concept of microscopic pathogenic organisms dates back to the sixteenth century, but it was not until the nineteenth that their role was defined. While Lister, Koch, and Pasteur played key roles in the emergence of bacteriology, they were able to capitalize on a host of previous discoveries and advances in a variety of areas. Chemistry, physiology, pathological anatomy, and clinical medicine all helped point the way to an understanding of the role of germs. In addition, the invention of the achromatic microscrope in the 1830s led to studies of infusoria, which in turn revived interest in the seventeenth-century "animalculae" theory of disease. By the 1840s minute parasites and fungi had been identified as causes of disease in humans and animals. The culmination of all of this work came in the 1880s, the decade that saw the identification of the organisms responsible for most of the great killer diseases. Once the precise organism was identified, it became possible to discover how it was transmitted and the role of carriers in its spread. It was possible, too, to create antitoxins and vaccines, thus opening up new fields for public health.

Aside from the work of men such as Theobald Smith, George M. Sternberg, William Welch, and a few others, in the nineteenth century Americans contributed little to the development of bacteriology; but by the 1890s laboratories were springing up in medical schools, universities, hospitals, and health departments, and privately endowed laboratories were appearing. The first health department laboratories were designed to do elementary analyses of milk, water, and other substances. Charles F. Chandler was appointed analytical chemist for the New York Metropolitan Board of Health in 1869, and in 1881 the New York legislature established a state chemical laboratory. In the meantime, Dr. Charles N. Hewitt, the mainstay of the early Minnesota Board of Health, established another small chemical laboratory in 1873.[1]

As noted in chapter 10, Massachusetts established a hygienic laboratory in 1886, and Michigan followed suit in 1887. Both of these laboratories were intended to perform chemical analysis, but the association of drinking water with typhoid fever soon led them into the field of bacteriology. Using the facilities of the Lawrence Experiment Station of the Massachusetts Board of Health, William T. Sedgwick pioneered in the application of bacteriology to sanitary science, and, as a professor at the Massachusetts Institute of Technology, offered one of the first courses in sanitation and public health. Frederick G. Novy, another pioneer in American bacteriology, and his colleague on the University of Michigan Medical School faculty, Victor C. Vaughan, in 1889 organized what was probably the first formal laboratory course in bacteriology offered by an American university. Vaughan later became a dominant figure in American public health.

The dynamic leadership of Charles V. Chapin was responsible for the city of Providence establishing another of the better laboratories in 1888. As with many of the early laboratories, the Providence laboratory began investigating the city's water supply, but, under the stimulus of a typhoid epidemic, it quickly turned to studying microorganisms.[2] Claims to priority in establishing laboratories have been made by local historians for several cities and states, but the issue is not important since it is clear that in the 1880s a number of laboratories had come into existence and that by 1890 work in chemical analysis and bacteriology was well under way.

The nation's greatly exaggerated fear of Asiatic cholera was responsible for the first diagnostic public health laboratory, which was in New York City. Drs. Hermann M. Biggs and T. Mitchell Prudden in the fall of 1887 were able to isolate cholera vibrio from passengers on an immigrant vessel. Biggs realized he had found a way to make a definite diagnosis of the disease, but he had to await a cholera scare in 1892 before he could convince the city health department to use this new technique. On September 9 of that year the department established the Division of Pathology, Bacteriology, and Disinfection under the direction of Dr. Biggs. He immediately began testing suspected cholera cases and was able to make a positive identification in a number of them.[3]

Diphtheria, a major problem in the second half of the nineteenth century, reached a peak in America in the early 1890s and was responsible for the first wide-scale application of bacteriology to public health. As the number of cases in New York City began to rise early in 1893, Dr. Biggs reported to the board of health that bacteriological testing of patients in the diphtheria hospital had shown that half of them had pseudo-diphtheria. He shrewdly pointed out that laboratory testing to make a positive diagnosis of all reported cases of diphtheria would be much cheaper than disinfecting and quarantining the homes of all suspected cases. The board acted on his advice and appointed Dr. William H. Park as "bacteriological diagnostician and inspector of diphtheria." At the same time Dr. Biggs had started routine laboratory testing of suspected tuberculosis cases. Although many physicians were dubious of this new diagnostic method, the profession, responding to public pressure, recognized its value, and the New York City Health Department was forced into a rapid expansion of its laboratory staff and facilities.

In his quest to keep informed of the latest developments in bacteriology, Biggs visited Europe in 1893. Learning of Emile Roux's technique for producing large quantities of diphtheria antitoxin in horses, he immediately cabled Park to begin producing the antitoxin. The health department promptly requested funds for the project, but when Biggs learned the money would not be immediately available, he assumed personal responsibility for buying the horses and laboratory equipment. The health department, which had been operating a smallpox vaccine laboratory since 1874, in 1895 turned production of the vaccine over to Dr. Biggs and his division. He and his assistant, Dr. Park, studied the best methods of production and began producing a high-grade vaccine the following year. In this same year the laboratory also began production of an antitoxin for tetanus.[4]

By October 1895 the laboratory staff had completely outgrown its quarters, necessitating a move. Despite this rapid growth, constant research and refining of production techniques steadily increased the quantity of vaccines and antitoxins produced and improved their quality. For example, within two years, the cost of diphtheria antitoxin was reduced from 80 cents per 100 units to 10 cents per 100. Some years earlier the smallpox laboratory had been given authority to sell its surplus vaccine; in 1895 Biggs was able to extend this authority to include the sale of antitoxins and other biologicals. By 1896 the health department's laboratories were supplying the city with ample supplies of vaccines and antitoxins and acquiring research funds through its sale of surpluses. More significantly, the widespread use of diphtheria antitoxin had drastically reduced the case fatality rate.[5]

The work of Biggs, Park, and their associates won immediate national and international recognition, and a stream of bacteriologists and health workers flocked to their laboratory. By 1895 ten other cities had already established diagnostic laboratories, and within a few years they had become essential to any effective health department.[6] The New York City Laboratory was not the first of its kind, but it was the first one to use laboratory testing for diseases on a routine basis, and in spearheading testing it provided public health workers with a radical new method for fighting disease. The advent of vaccines and antitoxins in conjunction with the discovery of the role of vectors and carriers provided a means for both preventing and curing contagious disorders. Science rather than sanitation now seemed to be the solution to sickness and disease.

The bacteriological revolution, along with other developments in medicine, immeasurably strengthened the position of the medical profession, and it also firmly ensconced physicians in charge of public health. The nineteenth-century view that laypersons had to control public health boards gave way to the assumption that community health was best left to professionals. The medical profession in these years was somewhat ambivalent about bacteriology and the development of public health agencies. If one can judge by newspapers and popular journals, the public was far quicker to accept the germ theory than physicians were. Most articles in medical journals supported the concept of bacteria, but many conservative physicians were unconvinced. An 1884 article in *JAMA* discussed the work of Robert Koch and others on the tuberculosis bacillus and concluded that a "too ready acceptance of the bacillus doctrine" was likely to do more harm than good and that "neither phthisis nor any form of tuberculosis [was] contagious."[7] When the New York Health Department began treating diphtheria patients with antitoxin, a leading clinician in the city asserted that he had seen 154 patients in the diphtheria hospital, not one of whom had benefited from the treatment.[8]

It is well to keep in mind that medical journals were written by and for a relatively small group of well-educated elitist physicians, the same group that dominated the AMA and state and local medical societies. Most physicians were poorly educated, did little to keep abreast of their profession, and spent their time struggling to make a living. The physicians who promoted public health and served in health departments represented the elite of the profession. Most came from middle- or upper-class backgrounds and had no financial worries. They tended to have a social awareness and to keep up with the latest developments in medicine. They advocated laboratory diagnosis of contagious diseases, compulsory reporting of cases, and isolation of patients. Their elitist colleagues in private practice, however, resented any interference with their patients. Reporting contagious diseases cases was seen as a breach of the confidential relationship between doctor and patient. And even those who were inclined to accept the findings of bacteriology still thought that disease among the poor was largely the result of their filthy habits.

While the better physicians generally gave strong support to the public health movement in the nineteenth century, the emergence of an institutionalized and professionalized public health movement at the end of the century, as indicated above, tended to divide physicians. Nowhere is this better seen than in the struggle to require the compulsory reporting of tuberculosis cases in New York City beginning in 1897. After gathering overwhelming evidence to demonstrate that tuberculosis was a communicable disease, Dr. Biggs and his associates persuaded the city's board of health to require all physicians to report their cases. Almost without exception medical journals and societies denounced the action. The *Medical Record* admitted that tuberculosis was somewhat contagious but called the ruling "dictatorial and defiantly compulsory." Both the Academy of Medicine and the County Medical Society of New York denounced the board of health, the latter calling its ruling "unnecessary, inexpedient, and unwise." When the board held its ground, the medical societies turned to the state legislature in an attempt to reduce its authority. Dr. Biggs and his supporters successfully upheld the board, but to do so they were forced to spend a considerable part of the next two years at the state legislature.[9]

The attitude of the New York physicians was in no sense unique. Philadelphia passed an ordinance requiring the reporting of tuberculosis cases in 1893 but repealed it the following year when faced by opposition from the College of Physicians. This latter body declared that registering consumptives would add hardship to their lives, "stamping them as outcasts of society." In any event, because "of the chronic nature of the malady," reporting cases "could not lead to any measures of real value." In Chicago the opposition was strong enough to prevent compulsory reporting of the disease until 1902. The St. Louis *Medical Review* expressed the hope that St. Louis would not emulate New York City, adding that it was sure the ordinance would have "but an ephemeral existence."[10] On behalf of the medical profession, it should be said that a diagnosis of tuberculosis was viewed by most laypersons as the kiss of death. Many insurance companies had clauses in their policies negating them in the event of death by the disease. Under these circumstances, patients and their families pressured physicians to avoid mentioning tuberculosis on death certificates. Physicians, in turn, realized that payment of their fees frequently depended on the patient's insurance.

Tuberculosis, which was so feared in the late nineteenth and early twentieth centuries, had drawn surprisingly little public attention earlier. It was even considered a slightly romantic disease, allowing delicate young females to decline to a tragic death; Mimi in *La Bohème* illustrates this poetic view. Yet it had been consistently a leading cause of death. Unlike the more dramatic infections, its victims often lingered for many years, making it a familiar sickness. The disease was generally assumed to be a constitutional disorder, resulting from an inherited tendency toward weak lungs or from some other condition undermining the respiratory system. Its significance as a major cause of sickness and death was not recognized until the development of improved morbidity and mortality statistics in the latter part of the nineteenth century. Ironically, although the tuberculosis bacillus was among the first pathogenic organisms discovered, the twentieth century was at hand before most physicians and laypersons were convinced that it was a communicable disease.

The idea that fresh air and rest could cure tuberculosis led many physicians to advise their patients to move to the country or to go West, advice which was responsible for a good part of the migration to the Southwest. This assumption was also the basis for the excellent work of Dr. Edward Trudeau, who founded a tuberculosis sanatorium at Saranac Lake, New York, in 1876. His success eventually led to the founding of hundreds of similar institutions over the next forty years and stimulated an entire fresh air movement. Among the states receiving the dubious benefit of an influx of immigrants seeking relief from tuberculosis were Michigan and Minnesota. Not surprisingly, health leaders in both of these states were among the first to recognize the seriousness of the tuberculosis problem. In the 1880s Dr. Victor C. Vaughan in Michigan and Dr. Charles N. Hewitt in Minnesota began pointing out that the disease was communicable. Their interest was aroused in part by the relatively high incidence of the disorder among cows. In Minnesota supervision of animal diseases was given to the state's board of health in 1885. Michigan in 1889 established a separate Live Stock Commission to work with diseases of animals and their relationship to humans, but it, too, was instructed to work closely with the state board of health.[11]

It is a commentary upon America's limited sense of social responsibility in the nineteenth century that the states and the federal government spent far more for medical research on the diseases of animals than for research on diseases of humans. By the 1890s a number of cities were beginning to inspect milk supplies. Dr. Hewitt persuaded the Minnesota Board of Health in 1895 to require testing of all dairy herds in the state and to condemn those with tuberculosis. The program was relatively effective, but the opposition it aroused undoubtedly contributed to Dr. Hewitt's removal two years later as secretary of the Board of Health, a position he had held for twenty-five years.[12] Most health boards moved far more cautiously, and it was well into the twentieth century before the practice of eliminating tubercular cows became general.

Within a few more years the exact relationship of tuberculosis between cows and humans was established. In 1896 Theobald Smith, at that time director of the Massachusetts State Laboratory, identified two different strains of the disease and indicated cows as a source of human tuberculosis. By 1904 M. P. Ravenel had shown that bovine tuberculosis could be transmitted to humans, and in 1912 William H. Park and Charles Krumwiede demonstrated that contaminated milk was a significant source of various forms of the disease among children.[13]

In addition to the pioneering work of Drs. Vaughan and Hewitt in stimulating health departments to tackle the problem of tuberculosis, men such as Theobald Smith and Dr. Hermann M. Biggs carried the fight into the twentieth century. Under prodding from Smith, the Massachusetts State Health Department made the disease reportable in 1901 and conducted one of the more successful campaigns to reduce its incidence.[14] Biggs lectured to medical school faculties, health departments, and lay groups, stressing the communicability of the disease and listing the means to control it. His department's tuberculosis program in New York City became a model for health departments throughout the country. Although a leading advocate of bacteriology, Biggs was also one of the first to realize that tuberculosis was to a large extent a product of the social environment. Unlike most of his contemporaries, who were carried away by their enthusiam for fighting germs, he urged health leaders to give attention to social and economic conditions.[15]

Any major step forward in public health is only possible when backed by a strong public demand—and effective health departments are those that create a public awareness of social evils. The sanitary movement did not gain momentum until hundreds of volunteer citizens' groups sprang up throughout the country and overrode vested interests and apathy to push through major reforms. The same situation held true for tuberculosis. The first of these volunteer groups was the Pennsylvania Society for the Prevention of Tuberculosis, organized in 1892 by Dr. Lawrence F. Flock and a few others. Interestingly, shortly before this time, Dr. Biggs had written to twenty-four prominent physicians in Philadelphia asking whether or not the local health board should take sanitary measures to reduce tuberculosis. Only five or six bothered to reply, and of these, only two agreed the local health board should take action. In any event, by 1904 twenty-three state and local societies had been formed, and in this year they joined to organize the National Association for the Study and Prevention of Tuberculosis.[16]

Either in conjunction with voluntary groups or on their own initiative, by the 1890s city and state health departments were beginning campaigns to educate the public on the danger from tuberculosis, diphtheria, and other communicable diseases. State departments sent educational literature to physicians and health officers, and pamphlets were issued to the general public warning them in particular that tuberculosis was spread by sputum. As the decade came to a close, anti-spitting laws were enacted, such as the 1897 one in Cincinnati, which prohibited spitting on the sidewalk.[17] The strength of the anti-spitting campaign at the turn of the century is exemplified by a brick stamped with the words "DON'T SPIT ON SIDEWALK," which was removed from a sidewalk in Hutchinson, Kansas, and is presently in the author's possession.

By 1910 most states had made the reporting of tuberculosis and other communicable diseases compulsory, and in major cities health departments were conducting bacteriological examinations of milk and water supplies. In 1897 Chicago became the first city to require pasteurization of all milk except for that from tuberculin-tested cows, although more than thirty years would elapse before this practice became general throughout the United States. Nonetheless, through conducting educational campaigns, controlling milk supplies, and isolating advanced cases in sanitariums, the incidence of tuberculosis was steadily reduced. A major step was taken toward reducing the number of tubercular cows when, in 1917, the United States Department of Agriculture began a national program of testing cows and compensating owners for the killing of their tubercular animals. Yet it was 1930 before Michigan, one of the most progressive states in this respect, could claim to have eliminated tuberculosis from its dairy herds.[18]

One of the more obvious lessons from public health history is that knowing how to prevent a disease does not necessarily lead to its control or elimination. Smallpox, for which a relatively effective vaccination had been available for almost two hundred years, was only eliminated in recent times. As discussed earlier, compulsory school vaccination and mass vaccination programs in times of epidemics only reduced the disease, making it one of minor importance. Later in the nineteenth century, aided by a strong antivaccination movement and public apathy, smallpox continued to flare up. In 1902 Michigan had a total of 7,086 cases, and between 1898 and 1905 Ohio had 29,457 cases and 890 deaths. In a commentary upon the medical profession, in 1900 twelve students in the Tulane University School of Medicine came down with smallpox, three of whom died.[19]

The antivaccination movement peaked in the 1880s and 1890s, but its influence continued for many years, helped in part by the failure to recognize that one vaccination was not necessarily good for life. It was led largely by irregular physicians and laypersons, and supported by the element in any population that will cling to traditional ideas at all costs.[20] The movement was most successful in opposing compulsory school vaccination, and its strength varied from state to state. The Kentucky State Board of Health reported in 1906 that smallpox, "which has so engrossed the time and energies of health officials," has now been practically elimi-nated. This same year the Washington State Board was urging that all schoolchildren be vaccinated—not just those in cities of 10,000 or more. In 1912 the California State Board of Health appealed for a more general vaccination law. Its failure to obtain one meant that between 1912 and 1917 California averaged almost 500 smallpox cases a year, and the total cases jumped to 2,053 in 1919, 4,497 in 1920, and 5,579 in 1921.[21]

The antivaccinationists successfully used the courts and legislatures to delay action. When a county in North Carolina ordered compulsory vac-cination of all schoolchildren in 1905, the health authorities had to do legal battle in order to have the order upheld. Eight years later, the state legislature specifically denied health boards the right to quarantine smallpox cases, whereupon the state board of health responded by making the disease reportable and posting notices throughout the state that the disease could be avoided by vaccination.[22] An outbreak of smallpox in Seattle in 1918–19 resulted in some 869 cases, an epidemic which the health department blamed on Christian Scientists and antivaccinationists who had pushed a bill through the legislature prohibiting compulsory vaccination.[23]

It is true that by 1900 the way was open for vastly reducing the inci-dence of the traditional killer diseases, yet progress was by no means rapid. Diphtheria remained a significant cause of death for many years despite the success of antitoxin. By 1915 an effective method of immuniza-tion had emerged through the use of toxin-antitoxin, and New York City began testing this new preventive. When it became evident by 1920 that the program was successful, the city began active immunization of chil-dren on a large scale. By 1940, when about 60 percent of the city's children had been immunized, the disease was virtually gone.[24] The New York success encouraged many other city and state health boards to move ahead in the fight against diphtheria. Typical of these campaigns was one conducted in Louisville, Kentucky, beginning in 1928. With the help of funds from the Rockefeller Foundation and the United States Public Health Service, the city health department adopted a slogan: "No Diph-theria in the City of Louisville by 1930."[25] Smaller towns and rural areas were slower to adopt immunization procedures, but the disease was gradu-ally brought under control.

The conquest of typhoid came in part from the sanitarians' quest for pure water and in part from the findings of bacteriology. In 1886, before the American medical profession was convinced that typhoid resulted from a specific bacillus, the Massachusetts State Board of Health established the Lawrence Experimental Station, essentially an engineering laboratory to measure water quality and study methods for improving it. In 1890 the town of Lowell requested the state bacteriologist, William T. Sedgwick, to investigate an outbreak of typhoid. Although he was unable to isolate the bacillus from the town's various water supplies, he systematically traced the epidemic to its source and thus pointed up the need to purify drinking water. Sedgwick's findings and the work already done by Hiram Mills, head of the Lawrence Engineering Laboratory, paved the way for the construction of the first open slow sand filter in 1893, an effective method for producing safe drinking water.[26]

Almost at the same time, studies in Providence, 1893–94, and Louisville, 1895–97, demonstrated that the addition of coagulants to a mechanical filtration system could remove bacteria. The net effect of this and other research was that filtration of water was rapidly adopted in European and American cities, with most American cities relying upon mechanical systems. By 1911 about 20 percent of America's urban population was using filtered water.[27] The next major step was the treatment of water with chlorine. It was used fairly extensively in Europe in the treatment of sewage in the late nineteenth century, but it was not until the early years of the twentieth century that it was used to purify water. In 1908 Jersey City, New Jersey, began treating its water supply, and within a few years chlorination was adopted by many cities. Chicago, which had one of the highest typhoid rates in the country, solved its problem, first, by draining its sewers away from Lake Michigan, its water source, and, second, through chlorinating its entire water supply by 1916. In consequence, the typhoid rate, which had averaged 67 cases per 100,000 people in the 1890s, fell to 14 by 1910, and to 1 per 100,000 by 1919, the lowest rate in the nation.[28]

The combination of safer water supplies and the use of typhoid immunization, although the latter was done on a relatively small scale in the early twentieth century, steadily reduced the number of cases and deaths from typhoid in the United States. The death rate from typhoid fell from 31.3 per 100,000 in 1900 to 22.5 in 1910 and to 7.6 in 1920. Only limited gains were made in the 1920s, a period of government inaction, but by 1940 the rate was only 1.1 per 100,000.[29]

The histories of tuberculosis and typhoid point up how much the improvement of community health depends not only on science but on technological developments, a rising standard of living, and a concern by citizens and government for the health and welfare of the people. Once science had identified the malaria parasite and explained the role of its vector, the anopheles mosquito, its conquest was largely a matter of drainage, insecticides, and screening. But drainage in many areas was an expensive project and required a willingness to spend tax funds, and screening presupposed a high enough standard of living for householders to afford screens. In the South it required the infusion of large-scale federal funds under the New Deal and massive outlays during World War II to break the cycle of poverty and relegate malaria to a disease of the past. The same situation was true, to a lesser degree, of parasitic diseases such as hookworm, in which case the wearing of shoes was a major requisite for disease control, and of the various nutritional disorders associated with impoverished diets. The many pockets of trachoma in Appalachia and other areas of the United States in the early twentieth century were also largely associated with poverty, and their elimination, too, required both medical resources and a willingness on the part of government and private groups to improve the social environment.

NOTES

1. Philip D. Jordan, *The People's Health: A History of Public Health in Minnesota to 1948* (St. Paul, 1953), 50.

2. Mazÿck P. Ravenel, ed., *A Half Century of Public Health* (New York, 1921), 91; James H. Cassedy, *Charles V. Chapin and the Public Health Movement* (Cambridge, Mass., 1942), 55–59.

3. C.-E. A. Winslow, *The Contributions of Hermann Biggs to Public Health* (New York, 1928), 8–9; John Duffy, *A History of Public Health in New York City, 1866–1966* (New York, 1974), 94–95.

4. Duffy, *Public Health in New York City, 1866–1966*, 97–100, 104–5.

5. Ibid., 102.

6. Howard D. Kramer, "History of the Public Health Movement in the United States, 1850–1950" (Ph.D. diss., University of Iowa, 1942), 209.

7. D. H. Leonard, "The Bacillus of Tuberculosis and the Aetiology of Tuberculosis—Is Consumption Contagious?," *JAMA* 2 (1884):463.

8. Winslow, *The Life of Hermann M. Biggs: Physician and Statesman of the Public Health* (Philadelphia, 1929), 117–18.

9. Duffy, *Public Health in New York City, 1866–1966*, 103–4, 241–42.

10. William G. Rothstein, *American Physicians in the Nineteenth Century: From Sects to Science* (Baltimore, 1972), 272; Winslow, *The Life of Hermann M. Biggs*, 139–44.

11. Ola G. Hylton, "A History of the Public Health Movement in Michigan, 1888–1913" (Ph.D. diss., University of Michigan, 1943), 62; C. B. Burr, ed., *Medical History of Michigan* (Minneapolis, 1930), 1:808–9.

12. Jordan, *The People's Health*, 72, 76.

13. George Rosen, *Preventive Medicine in the United States, 1900–1975: Trends and Interpretations* (New York, 1975), 29.

14. Barbara G. Rosenkrantz, *Public Health and the State: Changing Views in Massachusetts, 1842–1936* (Cambridge, Mass., 1972), 119–23.

15. Herman M. Biggs, "Sanitary Science, the Medical Profession, and the Public," Anniversary Discourse, November 18, 1897, in *Transactions*, New York Academy of Medicine (New York, 1903), 201.

16. Rosen, *Preventive Medicine in the United States*, 26–27; Winslow, *The Life of Hermann M. Biggs*, 86.

17. Reginald C. McGrane, *The Cincinnati Doctors' Forum* (Cincinnati, 1957), 188.

18. Ravenel, *A Half Century of Public Health*, 149; Burr, *Medical History of Michigan*, 1:815–16.

19. Hylton, "History of the Public Health Movement in Michigan," 204; *Twentieth Annual Report of the State Board of Health of Ohio for the Year Ending December 31, 1905*, 5; John Duffy, *The Tulane University Medical Center: One Hundred and Fifty Years of Medical Education* (Baton Rouge, La., 1984), 140.

20. For a good short account of the antivaccination movement see Martin Kaufman, "The American Anti-Vaccinationists and Their Arguments," *Bull. Hist. Med.* 41 (1967):463–78.

21. *Biennial Report of the State Board of Health of Kentucky, 1906–1907*, 1, Microfilm Records of the WPA Ky. Med. Hist. Research Project, reel 24; *Sixth Biennial Report of the State Board of Health of the State of Washington, 1905–1906* (Seattle, 1907), 19; *Twenty-second Biennial Report of the State Board of Health of California, 1910–12* (Sacramento, 1913), 2–3; *Twenty-sixth Biennial Report . . . 1918–20*, 14; *Twenty-seventh Biennial Report . . . 1920–22*, 17.

22. Benjamin E. Washburn, *A History of the North Carolina State Board of Health, 1877–1925* (Raleigh, 1966), 26–27.

23. *Report of the Department of Health and Sanitation of the City of Seattle, Washington . . . 1918–1919* (Seattle, 1920), 9.

24. Rosen, *Preventive Medicine in the United States*, 44.

25. Louisville *Civic Journal*, May 30, 1928, Microfilm Records of the WPA Ky. Med. Hist. Research Project, reel 25.

26. Rosenkrantz, *Public Health and the State*, 99–105.

27. Ravenel, *A Half Century of Public Health*, 80.

28. James C. Connell, *Chicago's Quest for Pure Water*, Public Works Historical Society (Washington, D.C., 1976), 15–18.

29. U.S. Bureau of the Census, *Historical Statistics of the United States, Colonial Times to 1957* (Washington, D.C., 1960), 26.

14

The New Public Health

By the turn of the century, most major cities had established health departments. Their effectiveness and quality varied widely, but nearly all of them included professionals on their staffs. The head of the department was usually a physician, and the staff included at least one bacteriologist, chemist, sanitary engineer, and statistician and an assortment of inspectors, many of whom had some professional training. During the early years of the twentieth century municipal health departments expanded rapidly, and the original handful of sanitary inspectors grew into divisions handling contagious diseases, food inspection, plumbing, and other matters. Within a short time these divisions became bureaus, and by World War I municipal health departments began to assume their present form.

By this date, too, health departments were beginning to spin off many of the former responsibilities of nineteenth-century health boards. The areas of garbage collection, water supply and sewerage, nuisance removal, and occasionally tenements and housing were now handled by separate municipal departments. This is not to say that health departments had shrugged off all responsibility for these matters, but that municipal governments now accepted administrative responsibility for them, and health departments were no longer involved in these areas' day-to-day work. Health officials, however, kept a wary eye on all sanitary affairs and constantly nudged and pressured other city departments and on occasion assumed temporary responsibility for their work. For example, when a garbagemen's strike in 1907 resulted in the accumulation of huge mounds of garbage in New York City, the mayor authorized the city health department to use its full authority to reduce nuisances. The city health commissioner promptly took charge, using departmental employees and others to collect garbage until the strike was settled.[1]

As noted in the last chapter, with the help of revolutionary developments in microbiology, health departments began a major assault upon contagious diseases. By utilizing diagnostic laboratories and preventive vaccines and by quarantining the sick in homes or hospitals, attacks were pressed home on diphtheria, scarlet fever, typhoid, and other killer diseases. An essential part of these campaigns was to educate the medical profession and the public. Many physicians, having received only minimal training and being conservative by the nature of their profession, continued to share with the public a belief in the traditional sanitarian's concept of miasma as a cause of disease. For example, in 1901 Dr. Walter Wyman proclaimed in the *Journal of the American Medical Association* that municipal cleanliness should be the foremost feature of municipal government, that quarantine was the wrong method to deal with certain epidemic diseases, and that a good sanitary environment was the best means of eliminating contagious disease.[2]

Developments in bacteriology and chemistry also helped to improve the supervision of municipal food and water supplies. As scientific advances provided more accurate laboratory tests for milk and other substances, food inspection staffs rapidly expanded, and inspectors were sent into dairies and milk-processing plants, restaurants, food stores and markets, meat-packing plants, and a host of other enterprises concerned with the processing and marketing of food. The rising concern for the health of infants and children resulted in the emergence of school health divisions, child and maternal health programs, and the licensing of midwives.

Armed with a new understanding of tuberculosis, health departments began large-scale educational campaigns, established special clinics and hospitals, and sent nurses into the homes of patients. Having become aware of the role of insect vectors, health officials were now in a position to move against yellow fever, malaria, and other disorders. Malaria, a perennial source of morbidity and death in America, was still a serious threat to health as far north as New Jersey and New York City. Municipal health departments, often in conjunction with the state governments, began antimosquito programs involving drainage, screening, and other measures designed to reduce the mosquito population.

As improved techniques made possible the routine confirmation of diagnoses of contagious disorders by laboratory methods, health department laboratories expanded rapidly. In addition, the leading ones were producing antitoxins and vaccines and, in the process, were making significant contributions to medical research. The remarkable successes achieved by bacteriologists enthroned science as the wave of the future. Whereas the sanitary movement had received a major impetus from civic groups and volunteer agencies, the public health movement was now firmly in the hands of physicians and other trained specialists. The proposals of the Progressive movement, with its emphasis upon environmental reform, required expensive social programs. Science, by providing new means for identifying, curing, and preventing contagious diseases, was thought to offer health departments a way to promote health without the cost of major social changes.

Yet even as public health officials began concentrating upon attacking pathogenic organisms, the nature of disorders such as tuberculosis and infantile diarrheas necessitated their taking steps to improve the social environment. Nowhere was this more evident than in child and maternal health, an area that was to be of major concern to health departments during the first twenty years of the century. The work of the Summer Corps and the many volunteer groups in the late nineteenth century now gave way to more systematic programs run by municipal health departments.

As late as the 1890s about 40 percent of all deaths in New York City were those of children below the age of five years. Fortunately, newspaper accounts of the appalling mortality rate among foundlings, cited in chapter 12, had the additional effect of creating public awareness of the excessive death rate for all slum children. It was obvious to physicians and laypersons alike that ignorance on the part of tenement mothers was a major cause of infant death; for instance, tenement babies were often swathed in layers of clothing in all seasons and fed improper food. In addition, because of inadequate washing facilities, the babies were rarely kept clean. The New York Association for Improving the Condition of the Poor (AICP) and other private child health agencies sought to educate mothers at volunteer-run summer camps and milk stations, but the task was too great for a purely volunteer effort.[3]

It is not clear whether the child health movement stimulated the drive for pure milk, or whether the pure milk movement promoted the cause of child health, but the two issues did go hand in hand. The nutritional value of milk had long been recognized, and in the 1890s bacteriology demonstrated the close connection between contaminated milk and the high infant mortality rate. The milk stations established by Nathan Straus in 1893 to provide free or low-cost pure milk to tenement families set a pattern that was followed in many cities. Other philanthropic individuals and groups adopted the idea, and within a few years no less than six associations were operating milk distribution centers. By 1911 private philanthropy was maintaining thirty of these milk centers in the tenement areas.

The AICP, the preeminent New York agency for caring for the poor, took the lead in using milk stations as a means to educate mothers. In 1905 it organized the New York Milk Committee, with the dual aim of improving the city's milk supply and educating mothers in infant care. The milk committee found a valuable ally in Dr. Josephine Baker of the New York City Health Department, a great American health reformer who was seeking municipal funds to establish child health centers. Her cause was helped, ironically, by a series of attacks on Nathan Straus in

1910 for providing pasteurized milk at his milk stations. When he threatened to close all seventeen of them, the resulting furor strengthened the city health department's hand, and in 1911 funds were appropriated for municipal milk stations. As these stations opened, the private ones were gradually phased out. By 1914 the city was operating fifty-six milk stations and providing assistance to the remaining seven still under the control of voluntary associations.[4]

In the meantime the health profession had acquired an important addition with the appearance of visiting nurses and district nurses. The idea for visiting nurses, the precursors of public health nurses, originated in 1877 when the New York City Mission employed a graduate nurse to work in a slum area. Voluntary associations in other cities picked up the idea, and by 1890 visiting nursing associations had been established in Boston, Chicago, and Philadelphia. By 1900 at least two hundred visiting or district nurses were employed, nearly all by business or private groups.[5] At about the turn of the century, municipalities began recognizing their value. The Los Angeles City Council, for example, employed its first district nurse in 1898, although New York City and Chicago developed the largest municipal nursing staffs. As of 1909, 10 percent of all visiting nurses were employees of the New York City Health Department.[6]

In the spring of 1908 Dr. Baker, who was well acquainted with the work of the visiting nurses, obtained the addresses of all newborn babies in a group of the worst tenements in New York City and during the summer sent thirty school nurses to visit the homes and advise the mothers there on the care of their infants. The success of the program led to the formation of the health department's Division of Child Hygiene under the direction of Dr. Baker in August of that year. Under her able leadership the division quickly expanded. At first the nurses worked with the milk stations and visited the homes of mothers with infants only in the summer. When the department opened its first fifteen milk stations in 1911, funds were provided for medical and educational services to be given on a year-round basis. The following year Dr. Baker prodded the various infant welfare groups into forming the Baby Welfare Association. The health department, which strongly supported the association, provided it with a central office and a secretary. The main purpose of the association, which was subsequently renamed the Children's Welfare Association, was to coordinate the activities of the department and the various volunteer groups.[7]

As equally important as the use of milk stations for baby health centers was the development of the Little Mothers' Leagues. Precisely when the term first came into use is not clear, although the AICP spoke of "little mothers" in its 1904 report. Among the purposes of the AICP's summer programs was to provide a recreational opportunity for older sisters who were compelled to take care of their siblings while their mothers worked. Although John Spargo denounced the idea of little mothers in his 1906 book, *The Bitter Cry of the Children*, Dr. Baker was a realist who decided it was far better to teach the older girls to care for infants and children than to simply criticize a system that was not likely to change. She broached the idea to the school authorities, who were unresponsive. In 1910 she persuaded one of the city's school principals to sponsor a Little Mothers' League, and several other schools immediately adopted the program. By 1912 some 20,000 girls over the age of twelve belonged to the four hundred-odd leagues. Each league was supervised by a physician and a nurse from the division of child hygiene, and the members met weekly for instruction in infant care. Although designed for the girls, the leagues proved equally valuable in educating their mothers.[8]

To reflect their changing function, in 1916 the milk stations were renamed "baby stations." An incidental result of World War I was a renewed concern for child health, and in 1918 the Children's Bureau and the National Council of Defense announced "The Year of the Child." One object was to urge physical examinations for preschoolers, a group that had been largely neglected. The New York Health Department, through its baby stations, had already started this work, and in 1918 it began vaccinating preschoolers for smallpox and administering Schick tests for diphtheria. Two years later the baby stations began immunizing children against diphtheria, a prelude to a large-scale national campaign against diphtheria, which began in 1928.[9] The Sheppard-Towner Act of 1921 provided for federal matching funds for maternal and child care. Unfortunately, the New York City Health Department was not able to take immediate advantage of the act since it was not until 1925 that the New York legislature passed the enabling legislation. By this date the department was maintaining seventy baby stations.

While New York City had one of the most innovative child health programs, every city of any consequence was following in its path. Within two years of the establishment of the New York City Health Department's Division of Child Hygiene, five states had organized childrens' bureaus at the state level, and by 1923 they existed in every state. Milk stations, baby stations, Little Mothers' Leagues, and visiting nurses, too, were basic to the better city health departments. Even those health departments with limited budgets often employed visiting nurses. In 1911 Memphis hired four white visiting nurses and one black visiting nurse. Los Angeles in 1913 had two maternity nurses, two infant welfare nurses, and another nurse at the city's milk station. In addition, it had six school nurses and one tuberculosis nurse. By 1916 its staff of public health nurses had grown to sixteen.[10]

Through the efforts of Drs. Helen C. Putnam, Charles V. Chapin, William T. Sedgwick, Josephine Baker, and others, in 1909 the American Association for the Study and Prevention of Infant Mortality was founded. Stimulated by the Child Health Year (1918), it expanded its work and became the American Child Hygiene Association. This same year Dr. L. Emmett Holt and Miss Sally Jean Lucas, aided by the New York Academy of Medicine's Committee on Public Health, brought together a group of kindred spirits and formed the Child Health Organization of America.[11] The Child Hygiene Association crusaded primarily against disease, whereas the Child Health Organization concentrated its efforts on health education and worked largely with schools. While seeking to make health education an integral part of schooling, it encouraged teachers and school systems to use imagination and originality in spreading the health message. (The author recalls his first theatrical role as a grade-school child in the 1920s. He was the third germ in a health play about tuberculosis.) The two national groups merged in 1923 under the leadership of Herbert Hoover to form the American Child Health Organization. The excellent work of the child health organizations at all levels was one of the brighter spots during the lean years for government agencies during the 1920s.

Along with the infant welfare program came a major expansion of the school medical inspection system, whose origins have been detailed in chapter 12. The effectiveness of school inspection programs in New York City or any other city depended largely upon political considerations. Where the school board and city administration operated on the basis of patronage, medical inspection was at best of limited value. Dr. Josephine Baker obtained her appointment as a school inspector in New York City by obtaining a letter from a local politician. She described the entire health program as reeking with negligence. Many of the physician inspectors, she wrote, never visited the schools, but simply telephoned them to ask if any children were sick.[12]

Happily for New York City, a new administration took over in 1902, and a revived health department quickly established a sound school program. Originally the school medical inspectors were to send all children with contagious disorders home, but they quickly discovered that this would have depopulated many of the schools. The prevalence of head lice and skin and eye disorders was so great that the health department decided not to exclude from school those children with pediculosis, contagious eye and skin diseases, and pulmonary tuberculosis. Out of necessity in

November 1902 nurses were employed on an experimental basis to treat these disorders in the schools. These early school nurses were noble spirits, indeed, since nearly all of them acquired head lice, and their visits to the filthy homes of their small patients must have tested to the limit their faith in humanity.[13]

Once school inspection in New York City was placed on a firm basis, the findings of the inspectors literally forced remedial work on the health department. In 1902 a group of ophthalmologists examined a large number of schoolchildren and found 12 percent of them with contagious eye diseases and 4.2 percent suffering from advanced cases of trachoma. Subsequently another 20 percent were found to have defective vision. So many children were sent home with trachoma that they swamped the city dispensaries, necessitating the opening of a special hospital to provide surgical treatment for advanced cases and outpatient care for the others. In 1905 the routine inspection of children was turned over to the school nurses, freeing the school medical inspectors to make cursory physical examinations of the students.[14] The result was to bring into even sharper focus the need for curative measures. Uncovering large-scale medical problems among poor children was pointless without positive action to remedy the situation.

When the health department learned in 1906 that the parents of many children who needed their adenoids and tonsils removed did not have carfare to take them to the city dispensaries, it organized a group of department and volunteer physicians to operate on the children in one of the schools. Rumors spread by so-called snip doctors, individuals who charged from twenty-five to fifty cents for removing tonsils or adenoids, caused a near riot by Jewish refugees from Eastern European pogroms who were convinced that the school doctors were slitting the throats of their children. The snip doctors' fear of losing patients, however, was a fear shared by most members of the medical profession. When School Superintendent William Maxwell recommended testing the vision of all schoolchildren and supplying free glasses to those who could not afford them, his suggestion was greeted with jeers and cries of socialism.[15] Despite considerable opposition, the department gradually opened a number of nose and throat clinics.

New York City's health department was fortunate in having Dr. Josephine Baker in charge of the Division of Child Hygiene, which was the first agency of its kind. A forceful and energetic individual, within two years she built the school health staff to a total of 142 medical inspectors and 137 school nurses. By 1912 when it became clear that considerable progress had been made in the fight against contagious diseases, Dr. Baker began asking for funds to deal with physical defects. A study in 1913 showed that only about one-third of all schoolchildren had been given physical examinations. Of the one-third examined, 72 percent had needed medical attention, but only slightly over a quarter of them had received any care.

The health department had already been criticized by the local medical societies for providing free medical care through its clinics. Removal of tonsils and adenoids was a major medical fad in these years, and the department was maintaining five nose and throat clinics for the poor. In 1914 the New York Academy of Medicine objected to them on the grounds that the surgery should be performed in operating rooms backed up by convalescent wards. In recommending that the department close these clinics, the academy's Committee on Public Health added that "the functions of the Department of Health should be restricted to the prevention of disease and that no therapeutic activities should be undertaken."[16] The health department bowed to the medical argument and closed the nose and throat clinics. Nonetheless, as of 1915 it still operated nine other clinics providing free medical treatment for schoolchildren.

By 1925 the Division of Child Hygiene, now called Bureau, was able to report that the major contagious diseases were no longer a serious problem among schoolchildren. It also reported significant gains in reducing eye disorders as a result of the work of eleven eye clinics, the teaching of eye hygiene, and programs of sight conservation. The true picture, however, was not quite as rosy as the 1925 report indicated. While serving as director, Dr. Baker was constantly fighting for funds, and the number of clinics was always far short of what was needed. After she resigned in 1920 the school health program became relatively stagnant. The political climate of the 1920s was not conducive to providing free medical services, and the evidence indicates a slight deterioration in the health of New York schoolchildren. A 1927 study of pupils in twenty-four schools showed 35 percent more health defects than the comparable health department figures for 1921. Another survey in 1929 once again reported that only about one-fourth of physical defects uncovered by school inspectors had been corrected.[17]

New York was well ahead of most other cities in caring for its schoolchildren, although not in all areas of school health. Chicago opened a public school class for crippled children in 1899, and as of 1914 only three other cities—New York, Cleveland, and Detroit—had followed Chicago's example. Detroit, one of the leaders in the school health movement, developed a relatively good inspection system by 1915, one supported by dental and eye clinics and a program of visiting nurses. In the 1920s the Detroit Health Department introduced the "squad system" of school inspection. Under this method, school examinations were conducted by teams of three physicians, each of whom specialized in a particular aspect of the examination.[18]

On the other hand, many towns and smaller cities had no school programs, and most had only limited ones. Seattle was probably more representative of the average urban area. In 1915 Seattle's health commissioner criticized the school board for employing only six nurses to inspect and provide care for some 38,000 children. Subsequently a corps of medical inspectors was employed, but in 1921 a court suit forced the department to reduce its medical inspectors from twenty-six to twelve, put its chief medical inspector on half-time, and turn its clinic over to the Red Cross.[19] Baltimore, with a population of well over half a million, began its school medical inspection system in 1905 with two physicians and one nurse under the supervision of the health department. By 1920 there were eighteen school nurses, but the inspection system was so ineffective that it did not even provide accurate statistics on the number of children with contagious diseases.[20] As indicated earlier, the 1920s was an era scarcely notable for government action in the area of social welfare. Nonetheless, it is safe to say that by 1930 most municipal officials had accepted the principle that they had some responsibility for the health of schoolchildren.

One of the more significant urban health developments in the early twentieth century was the health center movement. Its origins lay in efforts by volunteer social workers in the 1890s to improve the lot of immigrant slum dwellers. Jane Addams's Hull-House in Chicago and Lillian D. Wald and Mary Brewster's Henry Street Settlement in New York were the first organizations to start transforming the neighborhood dispensary into a community health and social service center. Their settlements provided help for the sick, but they also sought to become community agencies for preventing disease and improving the social environment. As mentioned previously, the successes achieved by bacteriology against contagious diseases shifted attention away from the physical environment, but health leaders never lost sight of the social environment as a cause of illness. Dealing with problem areas such as tuberculosis, venereal disease, child health, industrial hygiene, and mental health, to name a few, required far more than an understanding of pathogenic organisms. Solutions lay in education and community action. In consequence, as new health programs proliferated, health departments became larger and more complex.

Unfortunately, the compartmentalization of growing health departments into bureaus and divisions came at a time when health officials, relying on bacteriology, were beginning to focus on the individual. Aside from a measure of impersonalization inherent in large organizations, the multiplicity of bureaus and divisions resulted in much waste and duplication. Individuals seeking help often found it necessary to visit several clinics, dispensaries, or offices. Even worse, the immigrant poor, set apart by foreign language and customs, and suspicious of all government officials as a result of bitter experiences in their homelands, were often too confused by bureaucratic procedures to take full advantage of the limited health care opportunities available to them. At the same time, many private organizations engaged in health care were also duplicating each others' services. It was precisely these problems that the early advocates of health centers sought to remedy. They believed that it was essential to coordinate private and municipal health care and education, to bring it directly into the neighborhoods, and to involve the local residents in health center work.

Wilbur C. Phillips, while serving as secretary of the New York Milk Committee, was one of the first to recognize that milk stations could become centers for child and maternal health and, in addition, provide health education and social services for the immediate neighborhood. He was given a chance to put his idea into practice after he moved to Milwaukee in 1910. With his help, the Milwaukee City Health Department in 1911 began a health center demonstration project for maternal and child care in a Polish neighborhood of thirty-three city blocks. The neighborhood mothers were made an integral part of the center by being given a voice in its operation. Subsequently Phillips returned to New York City and established a group to promote public health and welfare through democratic neighborhood organizations. An experimental neighborhood group was established in Cincinnati in 1917. Despite a favorable response by the residents involved in the project, opposition from the local medical society and accusations of socialism during the post–World War I Red Scare led the city administration to cut off all support in 1920. Somewhat similar projects were tried in Pittsburgh and Philadelphia, but with little success.[21]

In New York, Boston, and Buffalo the health center concept gained a more permanent footing. In 1914 a distinguished medical leader and hospital administrator, Dr. Sigismund S. Goldwater, was appointed health commissioner for New York City. Recognizing the value of public support, Goldwater first appointed a citizens' advisory council, and then established a Bureau of Public Health Education, the first such municipal bureau. Goldwater believed that the department's administrators of bureaus and divisions were too far removed from the field workers. Earlier he had envisioned hospitals as community health centers, but he now proposed to establish a relatively self-contained experimental health district. In November 1914 Health District No. 1 opened on the lower east side of Manhattan in an area comprised of twenty-one blocks and 35,000 people.

A district office was established with a medical inspector and three nurses. Every home in the district was visited, and records were kept of each family. When diseases or physical defects were found in the course of examining babies or schoolchildren, the nurse assigned to the family saw that remedial action was taken. Instead of prosecuting food handlers and others for violations of the sanitary laws, the health inspector sought to win voluntary compliance with the regulations through persuasion and health education. The remarkable improvement in the health of the district's residents led Goldwater's successor as health commissioner, Dr. Haven Emerson, to divide the entire borough of Queens into four health districts and to create within the department's management structure a separate Division of Health Districts. Each district had a health officer, a clerk, and a supervising nurse and staff, medical inspectors, and clinic physicians.[22]

The exceedingly high rate of physical defects uncovered through draft examinations during World War I shocked the public into an awareness of the importance of health and gave an impetus to the health center movement. It was further strengthened when the Red Cross decided to support the health center concept. By 1920 some 72 health centers had been established in 49 cities throughout the country and another 33 were planned or proposed in 28 other communities. Their purposes varied widely, from child welfare centers to eye, ear, and nose clinics, but they all shared the common purpose of promoting health education and preventing health problems. By 1930 over 1,500 health centers of one type or another were in operation. Approximately half were supported by municipal funds, but, regardless of the basic funding, they all provided some measure of coordination between city and private health agencies operating within the district.[23]

In New York City, where the health district concept ultimately became embedded in the health department, an unsympathetic political administration during the 1920s abolished the municipal health centers. Fortunately, two demonstration health districts, one sponsored by the Red Cross and another by the Milbank Memorial Fund, successfully kept the idea alive. It was given new strength in 1934 under the administration of Mayor Fiorello La Guardia and Health Commissioner John L. Rice. Health districts had always been viewed as stepchildren by the health department's bureau and district chiefs, who resented their loss of authority. To solve this problem, Dr. Rice gave the district health centers equal status by creating a new Bureau of District Health Administration and by establishing seven health districts with full-time officers in charge. Subsequently, with the help of federal funds, new health center buildings were erected and additional health districts created. By 1936 the city was divided into twenty-two health districts.

The child and school hygiene bureaus were merged into the Bureau of District Health Administration, and each district was given a complete staff. To develop community support, two committees were organized in each district—one, a medical advisory committee consisting of physicians within the district, and another representing a wide range of civic, religious, and social groups within the area. The late 1930s saw the peak of the health district movement. Although health districts survived in New York City in a modified form, on the national scene the sharp reduction in immigration in the 1930s and 1940s, the rising standard of living, changes in social work patterns, and opposition from medical associations all brought a steady decline in the health district movement.[24]

In addition to the successful attack on contagious diseases by health departments and the emergence of the child health movement and the district health movement, the early twentieth century also saw the expansion of the health department's traditional role in disseminating public health information. Even the earliest temporary health boards issued broadsides and pamphlets during epidemics to inform the public on how to maintain good health and avoid the prevailing disease. As municipal health departments emerged, they began issuing notices to local newspapers and sending information to physicians. By the 1880s a few began monthly publications intended for health officers, physicians, and teachers. Within a few years these publications were directed to a more general audience. Whenever a major attack was mounted on any disease, pamphlets were written for general distribution. Health departments also worked with school boards to encourage health education classes and programs. The first municipal agency to give formal status to health education was the New York City Health Department, which established a Bureau of Health Education in 1914.[25]

Municipal health departments also took leadership in gathering vital statistics. The sanitary regulations affecting burials, introduced in the early nineteenth century, greatly facilitated the collection of mortality statistics in urban areas. Records of marriages and births were left largely to the churches and courts at first, but by 1900 city ordinances, sometimes supplemented by state ones, began increasing the accuracy of marriage and birth statistics. By this time, too, the employment of statisticians made it possible to conduct epidemiological studies and led to the emergence of the formal academic field of epidemiology.

In appreciating the foregoing picture of steady progress in municipal health, one should keep in mind the words of a great American "philosopher," Mammy Yokum: "Mainly it were true, but. . . ." Even in New York City, the leader in urban public health, inefficient administrations that were often also corrupt constantly alternated with effective ones, and these changes in administration were reflected in the city's health department. Yet some political machines, whose very names imply corruption and patronage, were not always unsympathetic to health needs. Charles F. Murphy, who took over Tammany Hall in New York, had been a patient of Dr. Hermann Biggs, and until 1918 his political machine generally gave strong support to the health department. Tammany Hall, as was the case with other political machines, mobilized the poor, and health was of vital concern to its constituents.[26]

Dr. Josephine Baker claimed that she found Tammany politicians easier to work with than reform administrators because Tammany got things done without delay. Nonetheless, Tammany constantly pressured the health department into providing jobs for its supporters. Dr. Baker was frequently urged to employ the cast-off mistresses of Tammany leaders as nurses, and she concedes that she did use those whom she thought could work with children. She admits, too, that she was fortunate in that the Bureau of Child Hygiene, unlike other city bureaus, had no favors it could sell.[27] Regrettably, the situation was far different for those New York City bureaus responsible for food and other matters.

Relations with local physicians became an increasing problem as the twentieth century advanced. Over and above the larger question of the boundary between private medicine and public health, health officials constantly complained of the failure of physicians to comply with disease reporting regulations. Venereal disease has always been a special problem in this regard, and it will be interesting to see if the same will hold true for AIDS (acquired immune deficiency syndrome). Partly in order to mitigate physician opposition, health departments frequently employed private physicians to perform routine physical examinations in schools and industries. Dr. Haven Emerson reported in 1916 that health department physicians examined 20,357 food handlers and found a tuberculosis rate of 1 per 1,000. Some 1,100 private physicians examined 26,300 in the same industrial group and reported a tuberculosis rate of only 1 per 3,700. A similar disparity was found in the rate of venereal disease cases found by the two groups of physicians.[28]

Intemperate denunciations of health departments in medical journals were not at all uncommon, particularly after World War I. An article in the *New Orleans Medical and Surgical Journal* in 1920 declared that health regulations were turning the physician into "little more than [a] stool pigeon, a clerk for the health boards." The author claimed that the health ordinances relating to venereal disease would increase seductions and hasty marriages, and he concluded with patriotic fervor: "The idea of government wet nursing is socialistic rot of the most dangerous type, is destructive of the very fundamentals of liberty, and in my opinion has no just place in a free country."[29]

Outside of major urban areas, in America's smaller cities and towns, the public health movement made only limited progress. The city of Covington, Kentucky, was typical of most smaller towns. As of 1902 it had a health officer and a sanitary officer. The main concern of these officials was sanitation and occasional epidemics. In 1904 school janitors were instructed to fumigate their buildings once a week, and the following year an ordinance required all factories and public buildings to equip their closets with disinfectants. The same year another resolution required the fumigation of all homes occupied by persons with contagious diseases before visitors were allowed.

In the following years Covington took a number of progressive steps. In 1909 the health officer was instructed to vaccinate all schoolchildren at city expense, and in 1912 all schoolchildren were inoculated against diphtheria. During these years the town's infant mortality rate remained high. In 1921, reflecting the growing national awareness of child health, the city health officer, in conjunction with the Red Cross, local churches, and school officials, opened a clinic for children of the poor. A good share of the funds for the clinic was raised by contribution boxes in the schools and by a series of charitable social affairs.

In the meantime, Covington's health department, convinced that the town's contaminated water supply was responsible for a good part of the infant mortality rate, in 1920 began a long fight for a plant to filter the town's water. In 1923 an outbreak of sixty-eight cases of typhoid fever brought state and United States Public Health Service workers into Covington. Yet, despite this outbreak and succeeding minor ones, it was 1936 before the town was supplied with safe drinking water.[30]

The effectiveness of urban public health departments varied widely from state to state, and this was especially true of America's small cities and towns. Nonetheless, by 1930 the general organizational pattern of health departments was well established. Increasingly, health officers, particularly those in the larger health departments, had received some formal training in public health. As the traditional contagious disorders were gradually brought under control and health departments began to shift their focus, new divisions and bureaus began to appear. The appearance of public health as a medical specialty, and America's vastly improved communication system, however, ensured a large measure of standardization among health departments.

NOTES

1. John Duffy, *A History of Public Health in New York City, 1866–1966* (New York, 1974), 258–59.
2. Walter Wyman, "Sanitation and Progress," *JAMA* 36 (1901):609–14.
3. Duffy, *Public Health in New York City, 1866–1966*, 208, 212.
4. Ibid., 466–68.
5. Richard H. Shryock, *The History of Nursing* (rpt., New York, 1959), 298; Lavinia L. Dock and Isabel M. Stewart, *A Short History of Nursing* (New York, 1938), 161; Mazÿck P. Ravenel, ed., *A Half Century of Public Health* (New York, 1921), 441–42.
6. *Monthly Bulletin of the Los Angeles Health Department* 4, no. 6 (May 1917):1–2; Karen Buhler-Wilkerson, "Left Holding the Bag: Experiments in Visiting Nursing, 1877–1909," *Nursing Research* 36 (1987):44.
7. S. Josephine Baker, "The Reduction of Infant Mortality in New York City," *American Journal of Diseases of Children* 5 (1913):1–5; id., *Fighting for Life* (New York, 1939), 82–84.
8. Baker, *Fighting for Life*, 132–34; id., "The Reduction of Infant Mortality in New York City," 3–4; Duffy, *Public Health in New York City, 1866–1966*, 468.
9. Nina Bleiburg, "The History of the Child Health Conference in New York City," New York City Health Department MS, pp. 7–9.
10. William D. Miller, *Memphis during the Progressive Era, 1900–1917* (Memphis, 1957), 116; *Monthly Bulletin of the Los Angeles Health Department* 4, no. 6 (May, 1917):1–2.
11. This material is based in part on the author's notes taken during oral interviews with Dr. L. Emmett Holt and Miss Sally Jean Lucas in the summer of 1963.
12. Baker, *Fighting for Life*, 54–57.
13. Duffy, *Public Health in New York City, 1866–1966*, 476–77; Baker, *Fighting for Life*, 77–80.
14. Duffy, *Public Health in New York City, 1866–1966*, 477–79.
15. Ibid.
16. Ibid., 480–83; New York Academy of Medicine, Summary of the Activities of the Public Health Committee . . . 1915, New York Academy of Medicine Library MS, p. 10.
17. Duffy, *Public Health in New York City, 1866–1966*, 488–89.
18. Romaine P. Mackie, "Crippled Children in School," United States Office of Education, *Bulletin*, 1948, no. 5 (Washington, D.C., 1948), preface; *Bulletin of the Detroit Board of Health* 5, no. 7 (January 1915):6–10.
19. *Report of the Department of Health and Sanitation . . . City of Seattle, Washington . . . Calendar Year Nineteen Hundred Fifteen* (Seattle, 1916), 19; Ragnor T. Westman, Annual Report and Survey, 1939–1943, Seattle Department of Health and Sanitation, Seattle, Washington, Health Sciences Library, TS, pp. 95–96, University of Washington.

20. William T. Howard, *Public Administration and the Natural History of Disease in Baltimore, Maryland,* 1797–1920 (Washington, D.C., 1924), 168–71.

21. George Rosen, "Public Health: Then and Now, The First Neighborhood Health Center Movement—Its Rise and Fall," *American Journal of Public Health* 61 (1971):1626–28.

22. Duffy, *Public Health in New York City, 1866–1966,* 266–69.

23. Rosen, "Public Health: Then and Now," 1629–30.

24. Ibid., 1632–34.

25. Duffy, *Public Health in New York City, 1866–1966,* 267.

26. C.-E. A. Winslow, *The Life of Hermann M. Biggs, Physician and Statesman of the Public Health* (Philadelphia, 1929), 187–88.

27. Baker, *Fighting for Life,* 92–97.

28. Haven Emerson, *Preparedness for Health,* Ether Day Address, Massachusetts General Hospital (1916), pamphlet, New York City Health Department, 13–14.

29. Louis G. Stirling, "Tendencies of the Times, Medical and Otherwise," *New Orleans Medical and Surgical Journal* 72 (1920):218–20.

30. Dr. James P. Riffe, "Health Department Minute Book," Covington Health Department, 4–10, Microfilm Records of the WPA Ky. Med. Hist. Research Project, reel 24.

15

State Health Boards and the Early Rural Health Movement

The size and diversity of the United States is evident in the almost haphazard development of state health boards during the early years of the twentieth century. At the regional level some pattern can be seen in the evolution of state health services, but even within regions wide variations occurred. In the Northeast, and to some extent the Old Northwest (the eastern Midwest of today), where a strong tradition of local or township self-government had always prevailed, state health boards tended to have little authority and to function largely as advisory bodies. Yet this was not true for all the northeastern states. For example, the Pennsylvania State Board of Health in 1915 was paying the salaries of some 670 district health officers and exercising direct control over them.

Although the method for selecting health boards and the requirements for board membership varied from state to state, the boards tended to be dominated by physicians. Some health boards were newly appointed by each incoming state governor; in the case of others, membership was staggered to ensure a measure of continuity. A number of states required that all board members be physicians; an equal number specified that physicians should constitute a majority of the members; and in two southern states, Alabama and South Carolina, the state medical society literally served as the board. In his survey of state health boards in 1915–16, Charles V. Chapin noted that six states required the presence of at least one physician on the board, and eight specified that one member must be an engineer.[1]

The leading state health official was usually the secretary or president of the board. Depending on the way the state organized its health agency, this official was known as the state health officer, superintendent of health, director of health, or commissioner of health. Whatever the title, the health officer was usually appointed by the governor or by the state health board, although even here the exact method varied. For example, in some cases medical societies nominated candidates. The terms of office for the health officer and board members ranged from two to seven years, frequently coinciding with that of the state governor. Few of the board members received any pay, and even state health officers often received only a nominal salary.

The first forty years of the twentieth century saw the transformation of state health boards from weak, ineffective agencies, staffed largely by volunteers, into relatively strong state departments run by permanent health professionals. As was true in the case of municipal health departments, societal changes—which included a higher living standard, improved roads and communication, and major developments in the biological sciences—all played a part in this development. The Progressive movement, with its concern for better government and an improved quality of life, also contributed to the strengthening of state health departments. Urbanization, which demanded that attention be paid to sanitation and health, was another factor in promoting statewide health measures. The existence of one or more major cities within a state's boundaries usually guaranteed that it would be among the leaders in developing an effective state board of health. New York City, for example, in its efforts to improve the quality of its milk, food, and water supplies, directly and indirectly promoted health and sanitary programs in towns and villages throughout its milkshed, watershed, and entire market area.

Another important factor in the emergence of state boards was the influence of strong individuals, many of whom established their reputations as municipal health officers and then moved into state government. Hermann M. Biggs of New York, George C. Whipple of Massachusetts, Charles V. Chapin of Rhode Island, Victor C. Vaughan of Michigan, John N. Hurty of Indiana, and Oscar Dowling of Louisiana were among the civic health leaders who influenced health reform at the state and national levels.

An equally important factor in the development of state health boards was the joint effort of private foundations and the federal government. Tuberculosis associations, whose work has already been mentioned (see chapter 12), did their most effective work in the northern and western states. The emergence of state health programs in the South was largely the joint work of the Rockefeller Foundation and the United States Public Health Service. As rural health became of increasing concern to the states and to the nation, other voluntary agencies and foundations such as the Red Cross, the Commonwealth Fund, the Milbank Memorial Fund, and the Kellogg Foundation also began making significant contributions to state and county health organizations.

Calamities and major emergencies have always stimulated community efforts to promote health. World War I and its accompanying influenza epidemics provided at least a temporary impetus to the public health movement and led to the reorganization and strengthening of most state health agencies. The same holds true for major floods. Disastrous floods always led governors to declare a state of emergency and caused the Red Cross, along with other voluntary associations and state and federal agencies, to swing into action. In the course of emergency relief measures, the inadequacies of existing health care programs were often revealed, and the resulting public pressure would force the state government into enacting some form of remedial legislation. A good example is the great Mississippi flood of 1927, which devastated hundreds of square miles in Louisiana. As of January 1, 1927, only ten of the state's parishes or counties had full-time health units. By the end of the year, when the state was recovering from the flood damage, the number of parishes with full-time health units had risen to twenty-two.[2]

Although the authority and influence of state health boards steadily increased in the early years of their rise, it was a piecemeal process in which state legislatures responded to specific crises. If the presence or threat of a particular disease or diseases was sufficient to arouse public apprehension, the state legislature might respond by voting a specific appropriation or by delegating further responsibility or authority to the board. Since smallpox was still a constant danger in the early years of the twentieth century—despite the availability of an effective preventive for over one hundred years—legislative appropriations enabled health boards to embark on large-scale vaccination programs that included both education and the distribution of vaccine material. In areas where typhoid fever was recognized as a problem, state boards were often able to obtain an appropriation of funds and the authority to regulate water supplies. In the southern states, the chief impetus to state action was provided by a growing awareness of the destructive effect of hookworm, pellagra, and malaria. The strong voluntary tuberculosis movement that emerged in the early twentieth century also contributed notably to strengthening the power of many state boards, although, as in the case of Michigan, the strength of the voluntary organizations was so great that some states tended to leave the battle to the private sector.[3]

The development of state health boards can be illustrated by a glance at the history of the Ohio State Board of Health, one of the better state health agencies at the turn of the century. Established in 1886, it gradually gained wider authority and a larger budget and staff. In 1893 a law required that the construction of new or improved water and sewer systems must receive the prior approval of the state board of health, and four years later an engineer was employed to inspect the state's water supplies.[4] The following year, 1898, saw two major steps forward. The board of health established a chemical and biological laboratory, and a Bureau of Vital Statistics was placed under the jurisdiction of the secretary of state of

Ohio. In 1901 the board helped to organize the Ohio Society for the Prevention of Tuberculosis and began an antituberculosis campaign. In response to pressure from the board of health and the state tuberculosis society, the legislature voted $210,000 in 1904–1905 to build a tuberculosis sanatorium.[5]

From its founding in 1886, the Ohio state board had encouraged communities of all sizes to establish local health boards, and its efforts in this direction were aided by a 1906 state law that provided that each city, village, or township should send a delegate to an annual meeting called by the state board.[6] An even more significant step was taken in 1908 when the Bense Act, designed to prevent pollution of the state's water resources, authorized the health board to require the purification of public water supplies and sewage. Since the Ohio River received pollutants from several other states, it was exempted from the act. The Ohio, however, was the state's main water resource, and the board promptly introduced a resolution into the legislature urging the cooperation of Pennsylvania, Kentucky, West Virginia, and Indiana in protecting the river. The following year the states involved organized the Ohio River Sanitary Commission, but many years would elapse before they would adopt uniform sanitary codes; it was difficult enough to persuade even one state to reduce water pollution. For example, in Ohio—one of the most progressive states in this respect— it was 1912 before the state board of health was able to overcome the legal obstacles to enforcing the Bense Act of 1908.[7]

Whether governments were concerned with the quality of food or water, as was the case with Ohio, or with reducing the incidence of a particular disease or diseases, as was true of the southern states, all of them either established public health laboratories or else expanded their existing facilities. The early laboratories concentrated on analyzing food and water, but increasingly they began providing diagnostic services. The next step was to provide antitoxins and vaccines against smallpox, diphtheria, typhoid, tetanus, and other disorders. As was the case with the better municipal laboratories, some of the state laboratories engaged in productive research.

The Ohio State Laboratory followed this general pattern. By 1910 it was making its free laboratory diagnostic service available to all Ohio physicians and was distributing silver nitrate gratuitously to physicians and midwives. By 1916 the laboratory was occupying an entire building on the campus of Ohio State University, employing fourteen staff members, and providing a wide range of services to the state.[8]

Ohio was one of the few states to move into the area of occupational health. The initial act creating the Ohio State Board of Health in 1886 provided for a division of industrial hygiene, but it was not established as

a separate division until 1912. The following year, 1913, the board required that all cases of industrial disease be reported.[9] With the addition
of the divisions of Industrial Hygiene and Tuberculosis in 1913, the board
then consisted of seven divisions—the two just named, and the Divisions
of Administration, Engineering, Hygienic Laboratories, Communicable
Diseases, and Plumbing Inspection. In 1915 a Division of Child Hygiene
was added.

The year 1917 witnessed a major reorganization. The board of health
was supplanted by a State Department of Health directed by a health
commissioner and a four-man advisory council. The council members,
two of whom were required to be physicians with experience or training
in sanitary science, were appointed by the governor, and the council in
turn appointed the health commissioner. The council members served
four years, but the health commissioner was appointed for five years.
Executive power was vested in the commissioner, and legislative and ju-
dicial authority were vested in the advisory council.[10] Allowing the advisory
council to appoint the health commissioner and extending the commissioner's term of office to five years reflected a growing national tendency
to try to remove politics from health affairs.

An equally important measure, the Hughes Act, reformed the entire
local health administration system. In 1918 Ohio had 2,158 independent
health units, representing cities, villages, and townships. The Hughes Act,
which went into effect in 1919, eliminated the village and township units
and based local health administration on cities and counties, reducing the
number of units to 80 city health districts and 89 general health districts.
A minimum of three full-time employees was required for each health
district—a health officer, a public health nurse, and a clerk. More significantly, the state agreed to pay one-half the cost of the three required
staff members, and the health department established a Bureau of Local
Health Organizations to assist in the establishment and operation of local units.[11]

Ohio, unlike a number of other states, welcomed federal assistance for
its health programs. When World War I helped lift the veil of silence about
venereal disease, the state health department established a Bureau of
Venereal Disease and happily accepted its share of federal funds made
available by the Chamberlain-Kahn Act of 1918. In addition to providing
free laboratory diagnosis, by July 1, 1919 it was operating thirteen clinics.
Since the department already had a child hygiene division, it was also able
to receive full benefit from the Sheppard-Towner Act of 1921, which
provided federal matching funds for state child and maternal care.[12]

At the onset of the Great Depression, Ohio's state public health program was one of the best in the nation. Ohio led the states in the number

of full-time county health units, had an effective statewide system of health districts, and boasted a health department consisting of nine divisions and seven bureaus. Its health department had been among the first to establish bureaus of industrial hygiene, child hygiene, local health organizations, and public health nursing. The department was provided with broad powers, but the advisory council and the health commissioners, recognizing the danger of antagonizing too many vested interests, used them sparingly. Instead, they relied largely on education and persuasion to carry out their policies. Although the department was active in promoting safe water, the regulation of food, milk, and drugs was left to local health departments and other state agencies.[13]

The board of health in Massachusetts, another state ranking high in terms of its success in promoting public health, presents a sharp contrast to the Ohio board. The Massachusetts board had only limited authority, and health prevention was left largely to its 355 township units. Moreover, a long tradition of local self-government meant that there was little uniformity among the many township health agencies. Fortunately, to compensate for this lack of unity, district health officers appointed by the state board had supervisory power over the area of communicable diseases and over other areas of concern. Although Massachusetts probably ranked first in the nation in the collection of vital statistics, its health department had no jurisdiction over them, nor did it have much voice in the state's excellent school health program, which was left largely to the state board of education or to local school boards. Fortunately, Massachusetts had a fine school system.[14]

The southern states, because they were predominantly rural and labored under the double handicap of racism and one-crop farming, lagged behind the rest of the country with respect to public health. Louisiana's health board dated back to 1855, but even in the early twentieth century it continued to be preoccupied with quarantine measures to prevent the introduction of yellow fever. It was reorganized in 1898, and a separate health board was created for New Orleans. The state board, following the general pattern of health boards, slowly expanded its activities, conducted drives against the major contagious disorders, and expanded into the usual bureaus and divisions. Judging by the board's annual reports, Louisiana was making remarkable progress. Unfortunately, Louisiana and the other southern states were held back by a large illiterate rural population of whites and blacks and an unresponsive white upper class. New Orleans, which might have been expected to provide leadership in health affairs, had one of the highest death rates in the country.

In 1910 Dr. Oscar Dowling took over as president of the Louisiana State Board of Health and immediately sought to infuse new life into the agency. At the first board meeting he proposed a traveling health exhibit that would carry the gospel of health to every community situated on a railway in Louisiana. A local railway line lent an engine, an exhibit car, and a car to house staff, and within about six weeks of Dowling's taking office, the health train left New Orleans for the state fair in Shreveport. The exhibit provided a wide range of health information and included literature on hygiene, pathological specimens from tuberculosis cases, enlargements of flies' feet, information on hookworm diseases, and a model of Dr. Charles W. Stiles's sanitary privy, not to mention model school desks, and displays on food, nutrition, dental care, dairies, and dairy equipment.

In the next seven and a half months the health train covered seven thousand miles in Louisiana and made 256 stops, visiting almost every town or village on a railway line. At each stop lectures were given on hygiene, and medical inspectors investigated dairies, stores, restaurants, food processors, and public buildings. They also tested milk, water, and foods, and rated the local arrangments for dealing with garbage and sewage. Dowling was appalled at the backwardness and poverty he found in the state, and he subsequently wrote a pamphlet in which he blamed Louisiana's high incidence of sickness and disease on ignorance and apathy.[15]

The train received nationwide publicity, and Louisiana's state health board received invitations to take the exhibit to California, Washington, and other states. On the way to Los Angeles, the train made three stops in Texas, and from Los Angeles it went to San Francisco. It returned to Louisiana after visiting Salt Lake City, Cheyenne, Denver, Omaha, Chicago, Memphis, and a number of other cities. Subsequently it toured several southern states. The train continued to travel around Louisiana until 1928 when Dowling fell afoul of Huey P. Long. Dowling and his health train performed wonders for Louisiana's national image, but, indefatigable as Dowling was, he had made only limited gains against the omnipresent malaria, hookworm, pellagra, and numerous contagious disorders plaguing Louisianians. Ironically, Huey Long, who politicized the board of health, made a major contribution to improving health conditions by building schools and roads, which helped to bring Louisiana's rural population into the mainstream of American life.[16]

The impetus for health reform in most of the southern states came first from hookworm. Charles W. Stiles, a zoologist, became convinced in the 1890s that hookworm was widespread in the South. In succeeding years he read a number of scholarly papers whose conclusions were picked up by northern newspapers. When the newspapers began suggesting that hookworm was the cause of southern laziness, many southerners were resentful, although a number of southern physicians suspected that there was some truth in the assertion. Stiles spoke on hookworm before the North Carolina State Medical Society in 1903, and the North Carolina State Board of Health recorded prophetically: "His visit is an epoch in the history of North Carolina and the South."[17] The following year the United States Army began a campaign against hookworm in Puerto Rico—one that served as a model for subsequent state programs in the South.

The first state to move against hookworm was Florida. It was the only southern state with a special tax for public health, and it had full control over local health officers. In addition, the state had three laboratories. In 1908 the state board of health, working in conjunction with the Florida State Teachers' Association, initiated the first major hookworm campaign in the United States.

In the meantime, Stiles's long struggle to create public awareness of hookworm culminated on October 26, 1909, when the Rockefeller Foundation organized the Sanitary Commission to Exterminate Hookworm Disease and provided it with one million dollars to be spent in the next five years. Florida, which was already well along with its own campaign, was the only state not eligible for foundation money. The commission, headed by Wickcliffe Rose, decided to work with local health authorities. Each state was to have a director of sanitation (appointed jointly by the state and the Rockefeller Commission), field inspectors, and a laboratory staff.[18]

By 1910 sanitary directors had been appointed in nine states and surveys were under way to determine the extent of the hookworm problem. A previous survey in Alabama had shown the presence of hookworm in all sixty-seven of its counties, with an infection rate in some areas of 62 percent.[19] One of the most shocking discoveries was that the majority of rural homes and schools did not even have privies. In Louisiana open dirt trenches were widely used, and the field inspectors in Arkansas reported that not a single sanitary privy was found outside of towns and cities. Not surprisingly, ignorance and apathy limited the combined efforts of the Rockefeller Foundation, the United States Public Health Service, and local officials. Lack of adequate statistics makes it difficult to assess the results of the five-year project, but about 43 percent of some 404,000 children inspected before 1914 were found to be infected. In 1915 an inspection of 549,000 schoolchildren for hookworm showed an infection rate of 39 percent.[20] Obviously hookworm was still a major problem, but, nonetheless, the initiative taken by the Rockefeller Foundation in these years laid the basis for a growing role for public health departments in the South.

The Rockefeller Sanitary Commission program in all states consisted of surveys, education, and treatment, with an emphasis upon educating local physicians. North Carolina, which had strengthened its health department in 1908 and had encouraged the organization of county units, developed the most effective program of those states receiving Rockefeller support. By the time the Rockefeller Foundation withdrew from the program in 1915, state and local health departments throughout the South showed considerable improvement. A few county health units had been established in nearly all the southern states, and the southern legislatures were beginning to provide larger appropriations for their health boards. There was also a growing awareness of the South's other two major medical problems, malaria and pellagra. As early as 1909 the North Carolina State Medical Society began studying pellagra and urging the use of federal funds to investigate the disease.[21]

Pellagra was first acknowledged to be a discrete disease in the United States in 1907. Subsequently, Dr. Joseph Goldberger of the Public Health Service established that it was a deficiency disease. Despite his demonstration in 1915 that the disease could be eliminated by proper diet, bacteriologists continued hunting for the pathogenic organism of pellagra until the late 1920s.[22] World War I temporarily brought prosperity to the South and reduced the incidence of pellagra. The postwar depression and the fall in agricultural prices in the 1920s, however, reduced southern living standards and brought a return of the disorder. When President Warren G. Harding, reacting to a letter from Goldberger, spoke of poverty and famine in the South, southerners resented the suggestion that their poor neighbors were not properly fed and derided Goldberger's claims. Southern politicians and their health officials closed ranks, denying the existence of pellagra and refusing all offers of help. Only Mississippi conceded that it had a pellagra problem and requested help from the Public Health Service.[23]

By the late 1920s the presence of pellagra could not be denied, and the evidence of its dietetic origin was overwhelming. Convinced at last of the need for action, southern health departments began distributing brewer's yeast, which Goldberger and his associate W. F. Tanner had found to be effective in curing the disorder.[24] Even more important, they began educational programs to improve the diet of poor southerners. Unfortunately, as with hookworm, there could be no permanent eradication of the disease so long as poverty was the lot of most rural southerners. This same situation held true for malaria. One of the greatest weaknesses of health agencies in the South was their lack of vital statistics. A few public health physicians recognized malaria as a problem, but they had little evidence to support their views. And even when the significance of malaria became known, there was little inclination to do much about it since blacks and poor whites were its chief victims. In consequence, the disease lingered on until World War II.[25]

Not a single southern state was admitted to the Census Bureau's death registration area until 1916, and it was 1921 before any of them were included in the birth registration area. It might be well at this point to explain the term "registration area." The Census Bureau first began publishing death statistics in 1850 based upon the census for that year. In 1880 it established a death registration area comprised of Massachusetts, New Jersey, the District of Columbia, and several major cities, all of which had a relatively effective system for recording mortality statistics. By 1900 ten states were included in the registration area. For admission to the area, the Census Bureau required that a state or city must have recorded approximately 90 percent of all deaths. The recording of births lagged far behind that of deaths, and it was not until 1915 that the Census Bureau created a registration area for birth statistics. At that date only ten states and the District of Columbia met the 90-percent requirement. By 1933 all the states were included in both the death and birth registration areas.[26]

The evolution of state health departments in the West closely followed developments in the older eastern states. California, as the largest and most populated state, had the best health department. The California State Board of Health was authorized to regulate plumbers and plumbing in 1885; and a factory sanitation act was passed in 1889, although the latter was enforced by the United States Bureau of Labor Statistics. As in most other states, the health board's powers were largely advisory and its budget small. In 1903 the appearance of bubonic plague in San Francisco provided the impetus for the board to be strengthened. In March 1905 the establishment of a Bureau of Vital Statistics enabled California to become the eighteenth state admitted to the national registration area. This same year a Bureau of State Hygiene was established complete with a chemical and bacteriological laboratory.[27]

In succeeding years the health department steadily expanded. By 1916 the California state board was administering some seven bureaus and, because of the state's sheer size, three laboratories, one each in Los Angeles, Fresno, and Sacramento. The same factor of geographic size led the board that year to recommend dividing the state into six health districts. An amendment to the health law was promptly enacted, called the Local Health Districts Act, but just two years later the board complained in its report for 1918 that despite the act's passage, not a single health district had been formed and only one county had a qualified health officer and staff.[28] In 1927 the board was reorganized into a State Health Department headed by a director and a six-member advisory council. Reflecting the national movement to establish county health departments, by 1930 California had fourteen full-time county health units.[29]

When Charles Chapin surveyed the state boards of health in the forty-eight states in 1916, his most scathing criticism was reserved for New Mexico, which had been admitted to the Union along with Arizona in 1912. "It is unfortunate," he wrote, "that a state with a population which now probably numbers nearly half a million should do nothing whatever for public health. It is the only state of which this can be said."[30] Although the report outraged a number of the state's citizens, reform Governor W. E. Lindsay, aided by influenza outbreaks and the discouraging results of the World War I draft physicals, requested Surgeon General Rupert Blue of the Public Health Service to survey New Mexico's health needs. Blue assigned the task to Surgeon J. W. Kerr, who began his work in September 1918.[31]

Kerr's report concurred with Dr. Chapin's. He found that the New Mexico State Board of Health had no legislative appropriation and that its sole source of income was the fees it received from licensing medical practitioners. There was virtually no reporting of contagious diseases, even to local health offices, and the state board had no records of cases or outbreaks. A wide range of state laws pertaining to sanitation, pollution, and food and drugs were on the books, but no money had been provided for their enforcment. Kerr's report, in conjunction with an equally critical one made a few months earlier by a representative of the United States War Department, provided the final impetus to public health reform.[32]

Despite considerable opposition, in 1919 a law creating an effective health department for New Mexico was pushed through the state legislature. To ensure the new department a good start, the governor requested the surgeon general of the Public Health Service to lend a health officer to organize and staff it, and the job was given to Surgeon C. E. Waller, who became the first director of the department. To help place the department on a firm basis, it was financed by a state property tax. Another law passed this same year provided that each county and municipality was to have a health office, and local officials were permitted to levy a tax for this purpose. The health reformers won still another victory in 1919 when the state legislature established a Department of Child Welfare.[33] Whereas state health agencies usually evolved over a period of time, in the case of New Mexico the health department sprang virtually full blown.

The steady growth of state health departments during the first thirty years of the twentieth century was of chief benefit to towns and cities.

Typically, a state provided a range of laboratory and consulting services, but these presumed the existence of health offices or departments. Since these agencies seldom existed in rural areas, the health needs of the rural population received little attention. The word "country" had a connotation of fresh and clean, and it was assumed that rural life was automatically healthy. A few observant individuals sought to dispel this illusion, but popular myths die hard. In 1899 Governor Daniel H. Hastings of Pennsylvania informed his legislature that it was a fiction to assume "that the country districts are naturally so healthy that there is no need for laws to prevent disease."[34] Virtually all states enacted laws requiring towns and villages to appoint health officers, but most of these laws were meaningless—either the community took no action or else funds were not allocated for the positions. In any event, no provision was made for rural areas.

The growth of municipal health agencies was not only instrumental in promoting the development of state health departments, but it was also responsible for the first rise of the county health departments. Precisely which county deserves credit for establishing the first health department is, as are so many "firsts" in history, a matter of debate. Whatever the case, the early county units grew in response to the needs of growing surburban populations. All three claimants to the title of "first" were counties containing sizable cities. In each instance the sanitary needs of the city's expanding suburban population forced the municipality to employ a full-time health officer with expanded jurisdiction over the entire county. Jefferson County, Kentucky, in which Louisville is located, found it necessary to employ a full-time health officer and staff of inspectors as early as 1908. In 1911 the city of Greensboro, North Carolina, seeking to improve its school health program, combined its health department with that of Guilford County. A devastating typhoid epidemic in Yakima County, Washington, this same year led the city of North Yakima, at the suggestion of the Public Health Service, to appoint a full-time health officer to serve both the city and county.[35] And if county health is to be equated with strictly rural health, then credit for the first county health unit should go to Robeson County, North Carolina. This county, with a population of only 52,500, did not have a single incorporated town of over 2,500, yet in 1912 its government appointed a physician to serve as a full-time health officer.[36]

Granting some merit to the claims of these counties, the major impetus to rural health came with the entrance of the Rockefeller Sanitary Commission onto the scene in 1910 and the Public Health Service in 1914. As noted in connection with the southern states, the commission's efforts to eliminate hookworm were responsible for stimulating the entire public health movement in the South. More important, they were responsible for the first health programs aimed specifically at America's rural population. In 1914 the Public Health Service, which was already becoming involved in rural health through its interest in pellagra, began studies on typhoid fever, which, as towns and cities developed safer water supplies, was becoming increasingly a rural or small-town problem. These studies, along with demonstrations of typhoid control in rural areas, encouraged the growth of permanent local health departments.

During this same decade, 1910–20, the National Tuberculosis Association was sponsoring programs in rural areas, the Red Cross was sending public health nurses into the countryside, and the United States Children's Bureau was beginning to promote infant and maternal care programs among rural women. The publication of Charles Chapin's survey of public health in 1916 led to some improvement in state health departments, but the rural health movement was barely under way at this time. The problems encountered in mobilizing millions of men during World War I that benefited the health movement generally also gave a slight lift to rural health. Early in 1917 the Public Health Service offered to promote sanitation and preventive health measures in areas containing military camps and defense industries, but no federal money was available. The service had no funds in its own budget for this purpose, but the Red Cross stepped into the breach and provided a limited sum to establish a Bureau of Sanitary Service. At the same time, Massachusetts and several other states provided some state money to aid community health programs in the vicinity of army camps.[37]

In May 1917 President Woodrow Wilson authorized the Army Medical Department to organize a sanitary corps to work with the troops, and the Public Health Service's appropriation was subsequently increased to enable it to expand its operations among both military and civilian personnel. Since most army camps and some defense industries were located in isolated or rural areas, the efforts to control diseases among the troops and civilian workers tended to strengthen health units in the adjacent countryside. The Public Health Service began a major antimosquito campaign to reduce the threat of malaria. Based on the army's experiences in Panama, the program sought to eliminate mosquitoes in a belt, one mile wide, surrounding camps and towns with defense industries. In consequence, although many camps were in the South, malaria did not become a problem.[38] An incidental benefit was the temporary reduction in the incidence of malaria among the civilian population.

In July 1918 Congress appropriated one million dollars to help state and local health authorities in their fight against contagious diseases. While most of the funds, along with those provided for antivenereal disease campaigns, went to cities and towns, rural areas adjacent to camps and defense plants derived some benefit from them. The end of the war dried up most government funds for health and sanitation, but the Public Health Service continued its interest in rural health, although on a much smaller basis. Even though most of the health work in rural areas had ended by 1920, the educational programs that had been no small part of it left a residual benefit, and a few of the wartime county public health units survived as permanent organizations.

The decade of the 1920s was one in which the government had only minimal concern with social problems. Nonetheless, the movement to improve rural health continued to make slow progress. The Rockefeller Foundation, based on its experience during the hookworm campaign, developed a policy of stimulating county health units through temporary grants. The funds were distributed through state health departments, which were also responsible for organizing and supervising the county units. By the 1920s the Public Health Service had a similar program. For the year ending in June 1928 the health service reported that it had participated in rural health demonstration projects in seventeen states.[39]

One of the better county health demonstration programs was underwritten by the Milbank Foundation. The foundation proposed to support health programs in three communities, one of which was to be a rural county in New York. Cattaraugus County applied and was accepted in 1922. In the next seven years a complete health unit was developed, with the foundation supplying over half of the budget for the first four years and then gradually reducing its contribution.[40] This and other demonstration programs showed that the initiative for rural health programs had to come from the outside, either from the state or federal government or else from private groups.

The disastrous floods in the Mississippi Valley during the spring of 1927 brought the Red Cross and other agencies into several states. In Kentucky, counties were encouraged to establish health boards in 1927 with the help of the state, the Public Health Service, and the Rockefeller Foundation. As a result of this outside help, twenty full-time county health departments were established in Kentucky by the end of the year.[41]

Kentucky was fortunate to be the home of a small but highly successful volunteer agency dedicated to improving the health of rural women. Mary Breckinridge, a well-to-do Kentuckian, following the loss of her two children, became interested in child health. Subsequently she served as a nurse in World War I and later took public health courses at Columbia University. On her return to Kentucky she became aware of the lack of medical care for rural women, and in 1925 she organized the Kentucky Committee for Mothers and Babies, later to become the Frontier Nursing Service. An energetic worker and successful fund raiser, by 1930 she had established a central clinic or hospital and six outpost centers in remote areas of the state. Each of her outpost centers was staffed with two nurse-midwives. The work she devoted her life to goes on today with an expanded Frontier Nursing Service still providing medical care to rural Kentuckians.[42]

In 1929 the Public Health Service reported that the number of county health agencies had increased from 280 in 1925 to 467 in 1929, most of the increase coming in Ohio and the southern states. Of the 467, 88 percent were receiving assistance from a state board of health, the Public Health Service, the Rockefeller Foundation, and the Children's Bureau. The service noted that approximately 2,500 counties in the United States were completely or largely rural, and that the net increase in the number of county health units between 1920 and 1929 had been forty per year. On this basis, the report added somewhat discouragingly, it would take fifty-one years to provide national service—a prediction that did not prove too far wrong.[43]

By 1930 state health departments bore little resemblance to the weak voluntary boards of health of 1900. They were largely managed by health professionals, and had much more authority, and they were providing a wide range of services to urban and rural areas. Their quality, however, varied widely, and political interference was always a threat. In Kentucky a clash between a new board appointed in 1918 by an incoming governor and the old board had to be settled in the courts. A similar struggle in Kansas in 1923 was finally decided in the state supreme court.[44] Health for the growing percentage of Americans living in urban areas was steadily improving, and some advances had been made in rural areas. Unfortunately, depressed farm prices in the 1920s and the onset of the Great Depression meant that rural Americans did not share equally in the rising standard of living. As of 1929 the Public Health Service estimated that 77 percent of the rural population had no health services.[45]

On the brighter side, the battle against the traditional killer diseases was largely won. Even in urban areas diphtheria, scarlet fever, tuberculosis, typhoid, and other fatal disorders were still present, but their incidence was sharply down. Health boards were beginning to think in terms of chronic, degenerative, and constitutional ailments and to turn their attention to automobile accidents and other threats to health and safety. The health problems of rural areas, particularly those in the South, awaited the rising standard of living that would come with the New Deal and the impact of World War II.

NOTES

1. Charles V. Chapin, *A Report on State Public Health Work Based on a Survey of State Boards of Health* (Chicago, 1916; rpt., New York, 1977), 67.

2. W. K. Sharp, Jr., "Modern Trends in Public Health Work in Louisiana," *New Orleans Medical and Surgical Journal* 90 (1937–38):10.

3. James Wallace, *The State Health Departments of Massachusetts, Michigan, and Ohio with a Summary of Activities and Accomplishments, 1927–28* (New York, 1930), 164.

4. Editorial, "The Development of Public Health Administration in Ohio," *The Ohio Public Health Journal* 10 (1920):105–6.

5. *Sixteenth Annual Report of the State Board of Health of . . . Ohio, . . . , October 31, 1901* (Columbus, 1901), 15–16; *Twenty-second Annual Report of the State Board of Health of . . . Ohio . . . December 31, 1907,* 12.

6. *Twenty-first Annual Report of the State Board of Health of . . . Ohio . . . December 31, 1906,* 10.

7. *Twenty-third Annual Report of the State Board of Health of . . . Ohio . . . December 31, 1908,* 12–14; *Twenty-fourth Annual Report . . . December 31, 1909,* 15; *Twenty-seventh Annual Report . . . December 31, 1912,* 10.

8. "Inception, History and Development of the Division of Laboratories," *Ohio's Health,* Laboratory Number, 14 (1923):51–55.

9. *Fiscal Survey of the State Department of Public Health, 1945–49* (Columbus: Ohio Public Expenditure Council, 1949), 31.

10. *Thirty-first Annual Report of the State Board of Health of . . . Ohio . . . 1928–29,* 197; Charles A. Sieck, "A Study of the Public Health Authority in Ohio" (M.A. thesis, University of Michigan, 1936), 26–27; Charles A. Neal, *State of Ohio, Department of Health, An Historical Review, Its Powers, Duties and Organization* (Columbus, 1929), 3.

11. Editorial, "The Development of Public Health Administration in Ohio," *The Ohio Public Health Journal* 11 (1920):110–12; *Thirty-first Annual Report of the State Board of Health of . . . Ohio . . . 1928–29,* 87–89.

12. Ibid., 182–83.

13. Neal, *State of Ohio, Department of Health, An Historical Review,* 9; Wallace, *The State Health Departments of Massachusetts, Michigan, and Ohio,* 161.

14. Wallace, ibid., 9, 18–19, 161.

15. *Biennial Report of the Louisiana State Board of Health to the General Assembly of the State of Louisiana, 1928–1929* (New Orleans, 1929), 19–49. The most complete account of the health train can be found in Jo Ann Carrigan, "The Gospel of Health on Wheels: Dr. Oscar Dowling and the Louisiana Health Train, 1910–1928," TS, pp. 1–9.

16. Carrigan, "The Gospel of Health on Wheels," 9–15.

17. Benjamin E. Washburn, *A History of the North Carolina State Board of Health* (Raleigh, 1966), 34.

18. Henry Frank Farmer, "The Hookworm Eradication Program in the South" (M.A. thesis, University of Georgia, 1966), 31–32, 72–78.

19. Shirley G. Schoonover, "Alabama Public Health Campaign, 1900–19," *The Alabama Review* 27 (1975):222–23.

20. Farmer, "The Hookworm Eradication Program in the South," 49–50; Mary Boccaccio, "Ground Itch and Dew Poison: The Rockefeller Sanitary Commission, 1909–1914," *J. Hist. Med. & All. Sci.* 27 (1972):52.

21. Washburn, *A History of the North Carolina State Board of Health,* 42.

22. Elizabeth W. Etheridge, *The Butterfly Caste: A Social History of Pellagra in the South* (Westport, Conn., 1972), chapters 1–3; John L. Carmichael, "Medical Reminiscences, Part I," *Alabama Medicine, Journal of the Medical Association of the State of Alabama* 16 (1984):25.

23. Etheridge, *The Butterfly Caste*, 146–62.

24. T. F. Abercrombie, *History of Public Health in Georgia, 1733–1950* (n.p., n.d.), 89.

25. James R. Young, "Malaria in the South, 1900–1930" (Ph.D. diss., University of North Carolina, 1972), 31–33.

26. James H. Cassedy, "The Registration Area and American Vital Statistics," *Bull. Hist. Med.* 39 (1965):221–31.

27. *Sixteenth Biennial Report of the State Board of Health of California, 1898–1900*, 115, 119–20; *Nineteenth Biennial Report of the State Board of Health of California, 1904–1906*, 9; *Twenty-first Biennial Report . . . 1908–1910*, 14.

28. *Twenty-fourth Biennial Report of the State Board of Health of California, 1914–1916*, 3; *Twenty-fifth Biennial Report . . . 1916–1918*, 10.

29. *Thirtieth Biennial Report of the State Board of Health of California, 1926–1928*, 7–8; *Thirty-first Biennial Report . . . 1928–1930*, 10.

30. Chapin, *A Report on State Public Health Work*, 41.

31. Myrtle Greenfield, *A History of Public Health in New Mexico* (Albuquerque, 1962), 13–14.

32. J. W. Kerr, "Public Health Administration in New Mexico," *Public Health Reports*, part 2, 33 (1918):1976–95.

33. Greenfield, *History of Public Health in New Mexico*, 21–23, 323–26.

34. "Biennial Message, Governor Daniel Hartman Hastings, January 1, 1899," *Pennsylvania Archives*, 4th ser., 12 (Harrisburg, Pa., 1902), 315.

35. Harry S. Mustard, *Rural Health Practice* (New York, 1936), 4–5.

36. Ibid.; Washburn, *A History of the North Carolina State Board of Health*, 60.

37. Bess Furman, *A Profile of the United States Public Health Service, 1798–1950* (Washington, D.C., n.d.), 314–15.

38. Ralph C. Williams, *The United States Public Health Service, 1798–1950* (Washington, D.C., 1951), 581–85.

39. L. L. Lumsden, "Cooperative Rural Health Work of the Public Health Service in the Fiscal Year 1928," *Public Health Reports*, part 2, 63 (1928):3149.

40. C.-E. A. Winslow, *Health on the Farm and in the Village* (New York, 1931), 1ff.

41. *The Club Woman*, April 27, 1927, in Microfilm Records of the WPA Ky. Med. Hist. Research Project, reel 25; John McMullen, "Public Health Service Cooperative Program in the Mississippi Flood Area," *Southern Medical Journal* 21 (1928):231–36.

42. Anne. G. Campbell, "Mary Breckinridge and the American Committee for Devastated France: The Foundations of the Frontier Nursing Service," *The Register of the Kentucky Historical Society* 82, no. 3 (1983):263–75. For an account of Breckinridge's life and career, see her autobiography, *Wide Neighborhoods: A Story of the Frontier Nursing Service* (Lexington, Ky., 1981).

43. L. L. Lumsden, "Extent of Rural Health Service in the United States, 1925–29," *Public Health Reports*, part 1, 44 (1929):1202, 1204.

44. Editorial, *Mississippi Valley Medical Journal* 25 (1918):233; *Twelfth Biennial Report of the State Board of Health of Kansas, 1922–24*, 5.

45. Lumsden, "Extent of Rural Health Service," 1207.

16

The Federal Government and Health Reform

Despite the federal government's active concern for the health of farm animals, before the twentieth century it evinced little interest in the welfare of human beings. In the 1870s the general fear of yellow fever that spread throughout the South and the Mississippi Valley led Congress to enact a weak national quarantine act and to create a relatively powerless national board of health to enforce it. Quarantine, however, still remained essentially in the hands of state and local officials, and the national board created in 1879 survived only briefly. The United States Marine Hospital Service, having fought off the threat of a national health department, slowly expanded its authority in the closing years of the 1800s. In this it was helped by a series of minor yellow fever outbreaks in the South, and the United States' acquisition of yellow fever–infested Cuba as a result of the Spanish-American War. Capitalizing on its responsibility for checking on the sources of pestilence overseas, the Marine Hospital Service moved into Cuba and Hawaii.

Walter Reed and his army associates rightly deserve credit for demonstrating the role of the *Aëdes aegypti* mosquito in spreading yellow fever, but their results were the culmination of about twenty years' work by several individuals. Carlos Finlay, a Cuban physician, had become convinced as early as 1881 that the mosquito was the source of the fever. Henry Rose Carter, the yellow fever authority for the Marine Hospital Service, in the 1890s recognized that a number of days had to elapse before yellow fever could be passed from one individual to another. He was assigned to Cuba in 1899 where he met Finlay, and the two men began testing the mosquito hypothesis, using methods similar to those subsequently adopted by Reed. Shortly after Army Surgeon General George M. Sternberg sent Reed to Cuba to study yellow fever, Carter was assigned to Key West, but before leaving Cuba he briefed both Reed and Jesse Lazear on his findings.[1]

Once the role of the *Aëdes aegypti* was confirmed, the way was open to eliminating one of the most terrifying and deadly diseases to strike North

America. The United States Army Medical Corps was soon able to eradicate yellow fever from Havana, and later its antimosquito work made possible the successful completion of the Panama Canal. When the last major yellow fever epidemic struck New Orleans in 1905, the Marine Hospital Service, working in conjunction with the Louisiana and New Orleans health boards, began an antimosquito campaign that stopped the outbreak by the end of August—marking the first time in the United States that a yellow fever epidemic had ended before the onset of cooler weather.[2]

Meanwhile the service was gaining further recognition through its role in combating outbreaks of bubonic plague on the West Coast. In January 1901 the hospital service quarantine officer in San Francisco, Joseph I. Kinyoun, attributed the death of a Chinese man to bubonic plague. The state authorities promptly denied the diagnosis, claiming the disease was syphilis and, with the help of newspapers, began a campaign of vilification against Kinyoun. Bear in mind that the very name, bubonic plague, evoked community memories of all the horrors of the dreaded Black Death, and even a rumor of its presence was enough to cause fear and panic. When a national committee of bacteriologists confirmed the presence of bubonic plague in San Francisco, California state officials had no choice but to concede its presence and cooperate with the hospital service. Governor Henry T. Gage, who had thought he could protect his state's good name by suppressing all information about the existence of the disease, vindictively insisted that Dr. Kinyoun be replaced. The hospital service, sensitive to both politics and states' rights, reassigned Kinyoun. Rightly feeling that he had not been given proper support, Kinyoun resigned from the service shortly thereafter.[3]

Kinyoun's successor, Dr. J. H. White, continued to encounter difficulties with state officials, but fortunately Gage was replaced in 1903 by Governor George C. Pardee who promptly appointed a new state board of health. Henceforth state officials cooperated fully with the hospital service and the San Francisco Health Board in improving the unsanitary conditions in Chinatown that had contributed to spreading the plague. The disease flared up again following the 1906 San Francisco earthquake, but health officers, under the leadership of Surgeon Rupert Blue of the hospital service, soon brought it under control.

Effective lobbying by Surgeon General Walter Wyman, and also the growing prestige of the Marine Hospital Service from its work with yellow fever and bubonic plague, resulted in a 1902 federal law reorganizing the service and renaming it the United States Public Health and Marine Hospital Service. The change in title marked official recognition that the Marine Hospital Service had become the de facto federal public health agency. The law listed the following administrative divisions of the service: Marine hospitals, domestic quarantine, foreign and insular quarantine, personnel and accounts, sanitary reports and statistics, and scientific research. One provision called for an annual meeting of state and territorial health officers with the surgeon general—a provision that legalized the supremacy of the federal government in public health affairs.

Equally important, the 1902 law strengthened the Hygienic Laboratory. In the previous year Surgeon General Walter Wyman had guided a law through Congress that officially recognized the Hygienic Laboratory by providing $35,000 for a new building and authorizing it to investigate "infectious and contagious diseases, and matters pertaining to the public health." The 1902 law instructed the Division of Scientific Research of the hospital service to coordinate all research within the service—the Hygienic Laboratory in Washington, the Plague Laboratory in San Francisco, and cooperative work with universities and states. An advisory board of scientists was established, and the Hygienic Laboratory was organized into four divisions. The original staff became the Division of Pathology and Bacteriology and three new divisions—chemistry, pharmacology, and zoology—were created.[4]

As Victoria A. Harden has pointed out, the 1902 law marked a watershed in the history of the Hygienic Laboratory; research was recognized as one of its legitimate functions; and, as a result of a provision providing for its orderly expansion, the laboratory entered the mainstream of biomedical research. Operating with a limited budget, its small staff made significant research contributions in the next thirty years. Two of its scientists whose work contributed most directly to public health have already been mentioned—Charles Wardell Stiles, the first director of the laboratory's Division of Zoology, who led the hookworm campaign, and the great epidemiologist, Joseph Goldberger, whose name is almost synonymous with pellagra. Other outstanding Hygienic Laboratory scientists were George McCoy and Edward Francis, who identified tularemia, and Alice E. Evans, who demonstrated that undulant fever in humans was the same disease as abortive fever in cattle.[5]

A major objective of the Progressives in this era was the conservation of national resources, and, among these, health ranked high on the agenda. Two economists, J. Pease Norton and Irving Fisher, both of Yale, took leadership in the movement for national health legislation. In 1906 a paper by Norton arguing for a national health agency stimulated the American Association for the Advancement of Science to appoint a Committee of One Hundred on National Health to investigate the subject. The committee, whose membership included prominent Americans from a wide range of areas, supported a bill introduced by Senator Robert L.

Owen of Oklahoma in 1910 to create a national department of health. The measure, which had the support of the American Medical Association, was immediately attacked by lobbyists for irregular medical sects, fringe groups such as the antivaccinationists and antivivisectionists, and representatives of the patent medicine industry. Their most strident spokesman was the National League for Medical Freedom, a body that encompassed most of the opponents to the health law.[6]

The most effective opposition, however, came from Surgeon General Wyman, who was determined to expand his own agency into a full-time health department. He initiated a series of bills extending the authority of the Marine Hospital Service and worked quietly to undermine the Owen Bill. Congress, always reluctant to commit itself on controversial issues, stalled for time. Late in 1911 Wyman died, and Congress, possibly out of respect for the deceased surgeon general, passed a compromise health bill in 1912. It changed the name of the United States Marine Hospital Service to the United States Public Health Service, authorized the service's publication of health information for the public, and extended the service's investigations into disease sources specifically to include sanitation, sewage, and pollution. An appropriation measure enacted the following year provided $200,000 for field investigations, $47,000 for the conquest of pellagra, and $25,000 for field work with trachoma and raised the Hygienic Laboratory budget to $20,000.[7]

By this date the Public Health Service was already investigating epidemics of typhoid and endemic trachoma, cooperating with the Rockefeller Foundation and local health boards in the fight against hookworm, beginning its work to eliminate pellagra, and initiating studies on occupational diseases. Under Surgeon General Rupert Blue, who succeeded Walter Wyman, the service extended its investigation of typhoid to interstate and international water bodies. The service had been given responsibility for building a leprosarium on Molokai Island, Hawaii, in 1905, and, when Congress established a National Leprosarium by taking over the Louisiana Leprosarium at Carville, it, too, came under the jurisdiction of the Public Health Service.

World War I greatly broadened the mandate of the health service. Its responsibility for the environment around camps and war industries required major antimosquito campaigns to reduce the threat of malaria and involved the service in widespread sanitary measures. One of the most significant developments was the creation of a division of venereal disease within the service. Since the subject was considered too delicate to be broached publicly, the bill establishing the division was simply called an army appropriation measure. An appropriation of $200,000 was made for the division, and another $2 million was given to the states on a matching basis for prevention and cure of the diseases. The service, which had already been operating venereal disease clinics in conjunction with the Red Cross, drew up a model code of laws for dealing with the problem and submitted it to the states, virtually all of which enacted some type of legislation designed to prevent the spread of venereal disease. With the end of war, the veil of silence once again fell over venereal disease. Congress reduced the funding for federal-state venereal disease clinics to $1 million in 1920, then to $546,345.30 in 1921, and finally cut off the appropriation completely by 1923.[8]

The pandemic of influenza that swept over the world in 1918–19 arrived in America coincidentally with the mass mobilization of manpower for World War I. A mild wave of influenza occurred in the spring of 1918, but it was not until September that the epidemic literally exploded in New England and the East Coast. The Public Health Service (PHS) had instructed its quarantine officers in August to be alert for signs of influenza, but the disease was not reportable, and quarantine under wartime conditions was impracticable in any case. As the seriousness of the outbreak became apparent, the Public Health Service, seeking to gather specific information, arranged with state health departments to submit daily reports and began a nationwide public information campaign.

The next step was to mobilize public health and medical resources. A director was appointed in each of the states—the state's health officer where possible or else a PHS officer. The major problem was the sudden demand for physicians and nurses. Boston, where the influenza first assumed major proportions, requested 500 physicians, and other cities, too, were calling for large-scale help. Fortunately, in the wave of patriotic fervor that accompanied the declaration of war, a large number of physicians who were ineligible for military service had organized the Voluntary Medical Service Corps (VMSC). When Surgeon General Blue asked this group for help, he was given the names of 1,900 doctors ready for immediate service. Appeals by the AMA eventually resulted in over 72,000 physicians joining the VMSC.[9]

Since medicine could do little about influenza and pneumonia in 1918, the most desperate need was for nurses, but these were in short supply. The Red Cross jumped into the breach, mobilizing all available trained nurses, and accepting thousands of untrained volunteers. As the cost of caring for literally millions of cases mounted, Congress appropriated an additional $1 million for the Public Health Service to fight influenza.

The precise cost of the 1918–19 influenza epidemic in terms of human suffering and lives lost cannot be determined. A PHS sample survey of eleven cities and towns throughout the United States showed that 28 percent of their residents had contracted the flu. If the figures are representative, then over a quarter of the American population caught the disease. Since the Census Bureau's death registration area at that time covered less than 80 percent of the population, the census statistics for deaths from influenza and its pneumonic complications are incomplete. In his excellent study of the influenza epidemic, Alfred W. Crosby, using the 1915 states' influenza and pneumonia death rates as a baseline, estimates total deaths from the epidemic at about 550,000. During the outbreak, bills were introduced into Congress to appropriate money for research on influenza, but public memory proved short. Once the epidemic was over, interest in influenza waned, and the measures died. The role played by the Public Health Service during the outbreak, along with its other wartime activities, undoubtedly helped its public image.[10]

Much of the credit accruing from the Public Health Service's wartime efforts, however, was lost in the battle over the care of war veterans. In October 1917 Congress established the War Risk Insurance Bureau in the Treasury Department and provided that medical care for war-connected injuries and sicknesses would be handled by the service's Marine hospitals. With the return of veterans, Congress provided funds for adding ten additional hospitals. Unfortunately, most of these were obsolete or dilapidated institutions, many of which were foisted on the service for political reasons. In 1921 President Warren G. Harding, notorious for his poor choice of officers, appointed Colonel Charles R. Forbes to head the War Risk Insurance Bureau. Forbes, an empire-building hustler, capitalizing on some of the legitimate complaints of veterans' organizations, managed to expand his agency into the Veterans Bureau. In 1922 all veterans hospitals were transferred from the Public Health Service to the Veterans Bureau.[11]

Although loss of responsibility for veterans' care was a setback for the Public Health Service—and of doubtful value to sick and wounded veterans—it may have allowed the service to focus more attention on its rural health program. As detailed earlier in chapter 15, for some years it had been working with private foundations and the Red Cross in promoting rural health. In accordance with this policy, in 1919 the service requested $500,000 to conduct cooperative demonstration rural health projects but received only $50,000. Despite this niggardly appropriation, within a few months the Public Health Service was working with state and local authorities in thirty-one counties, and over the ensuing years the service expanded this work in collaboration with private and government agencies.[12]

The effort to create a national health department or to strengthen the Public Health Service was only one aspect of the Progressive movement's fight for social justice. The Progressives, who advocated a wide range of legislation on such matters as child and female labor, workmen's compensation, public health, and health insurance, probably reached the peak of their success with the passage of the first federal child labor law in 1916. The event that may well mark the nation's turning point away from Progressivism was the movement's failure shortly thereafter to gain some form of government health insurance.

The passage of the British National Insurance Act of 1911 first stimulated American interest in compulsory health insurance. An editorial in *JAMA* the following year declared that the British Insurance Act marked a new era "for both society and physicians." Health insurance, the editorial went on, would eliminate the need for medical charity and "do away with any possible mercenary motive which might be alleged against individual physicians or the medical profession as a whole."[13] The American Association for Labor Legislation (AALL), an influential Progressive group representing many leading social scientists, in December 1912 voted to establish a Committee on Social Insurance. By this date the evidence uncovered by municipal health departments was making it clear that sickness was closely associated with poverty in urban areas, and the committee decided to concentrate specifically upon promoting health insurance.[14]

After examining the British and German social insurance systems and debating at length several drafts of a proposed law, in 1916 the committee proposed a model compulsory health insurance bill. It was to apply to laborers making $100 or less a month, and to cover medical, surgical and obstetrical care for workers and their families. The proposed insurance was also to provide cash benefits for twenty-six weeks, and pay up to $50 for burial expenses. The premiums were to be divided between the employee, employer, and the state.[15]

The immediate reaction to the AALL's proposed health insurance program was favorable. Editorials in *JAMA* were supportive, and the AMA Board of Trustees, convinced that a health insurance law was both necessary and inevitable, established a Committee on Social Insurance and instructed the committee to "secure such constructions of the proposed laws as will work the most harmonious adjustment of the new sociologic relations between physicians and laymen." The Public Health Committee of the New York Academy of Medicine also favored a health insurance law. After thoroughly studying the AALL's bill, the health committee recommended it but suggested that provision be made for periodic medical examinations and that the existing dispensaries be used for medical care under the proposed system.[16]

Confident of widespread support for health insurance, the AALL immediately introduced its model bill into the state legislatures of New York, New Jersey, and Massachusetts, and began campaigning for health insurance in several other states. The confidence of the AALL seemed fully justified. In New York and Wisconsin the state medical societies endorsed the bill in principle; the Massachusetts Medical Society remained neutral and suggested that further study was needed. Of the first four state health commissions appointed to study health insurance legislation, three reported favorably, and only the Massachusetts commission recommended delaying legislation until after the war. California under Governor Hiram Johnson had appointed a Social Insurance Commission to investigate health insurance in 1915. In 1917 the commission recommended a compulsory health insurance program paid for by contributions from individuals, industry, and the state. With initial support from the *California State Medical Journal*, the advocates of the commission's proposal were sure that a public referendum would win the day.[17]

At the national level, too, there was considerable enthusiasm for the movement. Surgeon General Rupert Blue of the PHS in his presidential address to the AMA in 1916 spoke of the excessive morbidity and mortality of unskilled workers, which he attributed in part to the fact that many did not make enough money to maintain a healthful living, "much less provide adequate medical care." "To meet the situation," he concluded, "there are unmistakable signs that health insurance will constitute the next great step in social legislation."[18] His views were shared by many national leaders in medicine. S. S. Goldwater, Michael M. Davis, Alice Hamilton, Haven Emerson, and General W. C. Gorgas were among the outstanding American physicians active in the fight. The American Public Health Association and a number of other national organizations also added their voices to the demand for health insurance.

On the other hand, despite the favorable view of the AMA's leadership, possibly a majority of its member physicians were either neutral or dubious of health insurance. A good many well-known physicians actively fought against it, and they had strong backing from Frederick L. Hoffman, president of the American Statistical Association, statistician for the Prudential Life Insurance Company, and one of the most influential figures in the area of health and medicine. Moreover, by 1917 the medical profession began turning against health insurance. Effective lobbying in state legislatures and well-financed public relations campaigns by medical societies and other vested interests soon ground the health insurance movement to a halt. In November 1918 California voters decisively rejected a compulsory health insurance program by an almost two-to-one vote. The only success achieved by the AALL and its allies came in the spring of 1919 when the New York State Senate passed a compulsory health insurance bill. Even this success was limited since the bill failed in the House.[19]

By 1919 Progressivism was on the wane, and the swing toward conservatism in the United States undoubtedly played a part in the failure of early health legislation. Equally important, insurance companies mobilized their lobbyists and public relations staffs to combat the threat that this legislation posed to their profits. More surprising was the opposition of organized labor, which preferred to concentrate on wages and hours and to keep out of health politics. The involvement of the United States in World War I was another significant factor since it had distracted public attention from domestic concerns and had enabled opponents of health insurance to brand it a German plot to destroy the American way of life. At the same time, the Russian Revolution had raised the specter of Bolshevism, and this, too, was seized upon as an argument against any form of governmental intervention in the medical area.

Probably more important than any of these factors was the rising opposition to national health insurance by the medical profession during the war. In the prewar years many physicians had enjoyed relatively low incomes, and health insurance was seen as a means of improving their economic status. According to Ronald L. Numbers, the war brought a sharp rise in physicians' income and a corresponding decline in their enthusiasm for health insurance.[20] Whatever the case, further efforts toward compulsory social legislation had to await the Great Depression.

The 1920s, the decade in which President Coolidge assumed that the chief business of government was to support business, was scarcely notable for social legislation. The most important federal health measure in these years was the Sheppard-Towner Act of 1921. The Nineteenth Amendment giving suffrage to women had passed the previous year, and women's organizations, using their new political power, provided the impetus to push the Sheppard-Towner Bill through Congress. The act provided an annual appropriation for five years of $1,240,000 for the "Advancement of Maternity and Infant Welfare." Of the annual sum, $50,000 was assigned to the Children's Bureau for administrative purposes, $5,000 was allocated to each state, another $5,000 was made available to states on a matching basis, and the rest was to be distributed to the states on the basis of their population. From the first introduction of the bill, the AMA was strongly opposed. An editorial in *JAMA* in February 1921 argued that advocates of the bill considered the federal treasury "an inexhaustible reservoir" and declared that, while every mother and child should receive food and medical care, the federal government was not responsible for providing them. A correspondent to *JAMA* insisted that pregnancy and childbirth were clearly medical matters and asserted that to assume social and economic matters were of more importance than medical ones was sheer nonsense.[21]

The Sheppard-Towner Act provided that state health departments receiving federal funds had to meet certain standards, and it created a "Federal Board of Maternity and Infant Hygiene" to pass on state programs. The states, however, were given wide latitude in their use of federal money. Forty states took immediate advantage of Sheppard-Towner money when the law became effective in 1922. In several other states the issue of whether or not to accept federal funds was heatedly debated. An editorial in the *New Orleans Medical and Surgical Journal* in July 1922 denounced the Sheppard-Towner Act as "paternalistic and socialistic in nature." Nonetheless, despite strong opposition from the state's medical societies, in July 1924 the Louisiana legislature voted to enter the program. Three states never participated—Massachusetts, Connecticut, and Illinois. In Massachusetts the Attorney General pronounced the Sheppard-Towner Act unconstitutional, and the state even went so far as to institute legal action, without success, against the United States Treasury Department.[22]

The amount of money appropriated for the Sheppard-Towner Act in relation to the millions of women and children needing help was negligible, but the act stimulated state funding, greatly increased the number of public health nurses, and provided a stimulus to health education. The Sheppard-Towner Act also reflected a strong national movement to improve child health. The year 1918, which had been proclaimed "Child Health Year" through the efforts of the Children's Bureau, saw the founding of the Child Health Organization by L. Emmett Holt and Miss Sally Jean Lucas. In 1923 this body merged with the American Child Hygiene Association and became the American Child Health Association.

Herbert Hoover, who had a genuine interest in child welfare, was elected president of the association in 1923 and made it an active force for child welfare. One of the association's first steps was to undertake a survey of 86 cities with populations ranging from 40,000 to 70,000. Of these cities, 41 had no full-time health officer; and of those with part-time health officers, 50 percent of the officers did not have medical degrees. Half of the 86 cities had no reliable birth or death records of children, and 17 made no provision for the medical inspection of schoolchildren. Reflecting the generally discouraging picture of child health, 44 percent of the children in the 86 cities had not even been vaccinated for smallpox. Although the problem of child health was well beyond the capacity of any volunteer organization to solve by itself, under the energetic leadership of Herbert Hoover, the Child Health Association raised several million dollars for health education and child health demonstration projects.[23]

During the 1920s all agencies concerned with the welfare of children made special efforts to train health educators and to make teachers and students aware of the need for personal and public hygiene. (The author recalls, as a grade-school student, hearing lectures on how to brush the teeth and on the need to wash hands and bathe, keep the hair and nails clean, and be aware of omnipresent germs.) It is safe to say that this decade probably marked the high point for school health education.

The medical profession continued to denounce the Sheppard-Towner Act throughout the 1920s, and the AMA almost succeeded in preventing its renewal in 1926. Although the act was extended for two more years, its opponents were steadily gaining strength in Congress. The act's chief beneficiaries, poor women and children, were not an effective political force, and the AMA and its allies won out in 1929 when the law was allowed to expire. In light of the general opposition to social legislation in the 1920s, it is surprising that a law providing federal money for maternal and child care was enacted at all. While the Sheppard-Towner Act helped set the stage for the massive matching grants of the New Deal, it did not establish a precedent. The United States Department of Agriculture had earlier used matching grants to promote agricultural education, and the Chamberlain-Kahn Act of 1918 had made a similar provision for dealing with venereal disease. Yet the Sheppard-Towner Act firmly established the principle of using matching grants for social purposes, and, more than that, it also made evident the idea that medicine could not be divorced from society—thus challenging the prevailing assumption of the medical profession that medicine was a science existing apart from the society in which it operated.[24]

At the same time that the federal government was becoming active in health concerns, private philanthropy began playing a more important role in public health. Influenced by the British humanitarian movement of the eighteenth century, voluntary charitable organizations and philanthropy have characterized American society for the past two hundred years. The many local health and sanitary associations of the nineteenth century helped bring the sanitary movement to fruition, and similar organizations continue to play a significant role today. During the early years of this century the most notable volunteer groups were the American Red Cross and the National Tuberculosis Association. The Red Cross is best known for its work during catastrophes and emergencies, but its local units consistently promoted health education. In rural areas the Red Cross became one of the main agencies providing public health nurses, thus helping in the formation of early county health units.

The National Tuberculosis Association and its local chapters played a major role in the drive to eliminate the disease. The association provided a wide range of educational programs, promoted tuberculosis hospitals and clinics, conducted mass screenings, and constantly pressured health departments and legislatures into taking firmer measures against the disease. The success of the tuberculosis association spawned a host of volunteer groups dedicated to curing and preventing particular diseases, disorders, or congenital conditions. One of the most effective of these was the National Polio Foundation. Since organizations and institutions, particularly those successful at raising money, have a viability of their own, the foundation merely shifted gears when polio was virtually eliminated and moved on to newer concerns.

The work of voluntary groups in the twentieth century was greatly aided by a tremendous expansion of large-scale philanthropy. In the field of medicine and health, the Rockefeller Foundation was the dominant philanthropic institution in the early years of this century. From its early pioneering work in combating hookworm and malaria, the foundation became a major force promoting rural health and the emergence of county health units. In the 1920s a number of other philanthropic foundations became interested in preventive medicine. Most of them financed health demonstration projects designed to encourage communities to maintain health departments. Among the better-known private agencies supporting public health projects were the Commonwealth Fund, the Milbank Fund, the Rosenwald Fund, the Phipps Institute, and the Kellogg Foundation.

A few enlightened corporations also recognized the value of a healthy population. The most effective one in this respect was the Metropolitan Life Insurance Company of New York. Haley Fiske, the company's vice president, firmly believed that profit and social responsibility were not incompatible. In 1909 he organized a welfare division in the company. Its director, Lee Frankel, considered starting an antituberculosis campaign until Lillian D. Wald convinced him that providing visiting nurses for the company's industrial policyholders in New York City was a far better plan. She pointed out that the cost of the nurses would be more than paid for by the reduction in the number of death benefit payments. The program was an immediate success, and Metropolitan soon extended the service throughout the country. Wherever possible, the company relied on visiting nurse associations; otherwise it employed its own nurses. Within three years from the program's inception, the company was paying for a million nursing visits a year at an annual cost of $500,000.

By the 1930s the nation's large immigrant population had been absorbed into American society and medical practice had changed, with the acutely sick increasingly being treated in hospitals. Moreover, state and local governments were assuming greater responsibility for public and private health. In 1939 critics of the Metropolitan Life Insurance Company argued that its policy of providing visiting nurses was merely a sales device. By this time the need for home nursing had become greatly reduced, and this factor, along with a sharp rise in nursing costs, convinced the company that the program had outlived its usefulness. In 1950 it announced that the visiting nurse program would cease, effective January 1, 1953.[25]

The public health leaders, or sanitarians, of the late nineteenth century evolved from a variety of professions, including physicians concerned with preventive medicine, engineers interested in water and sewer systems, and chemists involved in analyzing food and water. As the field of public health became institutionalized and professionalized, the need for specialized training became evident. Beginning in the 1870s, lectures in hygiene and state medicine were offered in several medical schools. The AMA also took up the cause of public health education, in part as a result of an address on "State Medicine" presented by Stanford E. Chaillé of Louisiana in 1879. Chaillé had been preaching before medical associations on the duty of the state to guarantee "the inalienable right of every human being to be supplied with uncontaminated air, water, food, soil, and personal surroundings." For several years he had been giving lectures on state medicine at the University of Louisiana Medical School (now Tulane), and in 1881 the school offered a course in public health.[26] The late nineteenth century also saw a strong movement to teach personal hygiene in the public schools—one that added to the demand for hygiene courses at the college and university level.

By 1900 public health was in the process of becoming a medical specialty, and the American Public Health Association appointed a committee to study the teaching of hygiene and to establish standards for degrees in that specialty. The committee recommended that M.D.'s who had been given six months' training in hygiene and had served six months as an assistant to a medical officer be given a "Diploma of Public Health." The D.Sc. was to be awarded after two years of specialized studies and the completion of a thesis. The committee further recommended that food and sanitary workers meet the standards of the British Sanitary Institute, which offered a certificate after the completion of twenty to forty hours of lectures and an examination.[27]

In the United States during the early 1900s—led by men such as Victor C. Vaughan of the University of Michigan, Alexander C. Abbott of the University of Pennsylvania, George Whipple and Milton J. Rosenau of Harvard, and William T. Sedgwick of the Massachusetts Institute of Technology—American schools began offering courses leading toward certificates and degrees in public health. The last three, Whipple and Rosenau of Harvard and Sedgwick of MIT, began a collaboration in 1909 that resulted four years later in the formation of a joint School for Health Officers. This institution eventually became the Harvard School of Public Health.[28]

The problem with developing degree programs was the lack of agreement on what constituted public health and on which group of professionals should have the dominant voice in the field. The main clash was between physicians, who insisted that public health was purely medical, and sanitary engineers, but tension had also developed between public health physicians working in the area of social medicine and medical practitioners who thought of medicine largely in scientific terms. Moreover, bacteriologists and chemists, too, began demanding a voice in public health education. Although by 1910, as noted above, a number of universities were offering courses in public health, the content of these courses depended largely on the department sponsoring them. The first step in resolving the question as to the direction of public health was taken by the Rockefeller Foundation General Education Board in 1914, when it called a conference under its auspices.[29]

By this date the demand for trained public health professionals was rapidly increasing. The fight to take public health departments out of politics had led New York and several other states to establish qualifications for health officers, but unfortunately there were few individuals who could meet them. When it became known that the Rockefeller General Education Board was interested in training public health workers, Harvard, Yale, Columbia, the University of Pennsylvania, and other schools immediately began asserting their claims to being the logical institution to do the job. Wickliffe Rose and Abraham Flexner of the Rockefeller Foundation agreed that educating public health professionals required a separate school.

The first issue—one that would shape the future of American schools of public health—was to determine the school's purpose. Rose envisioned a central school, supported by state schools, that would engage in some research but emphasize practical training and demonstration programs designed to educate both public health workers and the public. William Welch of Johns Hopkins, whom Flexner considered the ultimate authority on medical education, wanted an institution centered on scientific research rather than one designed to train health workers, and his views carried the day. Rose, Flexner, and Jerome D. Greene, secretary of the Rockefeller Foundation, in 1915 visited seven major cities (five of them on the East Coast), looking for the one with the best facilities for the new school. Suffice to say, Baltimore, which would appear to have offered the fewest advantages other than the existence of the Johns Hopkins Medical School and Hospital, won out. Flexner, a Hopkins graduate and an admirer of its medical school, needed little urging to choose Baltimore, and Welch, a dominant figure in American medicine and the Rockefeller Foundation's chief consultant on medical affairs, easily persuaded the other members of the committee.[30]

In 1916 the Rockefeller Foundation gave $267,000 to establish the Johns Hopkins School of Hygiene and Public Health—the word "Hygiene" representing Welch's idea of a place for basic research, and "Public Health" reflecting the foundation's intention to promote practical training. The planning took over two years, and it was not until October 1918 that the first permanent American school of public health opened its doors. It represented a compromise between the German concept of a research institute, which Welch had incorporated into his medical school, and the British system of providing practical training for health workers. And just as the Johns Hopkins Medical School set the pattern for American medical education in the twentieth century, so, too, the John Hopkins School of Hygiene established the formula for public health schools.

Tulane University, which pioneered in teaching hygiene and state medicine, had established a School of Tropical Medicine, Hygiene, and Preventive Medicine in 1913. Unfortunately, the school's first dean eloped with the daughter of a prominent New Orleans citizen the following year, and, although courses in hygiene and tropical medicine continued to be taught, the school, to all intents and purposes, disappeared.[31] By the time the Johns Hopkins public health school permanently opened, some fifteen other institutions were offering certificates or degrees in public health, and ten of them were granting doctorates.[32] Even so, the demand for trained public health workers far exceeded the supply being produced. The success of the AMA's Council on Education and the Flexner Report in raising standards of medical education had reduced the number of medical schools by almost half, drastically cutting down on the number of physicians precisely when the demand for their services was increasing. As private practice became more lucrative, fewer physicians were attracted to public health work.

An officer for the Rockefeller International Board in 1922 expressed fears about appropriating money for public health in the southern states "because we haven't the men to send to them to help them spend it wisely." This same year the United States Public Health Service called a conference of over one hundred leading university presidents, deans of medical schools, and sanitarians to consider the shortage in health personnel. Surveys of health departments showed that few of their administrators had any health training. Of 65 towns and cities in Massachusetts, only 5 had a health officer with a certificate or degree in public health. Another survey showed that less than 10 percent of health administrators in 72 cities throughout the United States had any special preparation for their work. Public health nurses were in particularly short supply.[33] The establishment of Johns Hopkins and other public health schools helped the situation somewhat, but unfortunately, the medical profession began a tradition of viewing public health in the same way that arts and sciences colleges have tended to look upon schools of education. The growing demand for trained public health professionals in the years between 1900 and 1930 resulted from a more active concern for public health at all levels of government. For the first time the federal government, working through the Public Health Service, the Agriculture Department, and other agencies, had started moving into the area. This same period also saw the emergence of large-scale philanthropic work in the public health field under the leadership of the Rockefeller Foundation and similar organizations. The net result was that by 1930 the field of public health had become both institutionalized and professionalized.

NOTES

1. Bess Furman, *A Profile of the United States Public Health Service, 1798–1948,* 159–60, 223–26, 235–36; Lawrence Altman, *Who Goes First? The Story of Self-Experimentation in Medicine* (New York, 1986), 129–58.

2. John Duffy, *The Rudolph Matas History of Medicine in Louisiana* (Baton Rouge, La., 1958–62), 2:433–36.

3. Ralph C. Williams, *The United States Public Health Service, 1798–1950* (Washington, D.C., 1951), 121–25; Furman, *A Profile of the United States Public Health Service,* 244–48.

4. Victoria A. Harden, *Inventing the NIH: Federal Biomedical Research Policy, 1887–1937* (Baltimore, 1986), 17–19.

5. Ibid., 20; Furman, *A Profile of the United States Public Health Service,* 352.

6. George Rosen, "Public Health, Then and Now," *American Journal of Public Health* 62 (1972):261–63; James G. Burrow, *Organized Medicine in the Progressive Era: The Move Toward Monopoly* (Baltimore, 1977), 100–102, 138–39.

7. Harden, *Inventing the NIH,* 35–38; Furman, *A Profile of the United States Public Health Service,* 288.

8. Furman, *A Profile of the United States Public Health Service,* 319–21, 341.

9. Alfred W. Crosby, Jr., *Epidemic and Peace, 1918* (Westport, Conn., 1976), 29ff.

10. Ibid., 51–53, 206–7, 322–24; W. H. Frost, "Statistics of Influenza Morbidity with Special Reference to Certain Factors in Case Incidence and Case Fatality," part 1, *Public Health Reports* 35 (1920):584–97.

11. Furman, *A Profile of the United States Public Health Service,* 344–47.

12. Ibid., 340.

13. Editorial, "Socializing the British Medical Profession," part 2, *JAMA* 59 (1912):1890–91.

14. Ronald L. Numbers, *Almost Persuaded: American Physicians and Compulsory Health Insurance, 1912–1920* (Baltimore, 1978), 15–18.

15. Ibid., 25; Burrow, *Organized Medicine in the Progressive Era,* 143–44.

16. Numbers, *Almost Persuaded,* 36; Summary of the Activities of the Public Health Committee . . . for January and February, 1916, New York Academy of Medicine MS, pp. 2–4.

17. Arthur J. Viseltear, "Compulsory Health Insurance in California, 1915–1918," *J. Hist. Med. & All. Sci.* 24 (1969):152–80; Numbers, *Almost Persuaded,* 37–51, 99.

18. Rupert Blue, "Some of the Larger Problems of the Medical Profession," *JAMA* 66 (1916):1901.

19. Numbers, *Almost Persuaded* 61–63, 91; Viseltear, "Compulsory Health Insurance in California, 1915–1918," 181.

20. Burrow, *Organized Medicine in the Progressive Era,* 153–56; Numbers, *Almost Persuaded,* 112–14.

21. Grace Abbott, "Federal Aid for the Protection of Maternity and Infancy," *American Journal of Public Health* 12 (1922):738; Editorial, "Federal Care of Maternity and Infancy—The Sheppard-Towner Bill," *JAMA* 76 (1921):383.

22. Editorial, "Medical Legislation," *New Orleans Medical and Surgical Journal* 75 (1922–23):90; Barbara G. Rosenkrantz, *Public Health and the State: Changing Views in Massachusetts, 1842–1936* (Cambridge, Mass., 1972), 154–57.

23. Harold L. Cavins, *National Health Agencies: A Survey with Especial Reference to Voluntary Associations* (Washington, D.C., 1945), 112–13; Herbert Hoover, *The Memoirs of Herbert Hoover: The Cabinet and the Presidency, 1922–1933* (New York, 1952), 97–99.

24. Rosemary Stevens, *American Medicine and the Public Interest* (New Haven, Conn., 1971), 143–44.

25. Diane Hamilton, "The Metropolitan Visiting Nurse Service (1909–1953)" (paper presented at the American Association for the History of Medicine, Philadelphia, May 1, 1987), 1–9; Karen Buhler-Wilkerson, "False Dawn: The Rise and Decline of Public Health Nursing in America, 1900–1930," in Ellen C. Lagemann, ed., *Nursing History: New Perspectives, New Possibilities* (New York, 1983), 91.

26. John Duffy, *The Tulane University Medical Center: One Hundred and Fifty Years of Medical Education* (Baton Rouge, La., 1984), 52–54.

27. "Report of Committee on Teaching Hygiene and Granting a Diploma of Doctor of Public Health," in *Selections from Public Health Reports and Papers Presented at Meetings of the American Public Health Association (1884–1907)* (New York, 1977), 87–90.

28. Jean A. Curran, *Founders of the Harvard School of Public Health, 1909–1946* (New York, 1970).

29. Elizabeth Fee, *Disease and Discovery: A History of the Johns Hopkins School of Hygiene and Public Health, 1916–1939* (Baltimore, 1987), 24–25. For this and the following material, I have relied heavily on this excellent study.

30. Ibid., chapters 2 and 3.

31. Duffy, *The Tulane University Medical Center,* 112–16.

32. "Public Health Education," *American Journal of Public Health* 8 (1918):600–607.

33. Harry H. Moore, *Public Health in the United States: An Outline with Historical Data* (New York, 1923), 390–93.

17

The Great Depression and the War Years

The first thirty years of the twentieth century witnessed vast changes in American life. Urbanization proceeded at an increasing pace, the automobile permitted the rise of suburbs and reduced the isolation of rural areas, telephones and radios marked the beginning of a communications revolution, and major strides were made in controlling the great killer diseases. Between 1900 and 1930 life expectancy for the average American increased from 47.3 years to 59.7, and the steadily rising standard of living brought a corresponding improvement in general health.[1] Yet the advances in medicine and public health did not benefit all Americans. Public health was provided largely by local governments, and the strength and effectiveness of the thousands of local public health agencies varied greatly. A few county health units were beginning to function in rural areas, but most rural Americans scarcely knew the meaning of public health, and a great many seldom if ever saw a physician. To make matters worse, falling agricultural prices during the 1920s depressed the farm economy. Even in cities the boom years did not bring universal prosperity. In Detroit, for example, where the expanding automobile industry had attracted thousands of blacks and whites from southern rural areas, employment was sporadic. The annual summer layoffs during the changeover from one automobile model to another ranged from two to four months—and there was no unemployment compensation for those dismissed.

For the majority of Americans the stock-market crash of 1929 had little immediate impact. The farm economy was already in depression, and employment in the urban areas decreased slowly at first and then at an accelerating rate. In terms of public health, the expiration of the Sheppard-Towner Act that same year marked a slowdown in government spending for health, although this was not universally true. According to the United States Public Health Service, the number of rural counties with health units increased from 467 in 1929 to 616 in 1932. The following year, as the Great Depression worsened, the number fell to 581.[2] Nonetheless, by 1930–31 the economic slowdown was affecting budgets of health departments at all levels.

The one encouraging note in these years was a growing public aware-ness of American citizens' health needs. The emphasis upon health educa-tion during the 1920s and the rising cost of scientific medicine were making many Americans conscious of the disparities in general health care. In 1926 a diverse group of leaders in medicine, public health, and the social sciences set the stage for establishing the Committee on the Costs of Medical Care. This body, supported by the Public Health Service, eight foundations, and various private groups, in 1927 began a five-year study of health facilities and health care in the United States. Its report in 1932 presented a discouraging picture, one that showed families at the lowest income levels receiving little medical attention and exposed the little incentive private medicine had to practice preventive medicine.[3]

While the committee was pushing ahead with its study, President Hoover, who was genuinely interested in child welfare and had served as president of the American Child Health Association (as mentioned in the last chapter), in 1930 called a White House Conference on Child Health and Protection. The conference brought no immediate changes in health policy; but the conference's reports, compiled by some 1,200 child ex-perts, contributed to a better understanding of child health. Although Hoover was constrained by his economic philosophy from using federal funds for relief purposes, the rising tide of unemployment in cities and towns and the continuing fall in agricultural prices by 1931 forced him to act. His major concern was to stimulate industry and agriculture, but in 1932 he supported the Relief and Reconstruction Act, which permitted the Reconstruction Finance Corporation (RFC), an agency designed to aid business and financial concerns, to lend $1.5 billion to state and local governments for public works projects. Since there was an acute need for water and sewer systems, these funds indirectly strengthened health de-partments. In Mississippi, for example, funds from the RFC in 1932 were used by the state health department to construct privies and other sanitary facilities.[4]

By 1932 diminishing tax receipts and the burden of rising welfare costs were rapidly increasing the indebtedness of governments at all levels, and the need for economy became a major theme in election campaigns. From Franklin D. Roosevelt to candidates for local offices, the promise was to reduce government expenditures. Indicative of the general reduction in government budgets, the secretary of the Kansas State Board of Health did not bother to make a summary statement in his biennial report after 1930, merely noting that the budget for 1932 had been reduced.[5] In 1933 the budget for the Indiana State Board of Health was slashed by $75,000, and its venereal disease and infant and maternal welfare divisions were eliminated. The state board's *Monthly Bulletin* justified the action on the grounds that it would place responsibility where it properly belonged—in the home community.[6]

Compounded by an American high-tariff policy, a European financial crisis, and other factors, the Great Depression brought the country close to complete economic collapse by the time Franklin D. Roosevelt assumed the presidency in March 1933. Although elected on a platform that included strict economy and reduction of the national debt, Roosevelt was a pragmatist who recognized the need for action at the federal level. Of the many agencies created during the first stage of the New Deal, from 1933 to 1935, the most significant in terms of public health were the Federal Emergency Relief Administration (FERA), the Works Progress Administration (WPA), and the Public Works Administration (PWA). In 1934 the FERA allocated $1 million to the Public Health Service for use in rural areas. In addition, all three agencies began providing nursing services and other public health services to state and municipal health departments. One of the major accomplishments of the FERA was a "Health Inventory," which consisted of a study of some 850,000 families in various cities, towns, and rural areas. Other federal funds were used to build thousands of privies and to attack malaria through extensive drainage programs. More important in the long run, the WPA and the PWA—the latter somewhat slowly at first, under the watchful eye of Harold L. Ickes—began building health centers, hospitals, laboratories, and municipal water and sewer systems.

By 1935, continuing high unemployment and the rise of extremism—in the persons of Father Charles E. Coughlin, Upton Sinclair, Dr. Francis E. Townsend, and Huey P. Long—pushed Roosevelt further to the left and led to the Second New Deal. Meanwhile, a nonpartisan Committee on Economic Security had drawn up a Social Security Bill, which was introduced into Congress in January 1935. With only minor amendments, this bill became the Social Security Act of 1935, marking the entrance of the federal government on a large scale into the area of social concerns.[7] Aside from establishing an agency for social insurance, the act immediately provided millions of dollars for maternal and child care and for public health services in general. Even more important, it opened the way for increasing federal expenditures on public health.

Of the eleven sections or titles of the act, Title V, which provided grants to states for maternal and child welfare, and Title VI, which appropriated funds for the Public Health Service to assist states and local governments, were of most importance to public health. Slightly over $8 million was appropriated for Title V and another $8 million was assigned to the Public Health Service in its role as administrator for Title VI. The funds were allocated to states based primarily on population but with allowance made for special needs.[8] Along with this money, large sums from other government agencies were made available to states and municipalities for constructing health and sanitary facilities. The immediate result was to give a sharp impetus to the public health movement and to raise the level of public health services throughout the entire country.

State historians of public health almost invariably mention the striking effect of the Social Security Act upon their states. A Texas historian, Howard E. Smith, declared that the "huge expansion of the Health Department" in 1935 was the result of the Social Security Act, the WPA, and the Public Health Service. Harriet S. Pfister, in her history of the Kansas State Board of Health, states that the board began a major expansion in 1935 with the help of the national government. In writing about public health in Georgia, T. F. Abercrombie wrote that health work "was stimulated beyond all previous anticipation." New Mexico, which had lagged behind in public health, in 1935 reorganized its health department in accordance with the standards set by federal agencies in order to gain access to Social Security funds. In so doing, according to historian Myrtle Greenfield, it emerged with a relatively sound state health program.[9]

In its biennial report for 1936–37, the Wisconsin State Board of Health reported that the Social Security Act had enabled it to expand rural health activities, by dividing the state into nine health districts instead of five, and had made it possible to immunize and test children for tuberculosis. Maternal and child care had improved with the assistance of funds from the federal Children's Bureau, and the WPA and PWA had allowed many cities and villages to build water filtration and sewerage plants. The Wisconsin state health board's report also noted that the Public Health Service had recommended that it establish an industrial hygiene unit.[10]

In Missouri federal funds made possible a major expansion in the child hygiene division of its state health department, the establishment of a new Division of Health Education, and, through a WPA grant, a new and improved system for collecting vital statistics. The state board of health reported at the end of 1937 that little progress had been made in establishing full-time health units during the previous fifteen years, but thanks to the Social Security Act, the percentage of Missourians served by full-time health workers had more than doubled in the past year. The following year the state board reported that federal funds had enabled the health department to start a venereal disease program and that all areas of public health were making progress. Significantly, the board asked for a larger state appropriation in order for the health department to take advantage of matching federal grants.

The Missouri state board had touched upon a nationwide problem when it mentioned the shortage of health personnel. Its report noted that Social Security funds had been allocated to the state university and to health centers for training purposes and that public health scholarships had been made available to physicians, engineers, and nurses. The increasing number of both state and federal scholarships for public health training in the 1930s stimulated the development of public health schools. By 1936 some ten universities were offering degrees or certificates in public health, and other institutions were offering courses in the subject. Nonetheless, the number of individuals graduating with public health degrees or certificates was still woefully short of demand. In 1934 a total of only 151 public health degrees and certificates were awarded by American and Canadian universities, and for the academic year 1935–36 the figure dropped to 134. Public health nursing fared a little better in 1936, with a total of 445 degrees and certificates granted. In addition to academic work, a variety of short courses in public health were offered by health centers and other agencies, but these provided only minimal training.[11]

New York State was in an enviable position when federal grants for public health purposes became available. The state had an outstanding health commissioner in Thomas Parran, and, with the election of Fiorello H. La Guardia, New York City gained a mayor highly sensitive to the health and welfare of its people. La Guardia had lost a child and wife to tuberculosis, and he not only chose a first-rate city health commissioner, in the person of Dr. John L. Rice, but backed him to the hilt. Beginning in 1934 WPA funds made possible a comprehensive mosquito-eradication program in and around the city, and the following year the city health department, with a staff of 91 WPA employees, began extensive field studies on air pollution. Aided by Federal Emergency Relief Administration (FERA) and WPA grants, the city's Bureau of School Hygiene extended its dental program to include all children from kindergarten to third grade, and with the help of the WPA, physicians were employed to examine those children about to enter school whose parents could not afford private physicians.[12]

Roosevelt's plans to create jobs through construction proved of immense benefit to the New York City Health Department. By the end of 1935 PWA and WPA funds enabled the department to move into its first permanent headquarters (the building it still occupies on Foley Square) and to begin construction on a new health center in the Bronx and the eight-story Willard H. Park Biological Laboratory. By 1937 nine new health center buildings had been completed or were under construction with the help of federal funds. The city's department of hospitals, under the direction of another outstanding commissioner, Dr. Sigismund S. Goldwater, also took full advantage of all available grants. Using PWA funds, by 1935 eleven hospital buildings were under construction, and authorization had been obtained to replace the chronic disease hospital on Welfare Island.

In this same year federal money enabled the New York City Health Department to start indexing and rebinding the statistical information in the Bureau of Records covering the years from 1847 to 1910 to make them conform with the system introduced in 1910. The extent of federal support can be gathered from the health department's budget for 1937. The city appropriated $4,725,818 for the year; in addition, the WPA spent $4,771,454 for projects under the department's direction, and another $109,145 came from the Public Health Service and the Children's Bureau. On top of these figures, the federal government provided $3,500,000 in loans and grants for the construction of health centers and other buildings.

Federal funds for the New York City Health Department peaked in 1938, but it received almost $2 million from the WPA between July 1, 1939, and June 30, 1940, and over a quarter of a million from the Public Health Service. Throughout the country federal grants were a major factor in promoting public health nursing. The Bureau of Nursing in New York City had 1,019 employees in 1937, 188 of whom were supported by federal agencies. In 1938 the number of employees increased to 1,582, of whom 698 were paid from federal grants.[13]

The multiplication of government agencies during the New Deal intensified the perennial problem of duplication of services. Recognizing this, shortly after the passage of the Social Security Act President Roosevelt created the Interdepartmental Committee to Coordinate Health and Welfare Activities. Partly in response to its recommendations, the Reorganization Act of 1939 sought to consolidate federal health, education, and welfare services into one federal agency. In consequence, the Public Health Service, which had been under the Treasury Department; the Food and Drug Administration, which had been under the Agriculture Department; and the Children's Bureau, which had been under the Department of Labor, were all transferred to the newly created Federal Security Agency. Although a step in the right direction, various public health activities were still carried on by other federal departments: the Bureau of the Census was occupied with compiling vital statistics; the Department of the Interior was responsible for the health of American Indians and sanitation and health services in the national parks; the Department of Agriculture was concerned with sanitary matters relating to dairy and meat products; and the Veterans Bureau and the armed services provided health services for literally millions of Americans.[14]

Private philanthropy, which had contributed so much to public health in the early years of the century, continued to give strong support. Illustrative of foundation support was a five-year Rockefeller grant in 1932 that opened the way to a collaborative program between the Johns Hopkins School of Public Health and the city of Baltimore. A metropolitan area with a population of about 60,000 surrounded the school and was established as the Eastern Health District. Faculty members, students, and city employees all worked together to provide clinical and public health services to the district, ranging from prenatal care to mental health care. Aside from providing the benefits to the residents, the district program served as a training and research area for health professions.[15]

Other foundations concentrated on rural and small town areas. Michigan had lagged in the development of county health units, and in the late 1920s the Children's Fund of Michigan, established by James Couzens, began assisting in the formation of district health departments in the northern section of the state. In 1931 the W. K. Kellogg Foundation decided to conduct a similar program in some of the state's southwestern counties. By 1935 it had established model health departments in five of them, and eventually its help was extended to a total of seven counties. The foundation also sponsored the first Rural Health Conservation Contest in Michigan in 1934. Due to the efforts of these two philanthropic organizations and extensive help from the federal government, by 1941 some 63 of Michigan's 83 counties had full-time health departments.[16]

By 1940 the Depression was receding into the past, and the threat presented by Hitler and Mussolini was turning American attention toward Europe. War preparations began absorbing larger shares of the national budget, and health departments were feeling the pinch as federal funding gradually diminished. Yet the first seven years of the Roosevelt administration had witnessed remarkable advances in public health. There was scarcely a city, town, village, or rural area that had not benefited from the New Deal programs. The drying up of federal money ended many health programs, but the residual effects were enormous. In addition to the many health centers, hospitals, laboratories, and administrative buildings that had resulted from the tremendous construction program, state and local health departments had expanded, and the number of permanent health units had literally multiplied. Of equal importance, advances in medicine during these years encouraged local officials to increase expenditures for public health. Bear in mind, however, that these remarkable improvements were relative and that many still remained for the future.

Over and above the leadership and concern for human welfare demonstrated by the federal government and the relatively enormous sums made available to state and local governments, the Depression years fostered a spirit of idealism, which permeated all of American society. Whether it was this factor or the exigencies of the Depression, public health departments throughout the country were able to recruit personnel of remarkably high caliber. It is true that economic conditions during the Depression were not conducive to private medical practice, thus encouraging young health professionals to move into public health; but it is also true that the sense of crisis stimulated idealistic young physicians, nurses, and others to work for the common good. Unfortunately, the remarkable advances in medicine and the improvement in the economic and social position of physicians in the post–World War II years has tended to draw many of the best and brightest young health professionals into research and private practice.

The 1930s not only saw a rapid development of public health institutions but also witnessed drastic changes in the nature of public health. In the early years of the decade the fight against the traditional communicable diseases was still continuing. Red placards on outside doors indicating the presence of diphtheria or scarlet fever were still not uncommon, and occasional outbreaks of smallpox, typhoid, and other disorders served as reminders of the need for diligence in applying preventive measures. Yet the battle against these disorders had essentially been won, and what remained was a mopping-up operation. Hence public health sought other fields to conquer.

During the first thirty years of the twentieth century, a great deal of progress had been made in the fight against tuberculosis, the Great White Plague. Educational campaigns, the removal of active cases to sanatoriums, and the rising standard of living all played a part in its decline, but the increasing use of pasteurized milk and the Agriculture Department's program to eliminate tuberculous dairy cows may have been at least as significant. In 1929 the department declared that 787 counties in thirty-three states had been declared "modified tuberculosis-free areas."[17] Despite all these efforts, the disease was still a ranking cause of death. The 1930s saw an intensification of the program to eliminate tuberculous cows, while at the same time health departments, aided by better and cheaper X-ray film, began conducting large-scale screening drives to identify cases and locate sources of infection. These programs, combined with health education and a rising standard of living, reduced the national tuberculosis death rate from 71.1 in 1930 to 45.9 in 1940.

By the 1930s health officials were also beginning to turn their attention to the two leading causes of death, cardiovascular disorders and cancer. Unfortunately, the public health field is always dependent on existing medical knowledge; thus, as of the 1930s, not a great deal could be done about either of these medical problems. The American Society for the Control of Cancer (presently the American Cancer Society) took the main initiative in creating public awareness of the obvious symptoms of cancer and the need for early detection.[18] Health departments, too, joined in this work, and they occasionally undertook limited screening programs. The only significant development with respect to cancer was the establishment of the National Cancer Institute in 1937. The word "cancer" had always carried a connotation of dread, and this fact may account for the appearance of a federal cancer research agency before the establishment of one for the ranking cause of death, cardiovascular disease. As with cancer, a limited understanding of the causes of cardiovascular disease precluded health departments from taking any significant preventive measures.

As we have seen, the need for an adequate supply of good food has always been recognized by responsible government leaders, and ensuring a good supply was one of the original responsibilities of health officials. Beginning in the mid-nineteenth century, in part because of the enormous rate of infant mortality, officials began concentrating on improving the milk supply. Later the bacteriological revolution demonstrated conclusively that milk was responsible for much of the infant diarrhea of the times and that it was also a major source of tuberculosis, brucelosis, and other diseases. By the 1930s pasteurization and the standardization of hygienic methods for protecting milk and dairy products were enabling major city health departments to turn over much of the administrative responsibility for sanitary regulations to other government agencies.

Improving the quality of milk had been a concern of health agencies almost from their inception, but in the twentieth century this concern was broadened to include a wide range of food and drugs. The first significant step, the Pure Food and Drug Act of 1906, applied not only to the regulation of food processing and handling but also to the health of food handlers. Shortly thereafter, two new developments added a new dimension to the relationship between food and health. First, Casimer Funk, E. V. McCollum, and others, in discovering vitamins (1911–12,) opened up the whole field of nutrition; second, Joseph Goldberger shortly thereafter was able to demonstrate that pellagra, which was scourging the South, was due to some nutritional deficiency. This is not to say that nutritional deficiencies had not been recognized earlier. The role of nutrition in scurvy, for example, had been noted time after time from the sixteenth century onward, but the discovery of vitamins brought the subject into sharper focus.

As early as 1906 the Association for Improving the Condition of the Poor in New York City had provided a nutrition service for the families it was helping. This service was designed to assist them in buying the best food at the lowest cost. Once the role of vitamins was identified, medical societies and public health agencies began reexamining the role of food in the maintenance of health.[19] In New York City, one of the leaders in public health, the Public Health Committee of the Academy of Medicine, prepared reports on "The Nutritive Significance of Food" in 1914 and distributed them to civic organizations. The following year the city health department opened a cafeteria for its employees in which the menu showed the nutritive value of the various food items. Subsequently the department published an official bulletin giving a sound weekly diet for a family of four.[20]

In the South Goldberger and the Public Health Service began a major campaign in 1921 to eliminate pellagra by changing the diet of poor southerners. Food habits are difficult to change, however, and southern governmental officials resented the implication that their people were poorly fed; hence progress was slow. Municipal and state health departments in other sections of the nation also began taking tentative steps in the direction of nutritional education, but it was not until the Depression years of the 1930s that much was accomplished. By this time the science of nutrition was well developed, and the better health departments began consulting with nutritionists. In a few instances nutritionists were employed on a full-time basis. The intermingling of government and private efforts in public health is demonstrated again in connection with nutrition. Many of the early food demonstration projects in the 1930s were supported by the Red Cross and other private philanthropic groups. The next impetus to the movement for better nutrition was supplied by the need to mobilize food and human resources during World War II.

Progress was also made in combating venereal disease. The history of venereal disease in the twentieth century is marked by clearly defined periods. The first occurred early in the century, when the conspiracy of silence about it was first broken by Dr. Prince A. Morrow and his associates in New York. They at least forced medical societies and public health professionals to consider the subject. The second arose from the mobilization of millions of young men during World War I. The resulting federal action to minimize infection among the troops stimulated municipal and state health authorities to open clinics, offer laboratory diagnostic services to physicians, and to begin studying the extent of the disorders. The gradual elimination of federal grants after the war led to closing most of the clinics, and by 1930 the veil of silence had once again descended, as mentioned in the last chapter. Reluctant to move into a sensitive area, public health officials contented themselves with performing laboratory diagnostic services.

The failure to deal with the venereal diseases was not for their lack of significance. Although K. S. F. Crede discovered in 1884 that the application of a 2 percent solution of silver nitrate to the eyes of newborn babies could prevent blindness caused by gonococcal infection, it was well into the twentieth century before its use became general in America. A survey of schools for the blind in 1907 showed that 28.2 percent of their residents were blind as a result of gonorrheal infections. Syphilis, too, was a costly disease from every standpoint. In 1920 it was estimated to be responsible for 14 percent of male patients admitted to mental hospitals for the first time.[21] These two disorders were responsible for a wide range of medical problems and were exceedingly costly to society. From a medical standpoint the chief difficulty in controlling them was the lack of an effective form of therapy until the advent of sulfa in 1937 and penicillin in the 1940s. For public health officials the main deterrents were society's veil of secrecy and the refusal of physicians to report their cases.

As Prince A. Morrow earlier had insisted on bringing venereal disease to public attention, in the 1930s Dr. Thomas Parran took the initiative in bringing the subject out into the open. The author recalls Dr. Parran telling him of the first occasion when, as health commissioner of New York State, he gave a radio talk on the subject. The announcer warned that if one person telephoned in to protest, Parran would be cut off the air. Fortunately, no calls were received. Later Parran, as surgeon general of the Public Health Service, had to insist, when he was quoted by the national radio networks or news services, that the word "syphilis" be used instead of a euphemism.[22]

Parran's appointment as surgeon general coincided with the passage of the Social Security Act, which, among its many provisions, established grants-in-aid to states for venereal disease control. Determined to promote a national drive against venereal disease, in December 1936 Parran called a National Conference on Venereal Work. Almost one thousand health professionals and other concerned individuals attended. With their support, and by arousing public interest, Parran was able to pressure Congress into enacting a National Venereal Disease Control Act in 1938. The act provided $3 million in matching grants to states for the first year, and successively increased the amounts for the next two years. Parran also pushed for additional research funds.[23] The major fruits of his work, however, were not harvested until the post–World War II years.

The twentieth century also saw the rise and growth of the mental health movement. This movement had its origins in the early part of the century when individuals and charitable groups began investigating the possibility of preventing mental illness. In 1909 the National Committee for Mental Hygiene was established for this purpose. The following year the New York Academy of Medicine cooperated with the Committee on Mental Hygiene of the State Charities Aid Foundation in holding what was called the "First Public Meeting in the Campaign for the Prevention of Insanity."[24] While a few able individuals and some of the better medical societies recognized that mental health belonged under the rubric of public health, there was little general interest in the subject. The public reaction to battle exhaustion, or shell shock as it was called during World War I, illustrates the prevailing view of mental illness. The *Monthly Bulletin* of the Indiana State Board of Health in 1918 carried an article claiming that shell shock occurred only in those subject to hysteria. It further explained that the "hysterical person is one burdened with a defective organization, which is an expression of biological inferiority." It concluded that human material like this—"unserviceable, contaminating and demoralizing"—should be excluded from the army.[25]

Representing the more rational line of thought on mental illness, Dr. Harry H. Moore in 1920 attributed about 14 percent of mental illness in America to syphilis and another 4 percent to alcoholism and suggested that heredity accounted for much of the rest. Recognizing the social causes of mental illness, he added that immigration, unemployment, congested populations, and child labor appeared to have an influence on the incidence of mental disease. Two years later Dr. Charles I. Lambert of Columbia University urged that the taboos surrounding mental illness be dropped and called for more intensive research on the subject. In 1929 Dr. Haven Emerson, in addressing a conference of social workers in California, stressed the social implications of mental illness, declaring that "public effort has not yet reached the stage where recognition is given to the social problems as a whole."[26]

Social workers were among the first to espouse the environment as a major factor in mental illness, and by the 1920s a number of private and government social agencies began concentrating on delinquent and disturbed children. Family clinics began employing psychiatrists, psychologists, and psychiatric social workers to counsel families in need of help. The onset of the Depression ended this happy collaboration, when psychiatrists, as physicians, sought to control the field and to relegate psychologists and paramedicals to a minor role, temporarily setting back the mental hygiene movement. Another clash developed in the 1930s between psychiatrists, who generally functioned on a one-to-one basis, and epidemiologists, who were attempting to study mental health on a community basis.[27] Health departments, always sensitive to public taboos and usually short of funds, were hesitant to take action until foundations and the federal government became involved. The Social Security Act marked the real beginning of federal support for mental hygiene programs. The majority of these programs were aimed at children, on the assumption that childhood was the best point at which to prevent mental illness. By 1940 child health divisions were beginning to employ the team techniques that had characterized the social work agencies of the 1920s. The rejection of hundreds of thousands of draftees for psychiatric reasons during World War II, combined with heavy federal involvement in community mental health programs, gave a major impetus to the movement in the postwar years.

As had been the case during the previous war, the outbreak of hostilities in 1941 disrupted all normal civilian activities. Its effect on public health was mixed, although on the whole the nation's health improved. The immediate result of the disruption was to add heavy burdens to health departments while at the same time causing them to lose personnel to wartime agencies. Medical and public health research became restricted largely to matters of direct concern to the war emergency, and basic research suffered. The extra demands for food arising from the mobilization of troops and the needs of our allies forced an easing of sanitary regulations with respect to food. The boom in restaurants and food-processing plants in cities and towns where troops and war workers were concentrated came at a time when the staffs of many local health departments were decimated, with the result that sanitary laws often were flagrantly violated.

The armed forces' recruitment of physicians, nurses, and other health professionals intensified the shortage of trained personnel, forcing health agencies to turn to volunteers. To make matters worse, as already noted, the loss of personnel came at a time when military camps and wartime industries were bringing thousands of workers and their families into new areas. The 1942 biennial report of the Missouri State Board of Health illustrated a familiar complaint. The board protested that its budget had not been increased despite greater responsibilities arising from the influx of troops. Federal grants were coming into the state, the board continued, but many required matching funds, and these had not been forthcoming.[28]

On the other hand, the war virtually ended unemployment and brought a general rise in the standard of living, while rationing and price controls ensured that the average American was probably better fed during the war than had been the case in the prewar years. No section of the United States benefited more than the South. The huge influx of troops into army camps located in southern rural areas infused large amounts of cash and created thousands of jobs and opportunities for merchants and businessmen. Fearful of the South's endemic malaria, the armed services, in conjunction with the Public Health Service, began extensive anti-malarial programs. At the same time, efforts to prevent venereal disease among the troops required extensive screening and case finding among the civilian population. Since military personnel from army bases flooded into adjacent cities and towns, the Public Health Service out of necessity began inspecting restaurants, food processors, and general sanitary facilities.

The net result was a general rise in the southern standard of living and much-improved health conditions. For the first time in history malaria was virtually eliminated from the southern states. Aside from the benefits of the antimalarial programs, a higher standard of living meant better homes with window screens for rural southerners. It also meant a more diversified diet and better food.

Moreover, across America the work of the Public Health Service and other government agencies improved the quality of local health units and stimulated the creation of new ones. It is true that hundreds of thousands of families were dislocated and that consumer goods and housing were in short supply, but unemployment and abject poverty virtually disappeared from America. It is ironic that spending for war was able to bring greater economic prosperity than the New Deal had. The 1980s have once again demonstrated that vast military expenditures can successfully bring temporary prosperity.

World War II gave the Public Health Service a major role in American health affairs. In 1941 the Division of Domestic Quarantine, renamed the States Relations Division, was given an appropriation of $4,470,000 to assist state and local health departments, $2,045,560 for general health and sanitation, $2,142,860 for malaria control, and another $250,000 for industrial hygiene. As the war dragged on, additional sums were appropriated. The Public Health Service was also given responsibility for medical and sanitary support for the Coast Guard and other branches of the armed forces. When, in response to war hysteria, some 110,000 Japanese-Americans were uprooted and interned for the duration of the war, their health care was also handed over to the Public Health Service. Another major contribution of the PHS was to institute a training program for nurses. As the armed forces increased their demand for nurses, Congress responded in June 1943 by enacting the United States Nurse Corps bill, which made it possible for the Public Health Service to recruit and train some 90,000 nurses in the next two years.[29]

While the war delayed much of basic research, it did speed up the application of existing medical knowledge. Through the National Institute of Health and its other laboratories, the Public Health Service produced an improved vaccine for yellow fever, developed an effective one against typhus, and carried on other wartime activities. In June 1941 President Roosevelt established the Office of Scientific Research to mobilize scientists on behalf of the war effort. One of its subdivisions, the Committee on Medical Research, deserves credit for a number of major medical advances. By the end of the war it was engaged in a wide range of medical projects, all of which were turned over to the Public Health Service with the coming of peace.

Among the many other wartime developments in the area of public health were the production of improved sulfa drugs on a large scale, the development and mass production of penicillin (a process that normally might have taken many years), and improved techniques for the use of blood plasma and whole blood. The shortage of quinine was compensated for by the development of synthetics such as atabrin and other derivatives. Desperately searching for an effective insecticide to protect troops from diseases carried by insect vectors, the army tested DDT and was able to produce large quantities of it by 1944. It proved immensely effective in antimalarial campaigns and is credited with preventing major outbreaks of typhus among soldiers and civilians during military activities in North Africa and Italy. Granting its potential for abuse and its danger to the environment, DDT was responsible for saving thousands of lives and preventing an immense amount of sickness during World War II.

As hundreds of thousands of men were called into military service, leaving many of their families with only limited resources, some form of state provision for medical care became necessary. In March 1943 the Emergency Maternity and Infant Care Act (EMIC) was enacted. It applied to servicemen in the lowest four pay grades and provided medical, hospital, and nursing care for their wives and infants during the first year of the infant's life. This program, one of the largest instituted by the federal government to that date, was administered by the Children's Bureau.

Surgery, as might be assumed, benefited from the wartime lessons learned in dealing with large numbers of seriously wounded men. World War I had provided the first impetus to the development of plastic surgery, but—partly as a result of the general advance in all biological sciences—major strides were made in this area and in other areas of surgery during World War II. The same held true for the treatment of shock, hemorrhage, and a wide range of injury-related medical problems. Developments in psychiatry meant that battle fatigue was dealt with more rationally, and the epidemiology of mental health began to come into its own. The effect of all these developments was that the public became convinced that medicine was the queen of sciences and its expectations were raised beyond what realistically could be accomplished. Fortunately, the prestige of medicine carried over into the area of public health. In consequence, whereas the post–World War I years had seen a letdown in public health activities, the reverse was true after World War II.

NOTES

1. United States Bureau of the Census, *Historical Statistics of the United States, Colonial Times to the Present* (Washington, D.C., 1960), 25.

2. L. L. Lumsden, "Extent of Rural Health Service in the United States, 1925–30," *Public Health Reports*, part 1, 45 (1930):1075; part 2, 48 (1933):1234.

3. Rosemary Stevens, *American Medicine and the Public Interest* (New Haven, Conn., 1971), 170–71, 183.

4. Lucie R. Bridgforth, "The Politics of Public Health in Mississippi: Felix J. Underwood and the Mississippi State Board of Health, 1924–1958," TS, p. 16.

5. See the sixteenth to the nineteenth biennial reports of the State Board of Health of the State of Kansas, 1932–38.

6. "The Board of Health," *Monthly Bulletin,* Indiana State Board of Health, 36 (1933):54–56.

7. For a good brief account of the New Deal see Arthur S. Link and William B. Catton, *American Epoch: A History of the United States Since the 1890s,* 3d ed. (New York, 1967), chapters 18–20.

8. Wilson G. Smillie, *Public Health Administration in the United States* (New York, 1946), 503–7.

9. Howard E. Smith, *A History of Public Health in Texas* (Austin, 1974), 15; Harriet S. Pfister, *Kansas State Board of Health* (Lawrence, 1955), 65; T. F. Abercrombie, *A History of Public Health in Georgia, 1733–1950* (n.p., n.d.), 137; Myrtle Greenfield, *A History of Public Health in New Mexico* (Albuquerque, 1962), 33–34.

10. *Thirty-seventh Report of the State Board of Health of Wisconsin for the Statistical Biennium Ending June 30, 1938* (Madison, 1938), 1–2.

11. *Annual Report of the State Board of Health of Missouri . . . for 1937* (Jefferson City, n.d.), 7–11; *Annual Report for . . . 1938,* 7, 10; "Public Health Degrees and Certificates Granted in 1936," *American Journal of Public Health* 27 (1937):1267–72.

12. For this and subsequent material see John Duffy, *A History of Public Health in New York City, 1866–1966* (New York, 1974), chapter 14.

13. Ibid., 353–54, 361.

14. Smillie, *Public Health Administration in the United States,* 420–22, 511; Bess Furman, *A Profile of the United States Public Health Service, 1798–1948* (Washington, D.C., n.d.), 409–10.

15. Elizabeth Fee, *Disease and Discovery: A History of the Johns Hopkins School of Hygiene and Public Health, 1916–1939* (Baltimore, 1987), 186ff.

16. The W. K. Kellogg Foundation, *The First Twenty-five Years: The Story of a Foundation* (Battle Creek, Mich., n.d.), 40–41; "News from the Field, Michigan Appraisals," *American Journal of Public Health* 25 (1935):633, 684–85; 31 (1941):291.

17. "Notes from the Field," *American Journal of Public Health* 19 (1929):1284.

18. For an excellent history of the public reaction to cancer see James T. Patterson, *The Dread Disease: Cancer and Modern American Culture* (Cambridge, Mass., 1987).

19. The New York Association for Improving the Condition of the Poor . . . , *Eightieth Annual Report, 1923* (New York, 1923), 12.

20. New York Academy of Medicine, Summary of the Activities of the Public Health, Hospital and Budget Committee . . . 1914, New York Academy of Medicine MS, p. 5; *New York Times,* May 11, 1915, May 7, 1916.

21. George Rosen, *Preventive Medicine in the United States, 1900–1975: Trends and Interpretations* (New York, 1975), 38; Harry H. Moore, *Public Health in the United States* (New York, 1923), 114.

22. John Duffy, conversation with Dean Thomas Parran, Graduate School of Public Health, University of Pittsburgh, April 3, 1966; Furman, *Profile of the United States Public Health Service,* 398–99.

23. Furman, *Profile of the United States Public Health Service,* 399–400.

24. New York Academy of Medicine, Minutes of the Section on Public Health, December 23, 1910, New York Academy of Medicine MS, p. 179.

25. Editorial, "Shell Shock and Hysteria," *Monthly Bulletin,* Indiana State Board of Health, 21 (1918):141.

26. Moore, *Public Health in the United States,* 114; *New York Times,* December 27, 1922; Haven Emerson, "Public Health and Mental Hygiene," *Hospital Social Service* 19 (1929):385, from the *Collected Works of Haven Emerson, M.D.* (New York City, 1962), vol. 2, no. 63.

27. For a good account of this clash see John C. Burnham, "The Struggle between Physicians and Paramedical Personnel in American Psychiatry, 1917–1941," *J. Hist. Med & All. Sci.* 29 (1974):93–106.

28. *Biennial Report of the State Board of Health of Missouri for the Calendar Years 1941–42* (n.p., n.d.), 9–10.

29. Furman, *Profile of the United States Public Health Service,* chapter 17.

18

The Postwar Years

The end of World War II brought a sense of exhilaration to Americans. First came tremendous relief at the cessation of hostilities and a feeling of exultation at the downfall of Hitler, the epitome of evil. Over and above this, the enormous output of war materials, the appearance of "miracle drugs," the major advances in medical and surgical techniques, and the successes in the applied sciences that made possible the atomic bomb and other breakthroughs seemed convincing evidence that science and technology could solve all problems. By 1940 bacteriology had opened the way to controlling the traditional killer diseases, and surely the new science, if given enough support, could solve the riddle of such major causes of death as heart disease and cancer. Penicillin seemed on its way to eliminating venereal disease in 1946, and apparently all that was required to handle other medical problems was adequate funds. In consequence, the federal government and private foundations began pouring money into medical research on an unprecedented scale.

Public health professionals could scarcely remain untouched by the prevailing enthusiasm for science. Their fight for status in the late nineteenth and early twentieth centuries had been achieved in part by separating themselves from the world of politics and emphasizing their role as specialists in the health sciences. The failure of some of the principal reformers in the American Public Health Association and their allies to win the battle for government health insurance—a fight in which it was arrayed against the American Medical Association in the World War I period, as we have seen—further convinced most public health professionals to avoid medical and political controversies. By 1940, however, changing conditions were forcing a redefinition of the role of public health professionals. Many of the newer medical problems, such as mental health and alcoholism, could not be prevented by immunizing the public through some new vaccine or by providing laboratory diagnostic services, and public health found itself being pushed into the area of social and behavioral concerns.

In the postwar years, the white-coated medical researcher came to symbolize all that was good and noble in the brave new world of science, and the vast amounts of money awarded for research in the health sciences were devoted primarily to basic research and medical technology. The predominant emphasis in medical training had always been on curative medicine, and in the postwar years research into preventive medicine received relatively short shrift. Prevention, as Arthur J. Viseltear has observed, was considered irrelevant by medical schools, and public health schools, too, tended to follow the Hopkins tradition of emphasizing basic research. Only a few individuals urged that society could gain far more from investing part of its resources in efforts to achieve a healthier environment and in attempting to understand the nature and causes of self-imposed risks than by devoting attention almost exclusively to therapeutic care and basic research. Relatively few studies were made on the cost-effectiveness of such topics as the value of low-fat diets, multiphasic screening, and annual physical examinations.[1]

While public health professionals generally preferred the relatively safe world of science and technology to the rough-and-tumble one of politics, the new community health problems were not encompassed by traditional biomedical concepts. Alcoholism, drug addiction, smoking, radiation, environmental hazards, and the problems of aging scarcely fitted the normal categories. And even heart disease and cancer were not specific disorders in themselves but rather classes of disease. Whereas maternal and child care had originally involved only the prevention of infection and a concern with physiological nutrition, the mental health movement introduced the issue of personality development. The concept of mental illness, an amorphous term at best, made the whole area of human emotions a legitimate sphere for public health. The virtual elimination of the major communicable diseases in the twentieth century had been relatively simple and cheap; solutions to the new public health problems, however, involved social reform and large public expenditures.

The contents of the *American Journal of Public Health* clearly show the changes in public health in the years from 1920 to 1960. In the 1920s and 1930s most articles dealt with topics such as communicable diseases, sanitation, public health administration, health education, and vital statistics. The era of social reform in the 1930s led to papers on medical care, but the general pattern remained much the same until the end of World War II. The postwar years saw a number of papers on the use and dangers of DDT and the value of fluoride in connection with dental caries. As might be expected, the attempt to establish some form of national health insurance during the Truman administration led to more articles on medical care. Other prominent issues discussed were food and nutrition and housing. Chronic diseases, problems of aging, and mental health, however, received scant attention.[2] The failure of public health departments to take the initiative with respect to the new health problems in the face of a growing public demand for action often led to the creation of separate government agencies.

The reluctance of many health officers to become involved in political issues is readily understandable. They were—and are—government employees, subject to political attacks, and their budgets and salaries are dependent upon political whims. Espousing a new or unpopular cause can have a disastrous impact on an entire health department and even cause the loss of the health officer's position. Moreover, for the past seventy years public health has been viewed with considerable suspicion by local physicians and medical societies, ever on the alert for any encroachment by health departments upon private medical practice. These factors, along with the rising political influence of the AMA and the tendency of public health professionals to claim the mantle of science, meant that by the 1950s the field of public health began finding itself at a crossroads. Its success in solving many former problems had only served to bring newer ones into sharper focus. Moreover, changes in society itself were creating a host of new challenges to community health. The growing awareness that all was not well with public health was reflected in the major theme of the annual APHA meeting in 1957: "Is public health in tune with the times?"

The one controversial issue in which public health professionals did become involved was that of government-supported health insurance. After the failure of the movement in 1918–19, the subject virtually disappeared from sight. A few individuals in the 1920s, such as Michael Davis, an authority on hospitals and health administration, and C.-E. A. Winslow of Yale, advocated comprehensive medical care programs and health insurance, but they had little support. In 1929 Baylor University Hospital adopted a hospital insurance plan. Its success led other hospitals to follow suit, and the program, despite strong opposition from the AMA, which equated it with socialized medicine, became the model for the present-day Blue Cross. In the 1930s insurance companies quickly recognized the opportunities that hospital insurance promised and began offering it. Voluntary insurance programs developed slowly in the 1930s and then began a rapid expansion during World War II.

In its final report in 1932, the Committee on the Costs of Medical Care recommended group medical practice and some form of health insurance, although it left open the question of how health insurance should be financed. Nonetheless, the AMA accused the committee of advocating compulsory health insurance, declaring that the real issue was "Americanism versus sovietism for the American people."[3] The Social Security Act of 1935 marked the real beginning of federal involvement in state and local public health, but the AMA and its allies managed to keep the act's provisions for medical care to a minimum. Nonetheless, support for comprehensive medical care programs was growing, even among the ranks of the AMA. Dr. John Peters of Yale in 1936–37 took the initiative in organizing a group called the Committee of Physicians for the Improvement of Medical Care. Its aim was to stimulate discussion on medical care problems and to show that the AMA's views on health insurance did not represent those of the entire profession.[4]

As public opinion became more sympathetic to some form of legislation on medical care, in 1938 President Roosevelt called a national health conference. Earlier he had appointed an Interdepartmental Committee to Coordinate Health and Welfare Activities, and this committee had appointed a subgroup, the Technical Committee on Medical Care. The technical committee's report, which surveyed the American health care system, was accepted by the interdepartmental committee and submitted to the National Health Conference. The report depicted health conditions among the poor in a grim light and showed that the level of health care was related directly to income. It recommended some type of health insurance program on the grounds that the nation's lower-income groups could never afford proper medical care under the existing system. The AMA promptly denounced the report, asserting that the American people were healthy and that there was no need for government action. The APHA, on the other hand, endorsed the recommendations of the report and resolved to help the government in carrying them out. In doing so, it declared that state governments were the best agencies for carrying out comprehensive medical care programs.[5]

In January 1939 President Roosevelt urged Congress to consider the various recommendations on national health, and the following month Senator Robert F. Wagner of New York introduced a national health bill. It was essentially an amendment to the Social Security Act, broadening its health powers and authorizing the states to provide medical care. The bill allowed the states broad discretion in determining the form of care and which groups should receive it. Although no funds were appropriated since the bill simply provided legislative authority, it was violently attacked. A spokesman for the Catholic Hospital Association was quoted in the *Journal of the American Medical Association* as stating that the bill would destroy the existing medical system and substitute "overpowering structures of huge bureaus, national councils and state organizations founded not on Christian inspiration but upon legal enactment." A *JAMA* editorial declared that the Constitution and the "American way of life are diametrically opposed to regimentation or any form of totalitarianism," and that Americans were not interested in testing "experiments in medical care which have already failed in regimented countries."[6]

Although the leading officers in the APHA supported the bill, Haven Emerson—representing the old guard, which opposed any interference with private medicine—spoke against it. Testifying before Congress, Emerson declared that there was no major shortage of health care in the United States and that public health should best concentrate upon prevention rather than medical care. [7] By this date economic conditions were improving and enthusiasm for reform was on the wane. In addition, Roosevelt was becoming preoccupied with security threats in Europe and the Far East and did not push the issue. In consequence, the bill died in Congress.

Several other bills were introduced during the war years, but they found little public support. As it turns out, the basic issue no longer concerned medical care for those who could not afford it, for this question had been settled: through the Veteran's Administration, the Social Security Act, the Emergency Maternal and Infant Care Act of 1943, and a variety of health care programs, the federal government was already subsidizing medical care for millions of needy Americans. The real issue was whether or not the government should become involved in medical care for those who presumably could pay for private medicine.[8]

In 1945 President Truman took up the cause of national health insurance in a strongly worded message to Congress. He called for the construction of hospital and health facilities, expanded maternal and child health and other programs, and, most significantly, for a national health insurance policy based on an expanded social security system. The Wagner-Murray-Dingell Bill embodying Truman's recommendations was introduced, but it encountered strong opposition from the AMA and the Republican Party. The editor of *JAMA* described the Physician's Forum, one of the organizations supporting the proposal, as "a group of several hundred physicians, most inclined toward communism and [possibly the ultimate insult from a Chicago-based journal] practically all living in New York."[9] This bill, like its predecessors, died in Congress.

In 1949, fresh from his electoral victory, and with a Democratic House and Senate, Truman once again called for national health insurance. The debate was bitter. The cold war had aroused fears of communism to a high pitch, and by labeling the bill socialistic or communistic, the bill's opponents easily carried the day. By 1951 Truman and other advocates of national health insurance realized there was little hope for a comprehensive law and decided to concentrate on securing a limited national health insurance program for the aged. It took fourteen more years of agitation before the law establishing today's Medicare system was enacted in 1965.

The two health areas that presented no threat to private medical practice or the free enterprise system were hospitals and medical research, and in the immediate postwar years Congress took decisive action to promote both of them. The Great Depression was conducive neither to building nor to maintaining hospitals, and the war years accentuated the general dilapidation of the nation's hospital system. President Roosevelt had recognized the need to subsidize the construction of hospitals in rural areas as early as 1940, and near the end of the war he and his public health advisors were contemplating a comprehensive system of medical care that involved rehabilitating the entire hospital system. In January 1945 a bill to promote hospital construction was introduced, and, with strong backing from President Truman, was enacted the following year as the National Hospital Survey and Construction Act, or the Hill-Burton Act.

The basic purpose of this act was to improve the quality and the distribution of hospitals. Rural areas had always been short of hospitals, and the growth of specialization, with its demand for laboratories and operating rooms, accentuated this shortage. The Hill-Burton Act first provided grants to the states to make statewide surveys and draw up plans for comprehensive hospital systems. In requesting federal funds, the states were to establish priorities based on the local areas in greatest need. When a state's plan had been approved, federal funds would be made available to the state's health department or some other agency. This agency would then provide one-third of the construction costs for public hospitals and for voluntary nonprofit hospitals. The sum of $3 million was provided for the surveys, and a total of $375 million was authorized for construction in the first five years. The distribution of federal grants was based on population and per capita income, with the states having the lowest per capita income receiving a higher per capita amount.[10]

Backed by the entire medical industry and enjoying strong popular support, the Hill-Burton Act was steadily broadened in the years succeeding its passage. In addition to general hospitals, almost every type of medical care institution was included within its purview—tuberculosis, chronic disease, and mental hospitals, rehabilitation facilities, and diagnostic and treatment centers. In the 1960s public health centers and other facilities offering medical care were added to the list. One of the earlier amendments had provided grants for research in hospital utilization, and subsequently Hill-Burton funds were made available for assisting in the development of regional and metropolitan plans for hospital services. By 1968 the Hill-Burton Act had channeled approximately $3.2 billion into the nation's hospital system.[11]

The Hill-Burton Act has proved most successful in stimulating the construction of hospitals and health centers in rural areas. The measure was originally conceived as part of a comprehensive medical care program, and in this respect, as Rosemary Stevens has shown, it has failed. The demand for hospitals in the postwar period resulted in a rapid growth of voluntary hospitals, most of which did not require federal assistance and were built in disregard of the state plans set forth under the Hill-Burton Act. In consequence, the haphazard construction of medical facilities resulted in an excessive number of beds in certain areas, shortages in others, and an enormous amount of duplication. Neither the states nor the federal government in the postwar years expressed much interest in making the growing medical care system an effective and efficient one. According to the National Advisory Council of the Public Health Service, in 1961 the amount spent on research in hospital administration and medical care represented less than .2 percent of the estimated $25 billion spent by the medical care industry.[12]

While government health insurance and medical care programs were an anathema to the AMA, that organization was more than happy to join in supporting and encouraging the popular demand for government-subsidized biomedical research. Acting on the advice of its scientists at the end of the war, the federal government decided to concentrate basic research funds at the National Institute of Health. This decision convinced Surgeon General Thomas Parran that there was need for a comparable center for applied research. A successful wartime agency, the office for Malaria Control in War Areas (MCWA), was based in Atlanta, and Parran was largely responsible for transforming it in 1946 into the Communicable Disease Center, now the Center for Disease Control (CDC).[13] The tuberculosis and venereal disease programs of the PHS were transferred to the new agency, and the strong cooperative relationships that the MCWA had maintained with state health departments were continued. The CDC also was authorized to help standardize laboratory techniques and monitor the production of vaccines. Its epidemiological division was strengthened and its staff greatly increased. In 1951 the Epidemiological Intelligence Service was organized to gather information on diseases in the United States and around the world. In addition, the services of its highly trained specialists were made available to any troublespots upon request.[14]

Spurred on by popular enthusiasm for medical science, the National Institute of Health began an enormous expansion. In 1948 the National Heart Institute, the National Institute of Dental Research, and the National Biological Institute were established by Congress. These new agencies were placed under the umbrella of the National Institute of Health, which then officially became the National Institutes of Health (NIH). The following year the National Institute of Mental Health was added to the NIH. By 1969 another seven institutes had been established by Congress. The explosive growth of the NIH can be seen also in the multiplication of its appropriation. Its entire budget in 1948 was $29 million; by 1967 its annual budget had grown to $1.4 billion. More significantly, in 1950 research expenditures by the NIH represented 18 percent of the total national outlay for medical research; by 1960 this figure had climbed to 40 percent.[15]

By the late 1940s the major medical disorders that had plagued the United States throughout nearly all of its history had virtually disappeared. The California State Board of Health, for example, reported only 42 cases and 2 deaths from diphtheria in 1955 compared to 11,000 cases and 700 deaths in 1924. Whooping cough, which had caused 894 deaths from 1930 to 1934, was responsible for only 89 in the years 1950 to 1954.[16] Typhoid, typhus, scarlet fever, and malaria were no longer of any real consequence since occasional cases or minor flareups could be dealt with easily. Tuberculosis, one of the more difficult diseases to combat, remained a problem throughout the country, but the death rate from it had fallen from 113.1 per 100,000 in 1920 to 9.1 in 1955. By this date the disorder was found largely in the poorer sections of major cities and among certain minority groups. In New York City, where as late as 1960 tuberculosis was the eleventh leading cause of death, it was primarily a disease of those over forty-five years of age.[17] In general, those most susceptible to it were American Indians located on reservations. In 1955 tuberculosis was still the leading cause of death among them.[18]

Influenza remained a threat, although the introduction of sulfonamides and antibiotics, by providing effective forms of therapy for pneumonic and other respiratory complications of influenza, had greatly lessened its danger. Following the 1918–19 epidemic, minor outbreaks continued to flare up. A variant form of the disorder became pandemic in 1947, but by this date new therapeutics were available to mitigate its worst effects.

The perennial venereal diseases, against which little progress had been made during the first forty years of the twentieth century, began retreating in the 1940s. The nation's death rate from syphilis was 12 per 100,000 in 1900, rose to a peak of 19.1 in 1917, and then slowly fell to 14.4 in 1940.[19] The problem with these statistics is that advanced syphilis masquerades in many forms; that fact, combined with the tender regard physicians have always had for the sensibilities of their private patients, may have led to misdiagnosis or reluctance to report cases. In any event, no effective form of therapy for gonorrhea or syphilis was available for many years. The long course of treatment with bismuth and arsenicals for syphilis was both costly and painful, and few patients were willing to complete it. In 1939 three physicians writing in the *Archives of Dermatology and Syphilology* agreed that arsphenamine, an arsenical, was the most effective treatment, but added that its side effects and the difficulty of administering it made it impracticable for use by the general practitioner.[20]

The first major breakthrough came with the discovery in 1937 that sulfanilamide was 90 percent effective in curing uncomplicated gonorrhea. The second one was the discovery by Dr. John F. Mahoney of the Public Health Service in 1943 that penicillin was better than 90 percent effective against syphilis. Subsequently it was determined that penicillin was equally valuable in treating gonorrhea. These two "miracle" drugs, or variations of them, were used on a large scale beginning in 1945. With federal, state, and municipal collaboration, a nationwide system of rapid treatment centers was quickly established. They were so successful that the death rate from syphilis dropped to 5 per 100,000 in 1950 and to about 2.5 by 1955.[21]

By this date health officials were confident that the venereal disease problem had been solved. It was assumed generally that state and local officials, with only token help from the federal government, could reduce the incidence of syphilis and gonorrhea to an absolute minimum. Two factors dashed these bright hopes. In the first place, the indiscriminate use of sulfa drugs and antibiotics, penicillin in particular, inevitably led to resistant strains of gonorrhea and syphilis. The second factor was the sexual revolution, which was made possible in large part by the success of the new drugs in removing the fear of venereal disease and by the introduction of effective birth control methods. A third factor may have been the general permissiveness that characterized American society in the affluent postwar years.

Beginning in 1957 the incidence of venereal disease throughout the entire country began to rise. A task force on syphilis appointed by the Surgeon General in 1961 found that the number of reported cases had tripled since 1957. Probably reflecting changes in sexual mores, between 1956 and 1960 the number of cases of syphilis among the 15-to-19-year-old age group increased by 136 percent and gonorrhea by 21 percent.[22] The 1960s saw the number of cases increase at a startling rate. The annual reports of the San Francisco Department of Health show that in 1956–57 it diagnosed and treated 1,818 cases of venereal disease; in 1960–61 the figure increased to 3,869; and in 1970–71 it climbed to 17,928.[23] The succeeding years were to see the venereal disease problem become even more acute with the appearance of resistant strains of old infections and the introduction of new ones.

One of the greatest medical successes of the nineteenth century was the virtual conquest of poliomyelitis. Although occasional cases and scattered epidemics were recorded in the eighteenth and nineteenth centuries, the disease was not recognized as a threat until the early twentieth century. The earliest outbreak in the United States was noted by Dr. George Colmer, a country practitioner in Louisiana. In an article entitled "Paralysis in Teething Children," published in 1843, he described a case he had treated, and reported hearing of eight or ten others in the neighborhood.[24] By the end of the century more references to individual cases and minor epidemics could be found in the medical journals. The first significant epidemic in New York City, which occurred in 1907, was not even noticed by the city health department until welfare officials the following year reported that many individuals with paralytic disorders were asking for help. The health department then traced some 800 cases and discovered there had been an epidemic the previous year. On the basis of the known cases, the total number of polio victims was estimated at about 2,000.[25]

As the more common communicable diseases were brought under control and the environment made safer from bacterial disorders, the incidence of polio began rising. As with some of the earlier diseases, it could prove fatal or else might leave its victims horribly disabled. By the late 1940s it had become the most feared disease in America. Fortunately, the development of virology in the 1930s opened the way to its control. The most prominent early victim of polio was Franklin D. Roosevelt, and his immense personal influence was largely responsible for the formation and success of the National Polio Foundation. This foundation collected large sums of money, a good part of which was poured into research. Meanwhile, scientists were moving against the disease on many fronts, seeking to understand its cause and its means of spreading and to devise a vaccine. Suffice to say, Dr. Jonas Salk of the University of Pittsburgh, capitalizing on the work of John F. Enders and his associates and the findings of dozens of other researchers over the previous years, was the first to develop an effective vaccine.

In the spring of 1954 a large-scale trial of the vaccine was made with several hundred thousand children in eleven states. The results were successful, although further testing was delayed temporarily when cases of polio appeared among those vaccinated. An investigation soon revealed that the vaccine produced by one laboratory had been defective. Testing was then continued on an even wider scale, and by 1960 the Salk vaccine was coming into general use. A number of investigators had been convinced from the beginning that a vaccine made from attenuated rather than inactivated poliovirus would be more effective in producing immunity and, since it could be taken orally, more acceptable to the public. Of the three men working on oral vaccines, Dr. Albert B. Sabin was most successful, and after thorough testing in 1961 his oral vaccine, made of attenuated virus, was licensed by the Public Health Service.[26]

The 1960s saw massive drives to immunize the entire population using the oral vaccine. Although one or two minor problems developed, the program proved immensely successful, virtually banishing paralytic polio from the advanced Western countries. In 1974 only seven cases were reported for the entire United States.[27] Public memory, unfortunately, was short, and, as the polio epidemics receded into the past, more and more parents neglected to have their children vaccinated. The situation calls to mind the case of smallpox at the beginning of the nineteenth century, when the public's ready acceptance of vaccination sharply reduced the incidence of the disease. A generation later, as vaccination was neglected, smallpox again became epidemic and was not controlled until the twentieth century. In recent years health departments are finding it necessary to reeducate the public on the need for polio vaccination.

The elimination of the more fatal communicable diseases also threw the more common childhood diseases into sharper focus. For centuries measles had been accepted as a normal occurrence of childhood, seldom even requiring the services of a physician. In a very small percentage of cases, however, serious complications could arise. For example, in 1963 there were an estimated 4 million cases of measles, 4,000 cases of measles encephalitis, and 400 measles deaths recorded. Efforts to produce a vaccine against measles began soon after the introduction of smallpox inoculation in the early eighteenth century, but it required the emergence of virology in the 1930s before any real headway was possible. Almost simultaneously with the development of an attenuated polio virus, the work of J. F. Enders, S. L. Katz, M. J. Milanovic, and others resulted in the discovery of an effective measles vaccine.

In 1963 two vaccines were licensed, and massive drives to immunize all children were started. Within five years the annual number of cases had dropped from about 4 million in 1963 to only 22,231 in 1968. By this date, health leaders, forgetting the lessons of the past, were confidently predicting the elimination of measles. Unfortunately for their predictions, once popular enthusiasm for the new preventive had waned, the number of measles cases began to rise. In 1970, 47,363 cases were reported, and the following year the total had reached about 75,000. Complete success is rarely achieved in public health, and to reach even a high level requires the utmost vigilance.[28]

The significance of heart disease, cancer, and chronic complaints was starting to be recognized by the late 1930s, but public health officials were hesitant to move into what was considered the domain of private medicine. A few major health departments established diagnostic clinics for cardiovascular complaints and cervical cancer, but these serviced only a limited number of poor. For example, in 1947 New York City opened a cancer-detection center in one of its clinics, and in 1956 some of the social hygiene clinics began routinely testing for cervical cancer.[29] Aside from joining with private cancer and heart groups in seeking to educate the public, health departments did little more than provide minimal diagnostic services.

The rejection by the military of about 1,750,000 men for neuropsychiatric reasons during World War II drew attention to the need for government action on behalf of the mentally ill. The steps taken by the government were largely influenced by two major developments in mental health. The first of these was the community health movement, and the second was the introduction of tranquilizers. The latter had two direct effects. In the first place, tranquilizer chemotherapy strengthened the position of those who argued that mental illness was largely somatic; in the second, along with the community health movement, it resulted in the discharging of thousands of patients. This large-scale release of mental patients was also aided by the movement for patient rights—one which, however laudable, was not without its negative side.[30]

Until the end of World War II, responsibility for the mentally ill was assumed primarily by the states and was usually not within the province of their public health departments. This situation changed in 1946 when several small groups working together were able to push the National Mental Health Act through Congress. Its three goals were to promote research, train psychiatric personnel, and provide grants to states to establish clinics and treatment centers and to fund demonstrations in prevention and care. Until the passage of this act, the federal government had given only small grants to the states to help with children's mental and emotional problems; now it was prepared to enter the entire field of mental health. In 1949 the National Institute of Mental Health was established to conduct the research specified by the act. As with other federal programs in these years, federal spending for mental health increased rapidly. The budget for 1948 was $4,250,000; by 1964 it amounted to $176,374,000.

The states up to the 1950s were still following the traditional policy of institutionalizing the mentally ill. The new policy established by the National Mental Health Act involved using federal grants to encourage community mental health programs and the growth of community clinics. It was based on the belief that prevention and early treatment would drastically reduce the need for hospitalization. In addition to federal funds, community health programs were strongly supported by the Milbank Fund. Stimulated by the prospect of outside funding and rising public interest, many states, led by New York and California, began developing community health programs. In New York a Mental Health Services Act enacted in 1954 authorized cities and counties to establish mental health boards and provided state funds to them on a matching basis. Within two years mental health boards were functioning in areas representing 85 percent of the state's population. California developed a similar program under the jursidiction of its Department of Mental Hygiene. Community mental health units were usually administered separately from public health departments, although the California State Board of Health reported that it was working closely with the mental hygiene department.[31]

The community mental health movement made a brave start in the 1950s but soon found itself overwhelmed. The public has always looked askance at the mentally ill, much preferring to keep them hidden away, and local taxpayers were reluctant to contribute to community facilities. To make matters worse, a study in 1960 showed that only about 20 percent of state mental hospitals had introduced any of the new forms of treatment, with the remainder simply providing custodial care.[32] The new policy of deinstitutionalization thrust thousands of patients onto communities ill-prepared to handle them. Nonetheless, a significant start had been made; and, if the program has made only limited progress today, at least it appears to be moving in the right direction.

Since health departments were no longer devoting most of their time to such traditional responsibilities as preventing communicable diseases and checking on milk and water supplies and general sanitary conditions, they began looking for other threats to community health. The issues of *Ohio's Health* in the 1950s and 1960s clearly illustrate the new concerns of state and local health departments. In 1951 the editor sought to calm public fears aroused by the Cold War. One article explained that it was possible to live through an atomic attack without any special equipment, and a series of articles was entitled "What You Should Know About Biological Warfare." Several other articles also featured topics relating to civil defense.[33]

In 1954 one series of articles was concerned with the problems of senior citizens; another series dealt with the health of migrant labor; many single articles discoursed on mental health and fluoridation. In subsequent years an increasing number of articles discussed radiation hazards and environmental concerns. The early 1960s saw the appearance of papers on teenagers, pesticides and environmental problems, and nutrition. In the year 1967 the following topics were discussed: the challenge of sex education, infants and preschoolers, crippled children, mental health, and speech problems. Subsequent issues carried more material on senior citizens and articles on dental care, drugs, hypertension, and breast cancer.[34]

The changing focus of public health can be seen, too, in the *Monthly Bulletin* of the Indiana State Board of Health. In 1963 one issue was devoted to the new programs developed during past years. These programs concerned a variety of subjects, including phenylketonuria, migrant labor, retarded children, hospital licensing, home care services, preventive medicine (tuberculosis and other disorders), milk sampling, radiological health, industrial waste, water pollution, air pollution, recreational area sanitation, and so forth.[35] The California Board of Health announced three years later that it was now concerned with sick people as people— not just with the illnesses affecting them—a rather startling new concept of public health. It then declared that its three major aims were, first, to attack the problems of liquid and solid waste disposal, air pollution, vector control, and the reuses of water; second, to provide personal health services, including health delivery to those "neglected under the segregated, income-limited system of health care"; and third, to convince people to maintain good health habits and to seek preventive health care.[36]

Equally revealing of the changes in public health is an almost nine-hundred-page, edited volume published in 1965 entitled *Health and the Community: Readings in the Philosophy and Sciences of Public Health*. Its collection of fifty-three articles, papers, and original essays covers virtually all aspects of public health. Several articles refer to chronic illness, but, aside from one paper on teenagers and venereal disease, two articles on coronary heart disease, and one on mass immunization for polio, there is nothing on communicable diseases.[37] Public health officers of the 1920s reading the book would find themselves in strange territory.

Before the twentieth century industrial and occupational health was an area to which neither the medical profession nor public health leaders paid much attention. As we have seen, the movement to regulate child labor in England and on the Continent was slow in reaching the United States, and it was late in the nineteenth century before a few state and municipal laws were passed that attempted to limit child labor and improve working conditions for women. The Progressive movement of the early twentieth century was concerned with the general deterioration in working conditions, but its work to create a more efficient and humane society was only one factor in helping to improve the health and safety of workers. Another was the growth of unions, which sought, among other aims, to improve working conditions. The third factor was the emergence of responsible business leaders, motivated in part by fears of labor and political unrest and in part by a sense of community responsibility.[38]

One of the key figures in exposing and remedying the worst abuses in industrial plants was Dr. Alice Hamilton (1869–1970), whose studies on the health of men and women working with phosphorus, lead, radium, and other dangerous substances are landmarks in occupational health.[39] Well before Hamilton's time, physicians had been employed by companies in mining, lumber, and other extractive industries, but company physicians tended to accept the assumptions of their employers—that health and safety were the responsibility of the individual worker—and the medical profession itself evidenced little interest in occupational health. Fortunately, a small group of socially conscious physicians joined with Hamilton in investigating working conditions, and their studies supplied ample material for the reformers. More important in arousing the public conscience was a series of labor disasters in the early years of the twentieth century, including explosions in mines and industrial plants, the New York Triangle Shirtwaist fire, and the grim deaths from phosphorus necrosis among matchworkers.

The initial step toward reform was taken in 1910 by a liberal group, the American Association of Labor Legislation, when it held a National Conference on Industrial Disease. The following year business leaders created the National Safety Council. Three years later, in 1914, the American Public Health Association belatedly organized an industrial hygiene section, and in 1915 the AMA finally came into the picture by holding its first symposium on industrial hygiene and medicine. There was general agreement among all concerned on the need for workmen's compensation laws, and, between 1911 and 1921 some twenty-five states passed legislation guaranteeing financial compensation for injured workers and their families. These same years also saw the establishment of several agencies in the federal government involved in promoting the health of workers— the Bureau of Mines in the Interior Department (1910), Children's Bureau (1912), Department of Labor (1913), and the Office of Industrial Hygiene and Sanitation, part of the Public Health Service (1914).[40]

Encouraging as these developments appear, they left a great deal to be desired. Workmen's compensation did not become nationwide until 1948, when Mississippi finally enacted its first law. Moreover, many of the early state laws were declared unconstitutional. This was the case in New York State, where a workmen's compensation law was passed in 1910 only to be voided by the courts. Three more years elapsed before a revised law managed to work its way through the legislature. Both state and federal courts were generally unsympathetic to any regulations affecting industry. For example, for the first thirty years of the twentieth century every federal child labor law that was enacted was declared unconstitutional.[41]

To make matters worse, the caliber of state laws varied widely, and many of them applied only to a few specified industries. In addition, the laws were subject to interpretation by courts that were too often unfriendly, and these courts further weakened them. In his study of American public health published in 1920, Harry H. Moore stated that help for injured workers was "often inadequate or slow in coming," and that workers were occasionally required to strike to get results. A consultant to the Ohio State Department of Health reporting on the health of coal miners reported: "Taking up a collection by passing around a paper or by 'passing the hat' was a frequent procedure to help out some sick or injured worker."[42]

Fortunately, the existence of compensation laws, which carried a potential for heavy liability, required most employers to carry insurance, and insurance costs became a major factor in promoting safer working conditions; in other words, safety devices lowered accident rates and reduced insurance premiums. The 1920s were scarcely conducive to labor legislation, and little further was accomplished until the New Deal. Although the National Industrial Recovery Act, which contained provisions concerning health and safety, was declared unconstitutional, the Social Security Act of 1935 provided funds for industrial hygiene research, and subsequent laws firmly involved the federal government in occupational health and safety. Stimulated in part by federal grants, state and municipal governments began moving into the area. As of 1936 only six states and one city health department had industrial hygiene divisions. Ten years later industrial hygiene units were functioning in thirty-eight states, seven cities, and two counties.[43]

Succeeding years saw steady additions to state and local regulations affecting working conditions, but perennial problems with these widely varying state laws and their lack of enforcement led to agitation for federal action. This agitation culminated in the passage of the Coal Mine Health and Safety Act in 1969 and in the enactment of the more comprehensive Occupational Health and Safety Act of 1970. The latter act authorized federal officials to enforce minimum standards and to provide research and training funds in the field of occupational safety. By this date the new interest in environmental concerns meant that the health of workers in a given plant had become closely interrelated with the welfare of the community.

One of the more interesting developments in the postwar years was the long—and often bitter—struggle over the fluoridation of water. Dental hygiene became of concern to the larger municipal health departments shortly after the emergence of the school health movement in the early twentieth century. One reason for this was that dental societies were always more willing to cooperate with health departments than medical societies were. For example, local dental societies, unlike medical groups, fully endorsed the New Deal program to provide dental care. This same interest in prevention led dentists to become the major advocates of the fluoridation of water supplies. Individual dentists first became interested in the subject while investigating the discoloration of teeth in certain geographic areas. By the 1930s fluorine was identified as the agent responsible for the discoloration, and at the same time it was demonstrated that children whose teeth were discolored had far less tooth decay than children with normal-looking teeth. In consequence, a number of dentists and researchers began suggesting the addition of fluoride to water supplies.

Additional research during the war years confirmed these findings and showed that the addition of limited amounts of fluoride was not deleterious to general health. In consequence, in 1945 the Public Health Service began conducting studies with water fluoridation in three American cities, using neighboring communities as controls. Two of the control groups withdrew from the study, leaving only Newburgh, New York, and its control city. It soon became apparent that Newburgh children's teeth were markedly better than those of children in the control community. After ten years of observation, in comparison with the control group, five times as many Newburgh children had all their teeth and were free of caries.[44]

In 1947 Madison, Wisconsin, fluoridated its water supply and was followed by a number of other cities. By 1951, when the AMA endorsed fluoridation, it had the support of the American Dental Association, the American Public Health Association, the Public Health Service, and virtually every scientific group. It appeared that fluoridation was on its way to general acceptance at this time, when opposition to it arose from widely divergent sources. These included conservative groups such as the Daughters of the American Revolution, extreme rightists, professional anticommunists, food faddists, naturopaths, opponents of any form of government regulation, and, as is usually the case, a number of dissenting scientists and medical and dental practitioners.[45] The climate of the Cold War era, a time when millions of Americans were fearful of communist plots, made the argument that fluoridation was a scheme to poison the American people acceptable to hundreds of thousands of Americans and created doubt in the minds of millions of others.

It was argued that fluoridation was unnecessary, unconstitutional, dangerous to general health, and an infringement on personal liberty. In vain the proponents of fluoridation mobilized the American Association for the Advancement of Science and every other reputable scientific body, along with such influential figures as Dr. Benjamin Spock, but, the majority of times that the issue was put to a referendum after 1942, it was defeated.[46] Slow progress was made, however, particularly after the advocates of fluoridation learned that it was much simpler to persuade municipal councils to take action on their own authority. New York City experienced some exceedingly heated and almost violent public meetings over the question until Health Commissioner George James, with the help of Mary Lasker, a prominent New York City philanthropist, persuaded the city council to go ahead quietly with fluoridation in the mid-1960s.[47] The debate over fluoridation is far from settled. In recent years only about one-third of the communities holding a referendum on the issue have voted in favor of it. Thus, after more than forty years of agitation, only slightly over half of the America people drink water naturally or artificially fluoridated.[48]

The case of fluoridation illustrates the difficulties health authorities often confront in persuading the public to adopt a beneficial policy. Matters involving technology and science are always a problem, since invariably a few reputable scientists or other professionals can be found to dispute the accepted scientific views in question, thus encouraging the doubtful and the many uninformed who object on completely specious grounds.[49] Moreover, parents did not perceive dental caries among their children as an immediate threat, and fluoridation promised only a future benefit. Earlier, school dentists had found it difficult to persuade children and their parents to practice oral hygiene, since most parents simply assumed and accepted tooth loss. The state of dental health was much improved by the time fluoridation was discovered, but, after over forty years of education, millions of Americans are still not convinced of its value.

Finally, the twenty years following World War II witnessed the revival of an interest in environmental conditions. In the nineteenth century the danger from air pollution was seen in terms of foul odors or miasmas emanating from putrefying organic matter. By the early twentieth century the concern was with belching smokestacks. In the postwar period attention turned to more subtle forms of water and air pollution, such as trace elements of lead, mercury, and arsenic and newly discovered chemical compounds. Leaded gasoline and lead paints were discovered to be sources of chronic lead poisoning among children in crowded tenement areas. While a few public health authorities had been warning against the massive use of insecticides, the appearance of Rachel Carson's book, *Silent Spring*, marked the beginning of a public demand for action. The dangers from these more subtle threats to public health were not easy to assess, and, as with chronic diseases, they required major legislation.

NOTES

1. Arthur J. Viseltear, "Health Education and Public Policy: A Short History of P.L. 94–317," *Preventive Medicine, USA* (New York, 1976):825–26.

2. For an excellent summary of the contents of the journal see George Rosen, "The American Journal of Public Health: Antecedents, Origin and Evolution," *American Journal of Public Health* 62 (1972):724–33.

3. Rosemary Stevens, *American Medicine and the Public Interest* (New Haven, Conn., 1971), 183–87.

4. Arthur J. Viseltear, *Emergence of the Medical Care Section of the American Public Health Association, 1926–1948* (Washington, D.C., 1972), 5–6.

5. Ibid., 5–8.

6. Editorial, "The Wagner National Health Bill," *JAMA* 112 (1939):1969.

7. For an excellent summary of Haven Emerson's views see his article, "Growing Pains of Public Health," *The Survey* 85 (1949):677–78.

8. Stevens, *American Medicine and the Public Interest*, 509–11. For a more complete account of the compulsory health insurance movement in the Roosevelt years see Daniel S. Hirshfield, *The Lost Reform: The Campaign for Compulsory Health Insurance in the United States from 1932 to 1943* (Cambridge, Mass., 1970).

9. Editorial, "The Wagner-Murray-Dingell Bill," *JAMA* 128 (1945):365.

10. Bess Furman, *A Profile of the United States Public Health Service, 1798–1948* (Washington, D.C., n.d.), 446.

11. Stevens, *American Medicine and the Public Interest*, 509–11.

12. Ibid., 510–12; Alfred H. Katz and Jean S. Felton, eds., *Health and the Community: Readings in the Philosophy and Sciences of Public Health* (New York, 1965), 279.

13. Furman, *A Profile of the United States Public Health Service*, 439–40.

14. Marshall W. Raffel, *The U.S. Health System: Origins and Function* (New York, 1980), 555–57.

15. Victoria A. Harden, *Inventing the NIH: Federal Biomedical Research Policy, 1887–1937* (Baltimore, 1986), 183; Dale R. Lindsay and Ernest M. Allen, "Medical Research: Past Support, Future Directions," *Science* 134 (1961):2018–19.

16. California State Board of Health, "Biennial Report for 1954–56," *California Health* 14, no. 10 (1956):89–90.

17. *Annual Report of the New York City Health Department, 1959–1960* (New York, 1960), 61.

18. Myrtle Greenfield, *A History of Public Health in New Mexico* (Albuquerque, 1962), 4–5.

19. United States Bureau of the Census, *Historical Statistics of the United States, Colonial Times to 1957* (Washington, D.C., 1960), 26.

20. Louis Chargin, W. Liefer, and T. Rosenthal, "Mapharsen in the Treatment of Early Syphilis," *Archives of Dermatology and Syphilology* 40 (1939):208.

21. Harry F. Dowling, *Fighting Infection: Conquests of the Twentieth Century* (Cambridge, Mass., 1977), 146–47.

22. *The Eradication of Syphilis*, Task Force Report to the Surgeon General on Syphilis Control in the United States, Leona Baumgartner, chairperson (Washington, D.C., 1961), 20.

23. *Annual Report of the San Francisco Department of Public Health, 1960–61* (San Francisco, 1961), 20.

24. John Duffy, *The Rudolph Matas History of Medicine in Louisiana* (Baton Rouge, La., 1958–62), 2:157–58; George Colmer, "Paralysis in Teething Children," *American Journal of Medical Sciences* 5 (1842–43):248.

25. John Duffy, *A History of Public Health in New York City, 1866–1966* (New York, 1974), 552–53.

26. Wesley W. Spink, *Infectious Diseases, Prevention and Treatment in the*

Nineteenth and Twentieth Centuries (Minneapolis, Minn., 1978), 197–206; Dowling, *Fighting Infection*, 202–19.

27. Dowling, *Fighting Infection*, 218.

28. Barbara Gastel, "Measles: A Potentially Finite History," *J. Hist. Med. & All. Sci.* 28 (1973):34–44.

29. George James, "Program Planning and Evaluation in a Modern City Health Department," *American Journal of Public Health* 51 (1961):1833–34.

30. For a first-rate account of recent mental health policy see Gerald N. Grob, "Forging Mental Health Policy in America," *J. Hist. Med. & All. Sci.* 42 (1987):410–46.

31. *California Public Health Report, Forty-third Report, July 1, 1950 to June 30, 1951*, 12.

32. Joint Commission on Mental Illness and Health, "Action for Mental Health," in Katz and Felton, eds., *Health and the Community*, 549.

33. *Ohio's Health* 3 (January 1951):11–18, (April 1951):17–24.

34. Ibid., see volumes 6 through 19, 1954–67.

35. *Monthly Bulletin*, Indiana State Board of Health 65 (1963):3ff.

36. California State Board of Health "Biennial Report for 1964–66," *California's Health* 24 (1966):3.

37. Katz and Felton, eds., *Health and the Community*.

38. For a good picture of occupational health and safety in the past one hundred years see David Rosner and Gerald Markowitz, eds., *Dying for Work: Workers' Safety and Health in Twentieth-Century America* (Bloomington, Ind., 1987).

39. Alice Hamilton, *Exploring the Dangerous Trades: The Autobiography of Alice Hamilton* (Boston, 1943); Barbara Sicherman, *Alice Hamilton: A Life in Letters* (Cambridge, Mass., 1984).

40. Jacqueline K. Corn, "Historical Aspects of Industrial Hygiene: Changing Attitudes towards Industrial Health," *Journal of the American Industrial Hygiene Association* 39 (1978):695–99.

41. Amasa Ford, *Urban Health in America* (New York, 1976), 53–55; *Thirty Years in Community Service, 1911–1941: A Brief Outline of the Work of the Committee on Public Health of the New York Academy of Medicine*, prepared by E. H. L. Corwin and Elizabeth V. Cunningham (New York, [1942]), 90–92.

42. Henry H. Moore, *Public Health in the United States: An Outline with Historical Data* (New York, 1923), 344; "Health of Ohio Coal Miners, Abstract of a Report by Emery R. Hayhurst, Ph.D., M.D., Consultant in Industrial Hygiene, Ohio State Department of Health," *The Ohio Public Health Journal* 10 (1919):167.

43. Corn, "Historical Aspects of Industrial Hygiene," 698.

44. Editorial, *The Journal of the American Dental Association* 65 (1962):578–85.

45. For an example of the scientific arguments against fluoridation see George L. Waldbott et al., *Fluoridation: The Great Dilemma* (Lawrence, Kan., 1978).

46. James Shaw, ed., *Fluoridation as a Public Health Measure* (Washington, D.C., 1954).

47. Duffy, *Public Health in New York City, 1866–1966*, 445–46. One of the first to point out to public health officers that it was much easier to sell fluoridation

to elected officials than to the public was Ruth Roemer. See her article, "Water Fluoridation: Public Health Responsibility and the Democratic Process," *American Journal of Public Health* 55 (1965):1337–48.

48. Tom Christoffel, "Fluorides, Facts and Fanatics: Public Health Advocacy Shouldn't Stop at the Courthouse Door," *American Journal of Public Health* 75 (1985):888–91.

49. For a solid study of politics and public health see Robert L. Cain, Elihu Katz, and Donald B. Rosenthal, *The Politics of Community Conflict: The Fluoridation Decision* (Indianapolis, Ind., 1969).

19

Public Health in a Changing World

In reviewing the past sixty years of American public health history two themes stand out. One is the steady fragmentation of health services and the other is the expanding role of the federal government. The fragmentation, as Ben Freedman observed over twenty years ago, has taken two forms. One is the assumption of responsibility for a particular health area by a state agency other than the state health department, and the other is the splintering of a specific health service among several state agencies.[1] This process, as indicated in the previous chapter, was hastened by the reluctance of public health officers to clash with the AMA and their inclination to withdraw from the political arena and retreat into research.

The New Deal in the 1930s with its emphasis upon social welfare, speeded the fragmentation process. Political leaders, impatient with the failure of health departments to press for needed changes, created new agencies or assigned health responsibilities to other departments or divisions. A Public Health Service study in 1950 showed that throughout the country about 60 state agencies were engaged in health-related activities. The number of state agencies concerned with some aspects of health within a single state ranged from 10 to 32. The high degree of fragmentation was further demonstrated by the number of agencies within individual states engaged in providing similar services. In one state 13 separate agencies were involved in accident prevention; in another, responsibility for health education was divided among 12 different state units. The study defined 36 categories of health activities and found that only 15 of them were either the part-time or full-time responsibility of all 48 state health departments. The rest were provided by some other agency or simply did not exist.[2] Apropos of the increasing role of state agencies in health matters, by 1953 the California State Board of Education was employing more public health nurses than the state board of health.[3]

The huge expansion of state and municipal health departments itself created major administrative problems. As of 1961 the California State Department of Public Health had eight divisions, twenty-two bureaus, seven laboratories, and five miscellaneous subdivisions.[4] The broadening scope of health responsibilities has also placed heavy burdens on state health boards. For example, by 1981 the Indiana State Board of Health had established twelve advisory committees, ranging from an Agricultural Advisory Committee to a Mobile Home Advisory Board, and including committees on topics such as serology, renal disease, and radiation control. In addition, the board had created four groups that dealt with specific programs, among which were a Commission for the Handicapped and a Vector Control Advisory Committee.[5]

In major cities, too, health departments found themselves confronted with a growing number of administrative subdivisions, many of which inevitably overlapped. Municipal administrative problems were also compounded by government decisions made at the state and national levels. A 1966 study of the New York City health services administration by an outside consulting firm showed that no less than 25 separate government agencies (6 federal, 5 state, and 14 municipal) were involved in distributing money for medical care within the city. The report spoke of the duplication of administrative services and the archaic handling of information and records and declared that the city had allowed vested bureaucratic interests to delay the proper decentralization of health care delivery.[6]

As health departments have been pushed into providing health care and other services for the aged and chronically sick, they have become more involved in providing social services. The Indiana health board, in addition to its Mobile Home Advisory Board, also had a Committee on Population Studies. The Michigan Department of Public Health in 1973, after surveying one hundred years of its history, pointed out that it was in a state of ferment, with some old programs being dismantled, others being transferred from the health department, and new ones being created. One of the questions the department posed was whether or not health functions should be combined with social services.[7]

This question had already been answered with the creation of the federal agency, the Department of Health, Education, and Welfare, in 1953, subsequently retitled in 1979 the Department of Health and Human Services. Indicative of the attitude of health leaders regarding the merging of the two functions, New York City Health Commissioner George James declared in 1965 that poverty was the city's third leading cause of death.[8] A 1983 editorial in the *American Journal of Public Health* entitled "Adoption: A Public Health Perspective" shows the degree to which the two fields of public health and social services have been merging. The editorialist spoke of the notable trend in public health toward closing the gap between public health and social welfare and pointed out the relationship between teenage pregnancy and adoption. She then urged a nationwide system to collect data on adoption in order to study the effect of adoption on both mother and child.[9]

Since living conditions are a major determinant of health, social services are an essential part of preventive medicine. As early as 1944 the American Public Health Association had resolved that a "national program for medical care should make available to the entire population all essential preventive, diagnostic, and curative services."[10] A House of Representatives committee studying a bill to provide community health services and facilities for the chronically ill in 1961 was informed that the United States was "woefully short of good diagnostic and ambulatory care clinics, good nursing homes, good home care, good referral services, and good rehabilitation programs."[11] While public health leaders have had only limited success in their effort to achieve a comprehensive medical care system for all Americans, in the past twenty-five years they have made some progress with respect to the aged poor and chronically sick.

Fortunately, the 1960s brought a new awareness of social deprivation to America and led to the establishment of several federal programs designed to assist needy groups. The Migration and Refugee Assistance Act of 1962 provided funds for clinics and health services to aid migrant workers and Cuban refugees. The 1965 Appalachian Regional Development Act authorized funds for health facilities for another impoverished group. Along with the creation of Medicare and Medicaid in that year, Congress enacted the Older Americans Act to assist in community planning and coordination of health and other services for the aged. The War on Poverty under President Johnson led to the Economic Opportunity Act of 1964. While some of the initial poverty programs included certain aspects of health, in 1965 the Office of Economic Opportunity (OEO), recognizing the intimate relationship between poverty and health, endorsed the development of comprehensive neighborhood health centers offering a full range of ambulatory services. By 1971 the OEO was supporting 49 of these health centers in various sections of the country. In addition, federal money was the mainstay of 298 mental health centers, 115 maternal and child health centers, and another 35 general health centers. Significantly, the OEO neighborhood health centers were also involved in job training and other areas of community development, thus combining both health and social services.

While the aims of the War on Poverty were commendable, they added to the fragmentation of government health and welfare services. The newer programs were designed to deal with individuals in special categories—war veterans, crippled children, migrant workers, American Indians, preschool children, the over-sixty-five age group, and so forth. In creating these programs, little consideration was given to the problem of overlapping functions. In the same way that most large municipal health departments have promoted fragmented services that compel individuals with multimedical problems to visit two or three clinics or health centers, so the federal government has encouraged the fragmentation and duplication of health services by setting up separate programs for such categories as veterans, migrant workers, and the aged.[12]

In the course of enacting a series of piecemeal public health laws in the past twenty-five years, Congress has taken tentative steps toward health planning and coordination. This limited action was stimulated by an excess of hospital beds resulting from the effect of the Hill-Burton Act, which had made over three billion dollars available for the construction of hospitals and health facilities during the postwar years (as detailed in the last chapter). Partly in order to solve this problem, the 1966 Comprehensive Health Planning and Health Services Act was passed. It sought to encourage states to coordinate all health services within their boundaries by offering grants for studies and health demonstrations. To qualify, each state was to submit a plan for coordinating its health services and to create a single state agency to serve as a coordinating body.

In 1974 this act was supplemented by the National Health Planning and Resource Development Act, which was designed to establish a nationwide network of health planning agencies. Although these acts were administered by the Public Health Service, their effectiveness depended upon state and local participation. Today, in a few areas state and local planning agencies have been able to reduce the number of hospital beds, but little else has been accomplished. A combination of vested interests and local pressures has largely nullified the intent of the federal laws. In the 1980s the Reagan administration's subordination of health and social services to military projects steadily eroded all health planning efforts until at present only skeleton agencies exist.[13]

The administrative problems for health officials at all levels have been compounded by the constantly changing nature of public health work. On the bright side, since World War II the emphasis in preventing contagious diseases has shifted from bacterial to viral disorders, and, due to the relatively large sums flowing into biomedical research through the National Institutes of Health, the Public Health Service, and other agencies, remarkable progress has been made. The virtual conquest of polio was noted earlier. In 1963 an attenuated live measles vaccine developed by John Enders and T. C. Peebles was licensed in the United States. Within five years reported measles cases, which had been averaging about half a million a year before the introduction of vaccine, were reduced to 22,231. As so often happens following the initial enthusiasm for a new preventive, measles vaccination was neglected, and by 1972 the annual number of reported cases had climbed to over 75,000.[14] A renewed campaign again brought a sharp reduction, but it was not until late in the decade that concerted drives within states and muncipalities reduced the annual number of cases by the 1980s to about 3,000.

Rubella, or German measles, which usually attacks adolescents and young adults, was generally classified along with measles as a mild disorder. Beginning in the 1940s studies began to demonstrate the association of rubella during pregancy with congenital malformations. Fortunately, a vaccine became available in 1969, the use of which has drastically reduced the incidence of the disease in recent years.[15] Mumps, another viral disease of childhood, was not reported nationally until 1968 when a total of 152,209 cases were recorded. The first live attenuated mumps vaccine was licensed in 1969. Due, at least in part, to the use of the vaccine, the annual number of reported cases fell to 32,850 in 1983.[16] Chickenpox, or varicella, is another of the disorders that formerly were considered to be harmless children's diseases but, as with the others in this group, were found to occasionally have serious and lethal complications. Unfortunately, at present no safe effective vaccine for it is available. However, varicella-zoster immune globulin is an effective prophylaxis for high-risk patients exposed to the disease.[17]

Influenza, one of the last great pandemic disorders, has long defied efforts to control it. Since the influenza virus is subject to frequent antigenic changes, efforts to achieve a vaccine effective against all strains have not been successful. The terrible influenza epidemic of 1918–19 made a permanent impression upon society's memory, and, when a strain appeared early in 1976 that resembled the so-called swine influenza of 1918, on the advice of his public health officials, President Gerald R. Ford began a campaign for a nationwide vaccination program. A host of difficulties were encountered. Not all virologists were convinced that the flu virus was identical with the 1918 one, and the vaccine manufacturers were apprehensive about the possibility of running afoul of federal antitrust laws or of being held liable for any problems associated with the proposed mass-immunization program. To further complicate matters, the *New York Times* attacked the whole program, calling it an election-year gimmick. After considerable debate Congress appropriated $135 million for the program, and it was initiated in October 1976.

After about forty million people had been vaccinated, in February 1977 the program was sharply curtailed. In the first place, no influenza epidemic had developed; in the second, a number of cases of Guillain-Barre syndrome, an acute paralytic disorder, occurred, about half of which were associated with the vaccine. The affair illustrated the difficulty of debating scientific issues before the public and in Congress. While the question as to whether or not a nationwide vaccination program was needed in this particular instance has not been decided, the events of 1976 showed that it was possible to undertake a nationwide vaccination program in a relatively short time. In addition, legislative and administrative steps have been taken to facilitate similar mass-immunization programs in the future.[18]

The reduced incidence of the traditional contagious diseases and the improvement in disease reporting have brought several disorders into sharper focus, one of which is hepatitis. In the past forty years a number of advances have been made in the study of this disorder, and two main types have been identified, the more dangerous hepatitis A, transmitted by food and water, and hepatitis B, usually contracted through infected blood or serum. As yet no safe vaccines are available, but immune serum globulin is relatively effective in the treatment of hepatitis A.

The transformation in sexual morality which began in the 1950s and the abuse of penicillin and other antibiotics in the postwar years, as indicated in the previous chapter, have made venereal disease one of the leading public health concerns. Although the trend of syphilis has generally been downward since peaking in World War II, the incidence of gonorrhea, which declined with syphilis in the immediate postwar years, has climbed steadily since the early 1960s. In the following decade genital herpes began to spread, and although it posed no serious threat to public health, it tended to discourage sexual promiscuity. Late in this same decade a much more serious disorder, acquired immune deficiency syndrome (AIDS), began appearing. As with some of the earlier epidemic diseases, AIDS is both horrible and highly lethal. At present its major ravages appear to be among drug addicts, homosexuals, prostitutes, and certain other high-risk groups, but it has aroused alarm in the general population. The public is always apprehensive about any new and deadly contagion, particularly one about which little is known. This fear has been intensified by the knowledge that AIDS can be transmitted through blood transfusions and other means, and that it can be spread through heterosexual activity.

The public reaction to AIDS has made its control exceedingly difficult. Syphilis and gonorrhea always have been underreported, but AIDS presents a special problem. Widespread public apprehension has resulted in turning AIDS victims into pariahs, thus compounding the difficulty of identifying and recording them. At this stage neither a cure nor a preventive has been discovered. By 1984 three laboratories had identified the virus that causes the disease, and subsequently diagnostic tests were devised. Congress and the White House administration, responding to public concern, are in the process of mobilizing scientific resources, and it is logical to assume that answers to AIDS will be found. Public health authorities, following the initiative of former Surgeon General C. Everett

Koop, presently are seeking to give the public a better understanding of the disorder, to provide screening for high-risk groups, and to encourage the use of prophylactic devices.

Granting that the above measures can reduce the further spread of AIDS and that an effective vaccine eventually will become available, there still remains the problem of those already infected. The best estimates are that from one to two million Americans fall into this category, a high percentage of whom will probably develop acute symptoms of the disease. The cost of health care for the present victims is rapidly increasing, and it can only go higher in the coming years. Since a high percentage of those infected are drug users and members of low-income groups, responsibility for their health care will fall upon government agencies. While local governments undoubtedly will carry part of the burden, the federal authorities probably will be forced to pick up the major share of the cost.[19]

A 1984 editorial in the *American Journal of Public Health* entitled "The Environment Returns to the Health Department" reflects a major shift in public health concerns.[20] In the nineteenth century the concerns of public health were essentially sanitation and quarantine. Public and personal cleanliness were equated with godliness and the advance of civilization itself. The bacterial revolution, while not denying the aesthetic value of cleanliness, placed the emphasis in the twentieth century on preventing the bacterial contamination of food and water. In the last forty years, as it became evident that industrial wastes were threatening our air, water, and food, public health authorities began to shift their emphasis from bacterial to physiochemical agents produced by industry. Toxic chemicals, radiation, and nuclear energy are increasingly preoccupying the attention of public health departments.[21] Unfortunately, the medical problems created by industrial wastes are frequently slow in developing, making it difficult in many cases to assess the risk.

Aside from the difficulty of determining the precise health effects of certain forms of pollution, the economic welfare of communities is often tied to the profitability of local industry. Consequently workers and local citizens frequently ally themselves with the offending industries, making it almost impossible, except in extreme cases, to remedy the abuses. Added to this is the strength of industrial lobbies. Since for much of the century the problem of pollution has been handled at the local and state level, a wide variation has existed in the effectiveness of antipollution laws and in the degree of their enforcement. Many states wishing to attract industries have enacted only minimal antipollution legislation and done little to enforce it. Closely allied to the industrial pollution issue has been that of occupational health, since toxic chemicals represented a direct threat to those working with them. It was not until the federal government began moving into the area that any effective steps were taken to prevent pollution at the workplace and improve occupational health.

One of the powers given to the early health boards was that of banning "nuisances." These were defined as anything causing foul odors or threatening health in other ways. Usually the board was empowered to take offenders to court, where they might be fined or ordered to cease and desist. This concept of "nuisance" carried into the twentieth century. Until 1970 the only legal mechanisms for dealing with pollutants were the enforcement of nuisance laws and private litigation. When a nuisance was successfully demonstrated, the offending company was fined or forced to pay damages to the injured party. These payments often resulted in the lifting of the injunction, thus permitting the pollution to continue. To make matters worse, in many cases it was cheaper for the offender to pay occasional nominal fines than to correct the abuse.[22]

California was one of the first states to attempt to deal with the rising threats from air pollution and radiation. Between 1956 and 1959 the health department established standards for air quality and motor vehicle exhaust emissions and initiated a comprehensive radiological health program.[23] In these same years the New York City Health Department adopted the first municipal legislation establishing a radiation control unit and requiring the registration of all places producing, storing, or using radioactive material. In 1961 the California Board of Health appointed a special committee to study air pollution. Four years later a separate air pollution agency was created with its own commissioner and a budget of $1,300,000.[24] Unfortunately, the California and New York City examples cited above were far from typical. Reluctant to pass stringent antipollution laws in a competitive economy, most communities and states enacted only nominal regulations.

In his presidental address before the American Public Health Association in 1983 Anthony Robbins pointed out correctly that most of the nation's environmental and occupational health legislation had been passed in the previous fifteen years.[25] The first of these measures was the Air Quality Act of 1967, which laid the basis for an ambient air quality standard. Local communities, however, were given the power to adopt their own standards of air purity. So poor was the response to the act that in 1970 Congress passed a Clean Air Act, which provided for a National Ambient Air Quality Standard to be promulgated by a federal agency.[26] Federal pressure, largely in the form of fines and the threat of withholding grants, has greatly improved air quality, but the problem of air pollution is far from solved.

These were the years when Congress enacted the Occupational Safety and Health Act, Mine Safety and Health Act, Toxic Substance Control

Act, Safe Drinking Water Act, and so forth. Significantly, the federal government has been taking an increasing role in protecting the quality of air and water. In part this increasing role reflects the fact that the healthiness of air and water in the Mississippi Valley or any other section of the United States cannot be controlled by local or state authorities. Yet, as in the case of occupational health, it also reflects the steady growth of federal involvement in health matters and the diminishing authority of official health agencies.

Occupational health, formerly a matter of industrial accidents and the overworking of women and children, has become closely associated with the issues of disability and chronic illness. More and more the medical problems of the workplace are the result of long-term exposure to carcinogenic materials, toxic compounds, and irritating substances. That coal mining contributed to respiratory disorders has long been recognized, but the medical profession has had problems in diagnosing and defining the precise effect of coal dust on the lungs. The consensus among medical investigators was that coal dust was only one factor contributing to the respiratory problems of miners. In the light of disputed medical testimony, company coal doctors tended to downplay the significance of coal dust.

The 1960s was a period of strong social concern, and the miners and their advocates argued that any respiratory impairment associated with coal mines should be attributed to black lung disease. In 1969 miners in West Virginia struck and demanded that the legislature permit black lung to be diagnosed by several methods, most preferably by impaired lung function. They also insisted that anyone who had worked in the mines for ten years or more and suffered from respiratory impairment should be presumed to have black lung disease. The miners had strong public support, and the state legislature that year responded by making their demands state law.[27]

While the West Virginia legislature was debating the problem of black lung, the issue was raised in Congress. The miners gained a partial victory in the Coal Mine Health and Safety Act of 1969, in which they were able to secure a more generous disability payment for black lung disease. The Senate, however, insisted on placing an eighteen-month limit on the provisions relating to black lung. When this time limit expired, the subject was reintroduced into Congress, where it was debated at considerable length. Supported by liberals and consumer advocates, the coal miners won the day and were able to supplant the medical definition of black lung disease with one of their own. An amended Coal Mine Health and Safety Act in 1972 stated that anyone who had worked in the coal mines for fifteen or more years and who suffered respiratory impairment would be assumed to have black lung disease. It also extended Social Security to anyone disabled by respiratory disease associated with mining. One of the more interesting aspects of this whole affair is that the legal definition of the disease, as Daniel Fox has pointed out, was determined not by physicians but by consumers and elected officials.[28]

With the obvious occupational hazards greatly reduced, attention has turned to the more subtle occupational diseases. As the black lung case has shown, there is often a great deal of scientific uncertainty and ambiguity insofar as the long-range effects of working with both natural and synthetic materials. Well over three hundred compounds have been classified as carcinogenic, but, because of the subtlety of their long-term effects, the degree of exposure necessary to cause harm is not clear. The Occupational Health and Safety Act of 1970 authorized the Occupational Safety and Health Administration (OSHA) in the Labor Department to gather information preparatory to establishing health and safety standards. Due to the subtle effects of most toxic materials, and in part to bureaucratic regulations and to the advent of the Reagan administration in the 1980s, as of 1983 OSHA had produced permanent standards for only twenty of the known carcinogens in the workplace.[29]

The long period of time that elapses before many occupational diseases manifest themselves makes it difficult to gather accurate statistics about them. While OSHA, the National Safety Council, and other agencies have excellent information on acute injuries, there is no accurate data available for the incidence or prevalence of occupational diseases. Chronic diseases are difficult to track, and statistics can easily be manipulated to justify reducing the budgets of health agencies. The establishment of OSHA was a major step forward in occupational health, but new synthetics are constantly appearing, and the agencies regulating them have never been adequately funded.[30] On a more encouraging note, the number of coal-mine deaths in 1987 was only 63, the lowest since coal-mine deaths were first recorded in 1869.[31]

The enactment of Medicare and Medicaid and the other social welfare legislation of the 1960s is significant since it marked the first time the federal government had moved to provide ambulatory primary medical care for the needy. Of course, as previous chapters have discussed, well before the federal government took this action, health departments had been involved in providing limited medical care for lower-income groups. The school health movement in the early twentieth century led to the establishment of a variety of specialized dispensaries and clinics to treat the children of the poor. These included various facilities for dealing with trachoma, tonsils and adenoids, and vision, hearing, and dental problems. Other clinics were established for adults suffering from such disorders as tuberculosis and venereal disease. These same years witnessed the beginning of the community health center concept, which was a step in the direction of comprehensive medical care. Health departments justified operating clinics on the grounds that their purpose was preventive medicine. Since in fact the clinics were providing medical care, they aroused opposition from local medical societies, leading in many instances to their curtailment. Valuable as these clinics are, they do not fill the need for primary medical care for those who cannot afford private medicine.

Several federal programs created during the ferment of the 1960s promoted community health centers designed to provide ambulatory comprehensive care for the poor and the medically underserved. Among them were the Office of Economic Opportunity, which funded a number of neighborhood centers, the Rural Health Initiative, the Health Underserved Rural Areas, the Appalachian Regional Commission, and the National Health Service Corps.[32] Congress set up the latter body to meet the problem of the growing shortage of health personnel and the maldistribution of practicing physicians. Its purpose was to supply physicians and other professionals to medically underserved areas. A community needing help had to provide clinic facilities and then apply to the Health Service Corps for personnel. The act establishing the corps stated that patients should be charged a fee, but specified that no one could be denied care because of inability to pay. At first physicians were sent into small communities and rural areas, but under the Carter administration they began to serve in urban centers.

Regrettably, little coordination developed between the many specialized local public health clinics and the comprehensive ones sponsored by the federal government. This failure was due in part to the belief of many of the sponsors of federal legislation that the states were either unable or unwilling to provide medical care for the poor. In the early 1970s many of the supporters of the National Health Service Corps envisioned that it would lead the way to a comprehensive medical care system covering all Americans who needed medical assistance. By recruiting physicians and providing scholarships to medical students, the corps rapidly increased in size during the 1970s, reaching a membership of 2,100 by 1980. The Reagan administration, which stressed private medicine and a reduced role for the federal government, soon ended any immediate hopes for a unified medical care system.[33]

The federal government, starting with the Marine Hospital Service in 1798, has long provided hospital care for a variety of special groups. The poor generally have been treated in state and municipal hospitals or in private hospitals at local government expense. With the establishment of Medicare and Medicaid, health officials came under pressure to recover expenditures for medical care from the federal government. The director of public health for the city of San Francisco reported that he had to expand his staff and hire specialized personnel to improve the fiscal management of his department.[34] In major cities with municipal hospitals, the city health department or a separate city department of hospitals is usually responsible for providing acute care for the poor. Unfortunately, many local officials have seized upon Medicare funds as an opportunity to further reduce the frequently underfunded budgets of municipal and state hospitals.

On the other hand, responsible voluntary organizations and conscientious state and local officials in many areas have promoted clinics and health centers for ambulatory patients and helped to support those needing hospital care. Even with this fragmented care provided by voluntary associations and government agencies, however, millions of Americans below the poverty level and millions more above it who are without medical insurance receive little or minimal medical assistance. The medical care given to the lower-income groups by public health departments and other agencies throughout the United States is so varied that it is difficult to make generalizations. It differs from group to group and from area to area—and can vary widely even within a given area. One of the most encouraging notes is that the AMA, which throughout most of this century has consistently denied that inequitable discrepancies existed in the American medical care system, resolved in May 1988 that a lack of national standards in the Medicaid program has led to "severe inequities" in the provision of health care benefits. Its house of delegates also voted to expand Medicaid to an additional twenty-seven million poor people.

The tragedy is that America, since the emergence of urbanization in the early nineteenth century, has had a permanent underclass. The economic group described in the 1830s as the dirty, immoral, and dissolute poor is still with us. And the average American is as confident as ever that one's economic position can be determined by hard work and drive, and although the poor are not judged quite so harshly as in the past, they are still inclined to be blamed for their poverty. In the past one hundred and fifty years a great many programs, both voluntary and governmental, have sought to solve the problem of poverty and improve the health of the poor, but with only limited success. As long as children are born in a ghetto environment, poorly nourished, provided with only emergency medical care, and given minimal education, the majority will follow their parents in becoming socially dependent adults. To correct this situation would take both large public expenditures and a paternalistic attitude toward the poor, neither of which is likely to win large-scale public support.

Despite the increasing activity of the federal government in health matters, public health is still largely in the hands of state and local authorities. The pattern established late in the nineteenth century still holds true for most states. In a few of them, public health is shaped largely by the state government; in the New England area it is primarily in the hands of local authorities; and elsewhere it rests with municipal and county governments or a combination of both. One significant development is occurring with respect to health board personnel. The public's skeptical view of the medical profession meant that for much of the nineteenth century health boards frequently were controlled by laypersons. Late in the century, as the profession gained knowledge and improved its public image, physicians successfully claimed the right to administer public health. Today, as public health is merging with social welfare and utilizing the services of dozens of professionals other than medical practitioners, state and municipal health boards, whose functions are policy making and administrative, are beginning to include more nonmedical members.

The principal role of the federal government is to set minimum standards of public health and encourage states and communities to meet or exceed these standards, to assist in training public health personnel, to gather statistics, to aid with emergency health problems, to provide advice and counseling, to help educate the public, and to promote all types of research in areas ranging from biomedicine to social welfare. The chief means by which the federal government promotes its health policies is a combination of carrot and stick. Various grants, usually requiring matching funds, are the major inducement to gain the cooperation of state and local governments. Since the concept of states' rights still carries a great deal of weight, most of the grants are made to the states, which then funnel the money to counties and communities. Some government agencies, such as the Environmental Protection Agency, have both grant money and the power to fine local governments for failing to meet minimum standards.

The entrance of government into the medical care area, which involves huge expenditures, has posed a host of new problems. For example, advances in medical science and technology have led to a flood of expensive and complicated medical machines. While these have immensely improved diagnosis and therapy, they have also contributed to rising medical costs. With manufacturers anxious to sell equipment and every health care institution insistent upon having the most modern instruments and technological aids, the result is excessive duplication and underutilization. Cost containment in this and other areas of medical care has become a necessity.

In addition, the medical problems of our aging population will require more home care programs, housing for the elderly, nursing homes, and hospice facilities. Studies are needed to determine how to achieve the best-quality care for the aged in the most cost-effective ways. And comparable studies will be needed to establish minimum standards for all of these facilities. While Medicare, Medicaid, and private medical insurance have relieved most Americans of major financial worries associated with accidents and illnesses, two serious problems still remain—the high costs of long-term hospitalization and nursing home care. Congress has just taken the first step in the area of catastrophic health insurance, but nursing home care can impoverish a high percentage of the elderly.

Public health departments at all levels of government have traditionally had a favorable public image, but in recent years they have lost a little of their sheen. Despite the wholesale acceptance of science, most people have little understanding of what it can and cannot do. Health officials, recognizing the limitations of science, tend to be hesitant about accepting the almost-daily newspaper reports of medical "breakthroughs" or "discoveries." The public, preferring simplistic answers, is much more likely to accept the optimistic word of a newspaper columnist or reporter than the more cautious assessment of a local health official. The environmentalists are a most commendable group on the whole, but there are extremists among them who criticize health authorities for not removing every conceivable threat to human health—an obviously impossible task.[35] We need a health-conscious population, but it must be an informed one.

The growing awareness of cancer and of the many dangers arising from the thousands of chemical compounds polluting the air and water has created a general sense of public unease. Probably more individuals are worrying about threats to their health than at any time in American history. And this has developed in the face of all evidence that the general population is healthier than in the past and that life expectancy is still increasing. It is true that the longer life span of Americans has resulted in more cataracts, arthritic complaints, cancers, Alzheimer's disease, and other disorders, yet older people on the whole are more active and healthy than ever before.

Periodically in American history physical fitness has become a major fad. The 1830s and 1840s, the reform period, was the first time an emphasis was placed on diet and exercise. The second health fad came late in the nineteenth century in conjunction with the dietary requirements of the Seventh Day Adventists and the appearance of the bicycle. Bernarr McFadden symbolized the next physical fitness movement in the 1920s, and America is currently in the midst of another one today. The present health movement is essentially beneficial, but its commercialization has contributed to public anxiety. To sell vitamins, health foods, weight-loss pills, exercise machines, and home air and water purifying devices, the manufacturers must first convince prospective customers that their health is in jeopardy. In addition to this deluge of advertising, the public is also confronted with newspaper and television stories and documentaries on the omnipresent danger from insecticides, industrial wastes, nuclear radiation, and other environmental threats. Unable to differentiate between valid warnings and lurid reports of unseen and unfamiliar dangers, small wonder that so many Americans today worry about their health.[36]

The widespread interest in health has also led to an outpouring of features and articles on medical topics in magazines and newspapers. Every discovery in the biomedical sciences is heralded as a major breakthrough, and medical terminology has become part of everyday speech. Controlling one's daily cholesterol level, blood pressure, weight, diet, caffeine and salt intake, and ingestion of fiber has become a major preoccupation for many individuals. For literally millions of Americans daily vitamins and calcium tablets are considered a necessity, and for an equal number of others only so-called natural foods are eaten. In a clear demonstration of the adage that a little learning is a dangerous thing, new medical "discoveries" are seized upon by the public and often turned into popular medical fads. Acquiring just enough medical knowledge to misunderstand health facts has undoubtedly been a major cause of much of the widespread public anxiety about health.

The economic principle that human wants are unlimited but economic goods are finite applies equally to medicine and public health. Preservation of human life at all costs is simply not feasible at the national level, nor is any preventative health measure completely risk-free. Using a vaccine that may result in serious complications for 5 or 10 individuals out of every 100,000 vaccinated is far better than permitting 1,000 to 10,000 cases of the disease to develop. Smallpox inoculation in the eigthteenth century resulted in 1 to 3 cases of highly fatal smallpox per 100 persons inoculated. Nonetheless, it was widely used, for the alternative was much worse. From colonial times, public health leaders have stressed the economic value of preventive measures, and in recent years researchers have moved into the area currently known as risk analysis. The role of public health promoters is to encourage the public to make rational health decisions.

Despite the fears of individual Americans and the jumble of public health laws and regulations, the federal government is slowly moving toward setting basic health standards, and state and local health departments generally are better funded than in any time past. Public health schools and universities are turning out larger numbers of professional health workers, and, along with private foundations and federal agencies, are engaged in more research than ever before.

The rising economic level and degree of health of the American people, however, in themselves create a demand for even greater efforts on the part of public health leaders. The rapid advances achieved so far in the twentieth century have set a standard that will be difficult to equal. It may be that any further significant increase in health and longevity can only come by returning to one of the chief aims of earlier health reformers. In the nineteenth century sanitarians made personal hygiene a moral crusade, and in so doing contributed enormously to improving public health. A comparable step forward can be made today by educating the public about self-imposed risks.

A prime example of what can be done in this area is the extraordinarily successful campaign started in 1964 with the *Surgeon General's Report on Smoking and Health*. Pushed ahead by successive surgeon generals, the campaign has sharply reduced smoking—a significant source of cardiovascular, respiratory, and other complaints. In the introduction to *Healthy People: The Surgeon General's Report on Health Promotion and Disease Prevention*, published in 1979, HEW Secretary Joseph A. Califano, Jr., asserted that the American people were killing themselves by carelessly continuing unhealthy personal habits, by carelessly polluting the environment, and by permitting the existence of harmful social conditions such as poverty, hunger, and ignorance. On the matter of personal responsibility, he cited a study showing that individuals who practiced seven simple health habits such as avoiding smoking and alcohol, keeping a proper diet, getting enough sleep and exercise, and wearing seat belts lived an average of eleven years longer than those who practiced none of them. In support of his position, an analysis of the ten leading causes of death in 1976 indicated that almost half of the deaths were due to unhealthy behavior or lifestyle.[37] Former Surgeon General Koop's commendable efforts to educated the public about AIDS illustrate the value of effective health education. Obesity, alcoholism, drug abuse, venereal disease, and automobile safety are all problem areas on which nationwide educational drives could have a major impact. The gospel of public health preached by the sanitarians, which taught both morality and personal hygiene, still has value today.

NOTES

1. Ben Freedman, "The Problem of Fragmentation of Community Health Services Operated by State Government," reprint from *Medical Times*, January 1944.
2. Joseph W. Mountin et al., *Distribution of Health Services in the Structure of State Government, 1950* (Washington, D.C., 1954), 14–17.
3. *California's Health* 11, no. 1 (July 15, 1953), 2.
4. Ibid., 19, no. 11 (December 1, 1961), 63.
5. Indiana State Board of Health, *Then and Now, 1881—A Century of Service—1981* (Indianapolis, 1981), 8–9.

6. New York City, Health Services Administration, Special Studies, Prepared for Library, System Development Corporation, 1966, Haven Emerson Library, TS, 1:21, 42–43.

7. *The First 100 Years: Michigan Department of Public Health,* (Lansing, 1973), 47–48.

8. New York City, Health Service Administration, Special Studies, 1:22.

9. Lorraine V. Klerman, "Adoption: A Public Health Perspective," *American Journal of Public Health* 73 (1983):1158.

10. American Public Health Association Subcommittee on Medical Care, "Preliminary Report on a National Program for Medical Care," *American Journal of Public Health* 34 (1944):984.

11. Leona Baumgartner, "Testimony on H.R. 4998," *Community Health Services and Facilities* (October 1961), 220–22.

12. For a good discussion of this subject see Rosemary Stevens, *American Medicine and the Public Interest* (New Haven, Conn., 1971), 520–22.

13. Milton L. Roemer, "I. S. Falk, The Committee on Costs of Medical Care, and the Drive for National Health Insurance," *American Journal of Public Health* 75 (1985):845.

14. Wesley W. Spink, *Infectious Diseases: Prevention and Treatment in the Nineteenth and Twentieth Centuries* (Minneapolis, 1978), 184–85.

15. Harry F. Dowling, *Fighting Infection: Conquests of the Twentieth Century* (Cambridge, Mass., 1977), 220–21.

16. Spink, *Infectious Diseases,* 192–94; C. C. White, J. P. Kaplan, and W. A. Orenstein, "Benefits, Risks and Costs of Immunization for Measles, Mumps and Rubella," *American Journal of Public Health* 75 (1985):739.

17. D. J. Weber, W.A. Rutala, and C. Parham, "Impact and Costs of Varicella Prevention in a University Hospital," *American Journal of Public Health* 78 (1988):19–22.

18. For two good accounts of the influenza affair, see Arthur J. Viseltear, "A Short Political History of the 1976 Swine Influenza Legislation," in *History, Science, and Politics: Influenza in America, 1918–1976,* June F. Osborn, ed. (New York, 1977), 29–58, and R. Neustadt and H. Fineberg, *The Epidemic That Never Was: Policy Making and the Swine Flu Affair* (New York, 1983).

19. On the subject of AIDS reporting see Daniel M. Fox, "From TB to AIDS: Value Conflicts in Reporting Disease," *AIDS: Public Health and Civil Liberties, A Hastings Center Report,* Special Supplement (December 1986), 11–16, and Katie Leishman, "A Crisis in Public Health: One City's United Efforts to Control AIDS . . . ," *The Atlantic* 256 (1985):18–41.

20. Charles Levenstein et al., "The Environment Returns to the Health Department," *American Journal of Public Health* 74 (1984):963.

21. Milton Terris, "Redefining the Public Health Agenda," *American Journal of Public Policy* 8 (1987):151–63.

22. Jacqueline K. Corn and Morton Corn, "Setting Environmental Standards for the Public: An Historical Perspective," *Proceedings of Life Sciences Symposium on Health Aspects of Energy Policy* (Los Alamos, N.M., 1975), 31–32.

23. "Report from Director to the Governor," *California's Health* 17, no. 6, (September 15, 1959): Introduction.

24. *Annual Report of the New York City Health Department, 1957–58* (New York City, 1959), 15–21; John Duffy, *A History of Public Health in New York City, 1866–1966* (New York, 1974), 429, 451.

25. Anthony Robbins, "Creating a Progressive Health Agenda, 1983 Presidential Address," *American Journal of Public Health* 74 (1984):779.

26. Corn and Corn, "Setting Standards for the Public: An Historical Perspective," 32.

27. Daniel M. Fox and Judith F. Stone, "Black Lung: Miner's Militancy and Medical Uncertainty, 1968–1972," *Bull. Hist. Med.* 54 (1980):43ff.

28. Ibid., 62–63.

29. Jacqueline K. Corn and Morton Corn, "The History and Accomplishments of the Occupational Safety and Health Administration in Reducing Cancer Risks," in *Reducing the Carcinogenic Risks in Industry*, Paul F. Deisler, Jr., ed. (New York, 1984), 176–77, 192–93.

30. M. Donald Whorton, "Accurate Occupational Illness and Injury Data in the U.S. . . . ," *American Journal of Public Health* 73 (1983):1031–32.

31. *Wall Street Journal*, May 15, 1988.

32. Marshall W. Raffel, *The U.S. Health System: Origins and Functions* (New York, 1980), 332–34.

33. Fitzhugh Mullan, "The National Health Service Corps and Health Personnel Innovations: Beyond Poorhouse Medicine," in *Reforming Medicine: Lessons of the Last Quarter Century*, Victor and Ruth Sidel, eds. (New York, 1984), 184–85, 190; Fitzhugh Mullan, "Rethinking Public Ambulatory Care in America," *New England Journal of Medicine*, 316 (1987):544–47.

34. *Annual Report, Department of Public Health, City and County of San Francisco, Fiscal Year, 1969–70*, 1–2.

35. David Harris, "Health Department: Enemy or Champion of the People," *American Journal of Public Health* 74 (1984):428–29.

36. Arthur J. Barsky, "The Paradox of Health," *New England Journal of Medicine* 328 (1988):414–18.

37. Department of Health, Education, and Welfare, *Healthy People, The Surgeon General's Report on Health Promotion and Disease Prevention* (Washington, D.C., 1979), viii–ix, 7–9.

Conclusion

While medical science has made major contributions to the control of contagious diseases in the twentieth century, one of the striking aspects of the history of these disorders is the fact that medicine played little part in the rise and fall of many of the great killer diseases of earlier days. For example, bubonic plague disappeared from Western Europe in the seventeenth and eighteenth centuries; typhus began declining later in this same period; and the incidence of tuberculosis, which seems to have peaked around the mid-nineteenth century, was diminishing well before the antituberculosis campaigns of the early twentieth century. Malaria, which ravaged all areas during most of the colonial period, had become primarily a southern disorder by the time the role of the anopheles mosquito was discovered.

Populations do tend to build up immunities over generations, and this undoubtedly played a role in reducing the incidence of the great killer diseases. Probably more important than this factor, however, have been the changes in environmental conditions in America. The sanitary revolution, based largely on the fallacious miasmatic theory of disease, was a major factor in eliminating much of the sickness of earlier times. The sanitarians' emphasis upon clean air, clean food, pure water, and personal hygiene undoubtedly helped to reduce typhoid and other enteric disorders. Personal hygiene also contributed to the eradication of typhus; and a rising standard of living, which permitted the screening of houses and other buildings, was a factor in eliminating malaria. It is not without significance that malaria did not disappear from the South until southern income levels were raised by the influx of federal money during World War II. And historically the gradual improvement in the quality of food and housing throughout the United States has been a major factor in reducing all forms of sickness.

It is a sad commentary upon the United States that, despite having the world's highest standard of living for most of the twentieth century, it ranks well below a number of other countries in terms of the basic measurements of public health. This fact can be accounted for in part by

America's firm commitment to rugged individualism and personal liberty and to the general suspicion of government controls. Only in America could a successful presidential candidate run for office on a program of reducing government to a minimum—or could legislatures enact speed laws and refuse to outlaw the use of radar detectors designed to nullify these laws. Public health regulations necessarily involve restrictions upon individual conduct and impose additional costs upon business. Although in the long run these regulations benefit both business and the community, they do not agree with the American concepts of individual liberty and free enterprise. In Britain and Europe, where vestiges of the old class systems still survive, the average citizen is far more likely than the average American to obey the laws and to accept the leadership of the better-informed members of society.

It is precisely for this reason that health education is so important in America. As even the briefest survey of history shows, laws and regulations in a democracy are only as good as public support for them. Where the public is informed, educated, and socially aware, the level of personal and community health is generally high. Unless the majority of citizens are convinced of the value of a particular law or regulation, it becomes meaningless. The Eighteenth Amendment (the Prohibition Amendment) is the classic illustration of this point. Before a health problem can be solved, the first step is to create enough public awareness of it to lead to a demand for government action. Voluntary associations play an important role in the education process, but the nature of environmental problems requires government intervention. Only when an informed public has been created is it possible to move toward effective regulation. Current health issues, such as those involving air, water, and radiation pollution, simply cannot be dealt with by the actions of individuals, private groups, or businesses alone. Regardless of one's philosophy about government, the sheer size and complexity of modern American society requires an increasing number of public health regulations.

One problem is that the public's attention span is short, and emergencies are soon forgotten. In addition, the benefits of preventive medicine are long term, and taxpayers are reluctant to invest in the future. Ironically, the more successful public health measures are, the less the public sees a need for them. All of this emphasizes the need for public health education, a process that should start in grade school and continue for life.

There are two areas where considerable gains can be made in public health. The first involves grappling with poverty, since it requires that all Americans be guaranteed decent housing, food, and medical care. The elimination of poverty has long occupied responsible Americans, and some limited progress has been made. Nonetheless, far too many American children are born to illiterate mothers who are often children themselves, are brought up in slums and run-down housing projects, deprived of adequate medical care and education, and bound in a vicious cycle of poverty. Whether poverty can be vanquished is questionable, but certainly the experience of Western European countries shows that a minimum general standard of health can be established. Although the medical care available to the majority of Americans ranks among the best in the world, that given to the lowest income groups rates from barely adequate to almost nonexistent. The many federal health programs depend largely upon matching funds from state and municipal governments. In consequence, the level of medical care provided by even such well-intentioned programs as Medicaid varies widely from state to state. The only solution is some form of a national health system.

In recent years historians have turned their attention to the history of minorities in the United States, and the picture they have presented is scarcely a cause for self-congratulation. By and large Americans tend to view the problems of poor minorities in the same way that they view those of poor whites, blaming their lack of good health on their way of life. Americans have always believed that hard work, thrift, temperance, and sound morals guaranteed a measure of economic success. On this basis, the logical assumption is that those living in poverty are responsible for their degraded way of life. If the health of Indians, blacks, Latinos, and other minorities has received little attention in this study, it simply reflects the fact that relatively little was done for them until quite recently.

The traditional attitude toward minorities is clearly demonstrated in the 1932 Tuskegee experiment designed to study the course of untreated syphilis in blacks. Beginning in that year, a select group of black males with syphilis was kept under close observation for many years but given no treatment. At the time the Public Health Service, state and local health officials, and even local black physicians and nurses at Tuskegee Institute raised no objection. In the 1930s few poor blacks with venereal disease would have received any medical attention; thus observing a number of them for presumed medical purposes seemed perfectly acceptable. The failure to treat them with penicillin in the 1940s cannot be justified, although present concepts of social justice were only beginning to permeate American society at that time.

While I am delighted that historians are beginning to delve into social history on a large scale, I think the tendency of a few of them to harshly condemn past generations for their medical treatment of the poor fails to consider the prevailing medical knowledge and ethical concepts they lived under. One understandably can be shocked to learn of the Tuskegee experiment, but no one condemned the experiment in the 1930s. At any time in American history much more could have been done to improve maternal and child care, school health, and all other matters relating to health. Having watched the political process for over fifty years, however, I am only happy that, due to the efforts of a relatively small percentage of dedicated individuals, so much has been accomplished in the past two hundred years.

The second area where health education can be of immense value relates to personal habits. Alcoholism, drug abuse, smoking, and diet to a large extent represent personal choices, and as such are amenable to education. The legal prohibitions against the sale of drugs have had only little more success than the Eighteenth Amendment. The hundreds of millions of dollars spent trying to enforce these laws in America and in bribing foreign countries to eliminate the production of marijuana and other drug crops would be far better spent on an extensive program of drug education. The campaign by federal and voluntary agencies to educate the public on the dangers of tobacco has drastically reduced the number of smokers in the past twenty-five years and demonstrates what can be done in the way of changing lifestyles.

The history of public health in America has not been one of constant and steady upward progress. One has only to glance at present public health statistics to realize how much still remains to be done. Yet public health, like politics, is the art of the possible. The problems of poverty, ill health, and drugs are inconsistent with American's self-perception and tend to be blamed on foreigners or racial and ethnic minorities. Americans much prefer trying to solve the drug problem by placing economic sanctions on certain drug-producing countries rather than by facing up to reality. By and large the American public has confronted public health problems only in emergency situations or when it has felt that the threat affected everyone. Had AIDS been restricted to homosexuals, drug users, and prostitutes, it would have received attention only from public health officers and a few physicians.

Americans have always been sensitive to individual hardship cases. A newspaper report of some child desperately needing money for medical treatment invariably brings an outpouring of public donations. The problem of poverty is that to most Americans the ghettos and slums are an abstraction, largely unseen. A highly contagious disorder threatening to spread to the general public attracts attention, but chronic health problems of the poor are largely ignored. In voting money for public health, legislators respond to pressure groups and are highly aware of the electorate's dislike of taxation. The economically deprived have few spokespersons, are seldom politically conscious, and are less likely to vote. Moreover, the average citizen is only concerned with immediate benefits—

a factor militating against public health policy, which often seeks to prevent future problems. Lastly, the more successful a public health program is, the more taxpayers are inclined to feel that it is not necessary.

Despite this pessimistic view, socially conscious citizens and responsible health personnel have worked in the past, and are working today, to improve the health and lives of all citizens. Medical ethics—which was largely medical etiquette for much of its history and which accepted medical experimentaton on the poor with but few questions until well into the twentieth century—has begun to emerge as a new factor in social values. Even more encouraging, the rise in the American standard of living has been accompanied by a corresponding improvement in the standard of social justice. The outpouring of books by young historians denouncing the historical injustices to labor, women, and minorities, and the shock that greeted the publication of James H. Jones's study of the Tuskegee experiment are themselves an indication of a higher moral standard and represent a hope for the future.

Bibliography

Basic to any study of public health history are the annual reports of state and local public health boards. These must be supplemented by the minutes and proceedings of the four national quarantine conventions from 1857 to 1861, the reports and papers of the National Board of Health, 1879–1883, and the many publications of the United States Public Health Service (formerly the United States Hospital and Marine Service). Other excellent sources are the papers and reports of the American Public Health Association and the American Medical Association, along with their respective journals, the *Journal of the American Public Health Association* (1891–) and the *Journal of the American Medical Association* (1886–). The *Transactions* of the New York Academy of Medicine (1847–1901) and the manuscript and printed minutes of the Academy's Committee on Public Health (1891–), along with comparable documents and publications of other state and local medical societies, are also invaluable.

The serious student of public health history will also want to examine the classic works of men such as Stanford E. Chaillé, John H. Griscom, Elisha Harris, Lemuel Shattuck, and Benjamin W. McCready. In addition, a host of special reports were issued by medical commissions appointed by local and state governments, many of them following major epidemics. For example, see the *Report of the Sanitary Commission of New Orleans on the Epidemic Yellow Fever of 1853: Published by Authority of the City Council of New Orleans* (New Orleans, 1854) and *The Sanitary Condition of Boston, the Report of a Medical Commission . . . Appointed by the Board of Health of the City of Boston . . .* (Boston, 1875).

Dissertations and Theses

The following is a list of dissertations and theses that were quite helpful:

Allen, Dotaline E. "History of Nursing in Indiana." M.S. thesis, University of Indiana, 1948.

Atkins, Gordon. "Health, Housing, and Poverty in New York City, 1865–1898." Ph. D. diss., Columbia University, 1947.

Bruton, Peter W. "The National Board of Health." Ph.D. diss., University of Maryland, 1974.

Carrigan, Jo Ann. "The Saffron Scourge: A History of Yellow Fever in Louisiana, 1796–1905." Ph.D. diss., Louisiana State University, 1961.

Donegan, Craig. "For the Good of Us All: Early Attitudes toward Occupational Health with Emphasis on the Northern United States from 1787 to 1870." Ph.D. diss., University of Maryland, 1984.

Ellis, John H. "Yellow Fever and the Origins of Modern Public Health in Memphis, Tennessee, 1870–1900." Ph.D. diss., Tulane University, 1962.

Farmer, Henry F. "The Hookworm Eradication Program in the South." M.A. thesis, University of Georgia, 1966.

Harstad, Peter. "Health in the Upper Mississippi Valley, 1820–1861." Ph.D. diss., University of Wisconsin, 1963.

Hylton, Ola G. "A History of the Public Health Movement in Michigan, 1888–1913. Ph.D. diss., University of Michigan, 1943.

Kirkpatrick, Robert L. "History of St. Louis, 1804–1816." M.A. thesis, Washington University, 1946.

Kramer, Howard D. "History of the Public Health Movement in the United States, 1850 to 1900." Ph.D. diss., University of Iowa, 1942.

Legan, Marshall S. "The Evolution of Public Health Services in Mississippi, 1865–1910." Ph.D. diss., University of Mississippi, 1968.

Plummer, Betty L. "A History of Public Health in Washington, D.C., 1800–1890." Ph.D. diss., University of Maryland, 1984.

Rooney, William E. "The New Orleans Marine Hospital, 1802–1861." M.A. thesis, Tulane University, 1950.

Sieck, Charles A. "A Study of the Public Health Authority in Ohio." M.A. thesis, University of Michigan, 1936.

Soraghan, Catherine V. "The History of St. Louis, 1865–1876." M.A. thesis, Washington University, 1936.

Young, James R. "Malaria in the South, 1900–1930." Ph.D. diss., University of North Carolina, 1972.

Because health, individually and collectively, is so basic to human society, evidence about it can be found in a wide range of historical documents. Newspapers, magazines, and national, state, and local historical collections provide a wealth of information on health matters from the earliest days of our nation's history. The many Works Progress Administration (WPA) collections of historical documents scattered throughout the United States are invaluable. One of the most useful of these is the Microfilm Records of the WPA Kentucky Medical History Project, University of Louisville Kornhauser Health Sciences Library.

State and Municipal Histories

A number of state and municipal histories of medicine touch on public health. The following are especially noteworthy:

Blanton, Wyndham B. *Medicine in Virginia in the Seventeenth Century.* Richmond, Va., 1930.

———. *Medicine in Virginia in the Eighteenth Century.* Richmond, Va., 1931.

———. *Medicine in Virginia in the Nineteenth Century.* Richmond, Va., 1933.

Bonner, Thomas N. *Medicine in Chicago, 1850–1950.* Madison, Wis., 1957.

Duffy, John. *The Rudolph Matas History of Medicine in Louisiana.* 2 vols. Baton Rouge, La., 1958–62.

Holley, Howard L. *The History of Medicine in Alabama.* Birmingham, 1982.

Waring, Joseph Ioor. *A History of Medicine in South Carolina, 1670–1825.* Columbia, S.C., 1964.

————. *A History of Medicine in South Carolina, 1825–1900.* Columbia, S.C., 1967.

Regrettably few good state or municipal histories of public health have been written. Although some excellent historical studies have been made of Massachusetts, there is no comprehensive public health history of the state. First-class examples are John B. Blake, *Public Health in the Town of Boston, 1630–1822* (Cambridge, Mass., 1959); Barbara G. Rosenkrantz, *Public Health and the State: Changing Views in Massachusetts, 1842–1936* (Cambridge, Mass., 1972); and George C. Whipple, *State Sanitation: A Review of the Work of the Massachusett State Board of Health* (rpt., New York, 1977). See also James Wallace, *The State Health Departments of Massachusetts, Michigan, and Ohio with a Summary of Activities and Accomplishments, 1927–28* (New York, 1930).

The following state histories were useful:

Abercrombie, T. F. *History of Public Health in Georgia, 1733–1950.* N.p., n.d.

Gillson, Gordon E. *The Louisiana State Board of Health: The Formative Years.* N.p., [1966].

————. "The Louisiana State Board of Health: The Progressive Years." TS.

Greenfield, Myrtle. *A History of Public Health in New Mexico.* Albuquerque, 1962.

Jordan, Philip D. *The People's Health: A History of Public Health in Minnesota to 1948.* Saint Paul, 1953.

Kendrick, John F. *Public Health in the State and Counties of Virginia.* Richmond, 1939.

Neal, Charles A. *State of Ohio, Department of Health, An Historical Review, Its Powers, Duties and Organization.* Columbus, 1929.

Pfister, Harriet S. *Kansas State Board of Health.* Lawrence, 1955.

Texas State Department of Health. *A History of Public Health in Texas.* Austin, 1950.

Smith, Howard E. *A History of Public Health in Texas.* Austin, 1974.

Washburn, Benjamin E. *A History of the North Carolina State Board of Health, 1877–1925.* Raleigh, 1966.

Among the better municipal studies are the following works:

Duffy, John. *A History of Public Health in New York City, 1625–1866.* New York, 1968.

————. *A History of Public Health in New York City, 1866–1966.* New York, 1974.

Galishoff, Stuart. *Safeguarding the Public Health: Newark, 1895–1918.* Westport, Conn., 1975.

————. *Newark, the Nation's Unhealthiest City, 1832–1895.* New Brunswick, N.J., 1988.

Howard, William T. *Public Health Administration and the Natural History of Diseases in Baltimore, Maryland, 1797–1920.* Washington, D.C., 1924.

Leavitt, Judith L. *The Healthiest City: Milwaukee and the Politics of Health Reform.* Princeton, 1982.

Smith, Stephen. *The City That Was.* Preface by John Duffy. Metuchen, N.J., 1973.

Other Historical Studies

Other historical studies bearing upon public health include the following:

Adams, George W. *Doctors in Blue: The Medical History of the Union Army in the Civil War.* New York, 1952.

Altman, Lawrence. *Who Goes First? The Story of Self-Experimentation in Medicine.* New York, 1986.

Beardsley, Edward H. *A History of Neglect: Health Care for Blacks and Mill Workers in the Twentieth-Century South.* Knoxville, Tenn., 1987.

Bell, Leland. *Treating the Mentally Ill: From Colonial Times to the Present.* New York, 1980.

Blake, Nelson. *Water for the Cities.* Syracuse, N.Y., 1956.

Brandt, Allan M. *No Magic Bullet: A Social History of Venereal Disease in the United States since 1880.* New York, 1985.

Breckinridge, Mary. *Wide Neighborhoods: A Story of the Frontier Nursing Service.* Lexington, Ky., 1981.

Burrow, James G. *Organized Medicine in the Progressive Era: The Move Toward Monopoly.* Baltimore, 1977.

Cain, R. L., E. Katz, and D. B. Rosenthal. *The Politics of Community Conflict: The Fluoridation Decision.* Indianapolis and New York, 1969.

Cassedy, James H. *Charles V. Chapin and the Public Health Movement.* Cambridge, Mass., 1942.

———. *Demography in Early America: Beginnings of the Statistical Mind, 1600–1800.* Cambridge, Mass., 1969.

———. *American Medicine and Statistical Thinking, 1800–1860.* Cambridge, Mass., 1984.

Cavins, Harold L. *National Health Agencies: A Survey with Especial Reference to Voluntary Associations.* Washington, D.C., 1945.

Chapin, Charles V. *A Report on State Public Health Work Based on a Survey of State Boards of Health.* Chicago, 1916.

Cosgrave, J. J. *History of Sanitation.* Pittsburgh, 1909.

Crosby, Alfred W., Jr. *Epidemic and Peace, 1918.* Westport, Conn., 1976.

Dain, Norman. *Concepts of Insanity in the United States, 1789–1865.* New Brunswick, N.J., 1964.

Dowling, Harry F. *Fighting Infection: Conquests of the Twentieth Century.* Cambridge, Mass., 1977.

Dubin, Louis I., and Alfred J. Lotka. *Twenty-Five Years of Health Progress . . . the Metropolitan Life Insurance Company, 1911 to 1935.* New York, 1937.

Etheridge, Elizabeth W. *The Butterfly Caste: A Social History of Pellagra in the South.* Westport, Conn., 1972.

Ettling, John. *The Germ of Laziness: Rockefeller Philanthropy and Public Health in the New South.* Cambridge, Mass., 1981.

Fee, Elizabeth. *Disease and Discovery: A History of the Johns Hopkins School of Hygiene and Public Health, 1916–1939.* Baltimore, 1987.

Furman, Bess. *A Profile of the United States Public Health Service, 1798–1948.* Washington, D.C., n.d.

Gillett, Mary C. *The Army Medical Department, 1775–1818.* Washington, D.C., 1981.

———. *The Army Medical Department, 1818–1865.* Washington, D.C., 1987.

Grob, Gerald N. *The State and the Mentally Ill: A History of Worcester State Hospital in Massachusetts, 1830–1920.* Chapel Hill, N.C., 1966.

———. *Mental Illness and American Society, 1875–1940.* Princeton, 1980.

Hirshfield, David S. *The Lost Reform: The Campaign for Compulsory Health Insurance in the United States from 1932 to 1943.* Cambridge, Mass., 1970.

Katz, Alfred H., and Jean S. Felton, eds. *Health and the Community: Readings in the Philosophy and Sciences of Public Health.* New York, 1965.

Lubove, Roy. *The Progressives and the Slums: Tenement House Reform in New York City, 1870–1917.* Pittsburgh, 1962.

Melosi, Martin V. *Garbage in the Cities: Refuse, Reform and the Environment, 1880–1980.* College Station, Tex., 1981.

———, ed. *Pollution and Reform in American Cities, 1870–1930.* Austin, Tex., 1980.

Moore, Henry H. *Public Health in the United States: An Outline with Historical Data.* New York, 1923.

Mountin, Joseph W., et al. *Distribution of Health Services in the Structure of State Government, 1950.* Washington, D.C., 1954.

Mustard, Harry F. *Rural Health Practice.* New York, 1936.

Neustadt, R., and H. Fineberg. *The Epidemic That Never Was: Policy Making and the Swine Flu Affair.* New York, 1983.

Numbers, Ronald L. *Almost Persuaded: American Physicians and Compulsory Health Insurance, 1912–1920.* Baltimore, 1978.

Okun, Michael. *Fair Play in the Marketplace: The First Battle for Pure Food and Drugs.* DeKalb, Ill., 1986.

Raffel, Marshall W. *The U.S. Health System: Origins and Function.* New York, 1980.

Ravenel, Mazÿck P., ed. *A Half Century of Public Health.* New York, 1921.

Rosen, George. *Preventive Medicine in the United States, 1900–1975: Trends and Interpretations.* New York, 1975.

Rosner, David, and Gerald Markowitz, eds. *Dying for Work: Workers' Safety and Health in Twentieth-Century America.* Bloomington and Indianapolis, Ind., 1987.

Rosenberg, Charles E. *The Cholera Years: The United States in 1832, 1849, and 1866.* Chicago, 1962.

Rothstein, William G. *American Physicians in the Nineteenth Century: From Sects to Science.* Baltimore, 1972.

Smillie, Wilson G. *Public Health Administration in the United States.* New York, 1946.

———. *Public Health, Its Promise for the Future: A Chronicle of the Development of Public Health in the United States, 1607–1914.* New York, 1955.

Spink, Wesley W. *Infectious Diseases: Prevention and Treatment in the Nineteenth and Twentieth Centuries.* Minneapolis, 1978.

Stevens, Rosemary. *American Medicine and the Public Interest.* New Haven, Conn., 1971.

Teller, Michael E. *The Tuberculosis Movement: A Public Health Campaign in the Progressive Era.* Westport, Conn., 1988

Williams, Ralph C. *The United States Public Health Service, 1798–1950.* Washington, D.C., 1951.

Index

Note on the Author

John Duffy is a distinguished scholar of public health and medical history and Clinical Professor Emeritus (History of Medicine) at Tulane University, School of Medicine. He is also Professor Emeritus at the University of Maryland, where he was the Priscilla Alden Burke Professor of American History, and he served as Professor of History of Public Health at the University of Pittsburgh, Graduate School of Public Health. Duffy's numerous published works include *The Healers: A History of American Medicine; A History of Public Health in New York City*, vol. 1, *1625–1866*, vol. 2, *1866–1966; Epidemics in Colonial America;* and *The Rudolph Matas History of Medicine in Louisiana* (2 vols.).